MADNESS, VIOLENCE, AND POWER
A Critical Collection

Edited by Andrea Daley, Lucy Costa, and Peter Beresford

Madness, Violence, and Power: A Critical Collection disengages from the common forms of discussion about violence related to mental health service users/survivors that position them as more likely to enact violence or become victims of violence. Instead, this book seeks to broaden understandings of the violence manifest in the lives of service users/survivors, consider the impacts of systems and institutions that manage "abnormality," and create space to explore the role of our own communities in justice and accountability dialogues.

This collection constitutes an integral contribution to critical scholarship on violence and mental illness by addressing a gap in the existing literature. In broadening the "violence lens," *Madness, Violence, and Power* invites an interdisciplinary conversation that is not narrowly biomedical and neuroscientific.

ANDREA DALEY is an associate professor and director in the School of Social Work at Renison University College (affiliated with the University of Waterloo).

LUCY COSTA is the deputy executive director of the Empowerment Council, an independent organization based in Toronto, Ontario, that advocates for the rights of clients/survivors of mental health and addiction services.

PETER BERESFORD is a professor of citizen participation at the University of Essex, emeritus professor of social policy at Brunel University London, and co-chair of Shaping Our Lives, a UK organization and network of user-led groups, service users, and people with disabilities.

WITHDRAWN TSALibraries

WITHDRAWN
TSA Libraries

Madness, Violence, and Power

A Critical Collection

EDITED BY ANDREA DALEY, LUCY COSTA,
AND PETER BERESFORD

UNIVERSITY OF TORONTO PRESS
Toronto Buffalo London

© University of Toronto Press 2019
Toronto Buffalo London
utorontopress.com
Printed in the U.S.A.

ISBN 978-1-4426-2996-7 (cloth)   ISBN 978-1-4426-2997-4 (paper)

♾ Printed on acid-free paper with vegetable-based inks.

Library and Archives Canada Cataloguing in Publication

Title: Madness, violence, and power : a critical collection /
    edited by Andrea Daley, Lucy Costa, and Peter Beresford.
Names: Daley, Andrea, 1963– editor. | Costa, Lucy, editor. |
    Beresford, Peter, editor.
Description: Includes bibliographical references and index.
Identifiers: Canadiana 20189067373 | ISBN 9781442629967 (cloth) |
    ISBN 9781442629974 (paper)
Subjects: LCSH: Violence – Social aspects. | LCSH: Violence – Psychological
    aspects. | LCSH: Mental illness – Social aspects. | LCSH: Mental illness –
    Treatment. | LCSH: Mental health services. | LCSH: Mentally ill – Care.
Classification: LCC HM1116 .M33 2019 | DDC 303.6—dc23

This book has been published with the help of a grant from the Federation
for the Humanities and Social Sciences, through the Awards to Scholarly
Publications Program, using funds provided by the Social Sciences and
Humanities Research Council of Canada.

University of Toronto Press acknowledges the financial assistance to its
publishing program of the Canada Council for the Arts and the Ontario Arts
Council, an agency of the Government of Ontario.

**Canada Council   Conseil des Arts
for the Arts   du Canada**

ONTARIO ARTS COUNCIL
CONSEIL DES ARTS DE L'ONTARIO
an Ontario government agency
un organisme du gouvernement de l'Ontario

Funded by the   Financé par le
Government   gouvernement
of Canada   du Canada

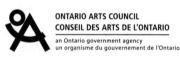

**Library
University of Texas
at San Antonio**

I dedicate this book to the people I only really knew as "clients," who were subjected to, and challenged in their own ways, the inhumanity and violence inherent in our institutions of "care," "support," and "justice," in which I participated. It is my intention that this collection serves, in some way, to acknowledge and honour your resistance and resiliency.

– Andrea Daley

To my god-daughter, Laura Lee, thank you for teaching me about love. Life is an adventure: never stop asking questions, believing in yourself, and fighting for a better world. Also, to my friends Terri Santos and Tristan R. Whiston, who have always supported me in overcoming the vestiges of my own experiences of violence.

– Lucy Costa

I would like to dedicate this book to Patricia Chambers, my lovely friend and colleague, working and smiling together for many but not enough years. You were always a beacon of survivordom for me, Patricia. Like many survivors, you may not be there when the good changes come, but when they do, it will be because of people like you. Thank you.

– Peter Beresford

Contents

Foreword

ROBERT WHITAKER

This volume – and I say this with admiration – demands much of its readers. It is intellectually challenging, and, at the same time, it makes a moral claim on one's emotions. By the book's end, the reader is left with a sense of duty to fight against societal wrongs that do great harm.

The writers bring a rich diversity of personal and professional knowledge to this text, which is a primary reason that it succeeds so admirably in fulfilling the editors' twofold purpose for commissioning the essays: "We want to broaden understandings of violence manifest in the lives of mental health service users/survivors," they write, and "to explore the role of our communities in justice and accountability dialogues." The first illuminates the depth of the systemic violence – politically, legally, medically, and by the societal discourse – inflicted on those we call "mad." The second challenges readers, who might see themselves as "reformers," to think about ways that they may unwittingly contribute to that systemic violence.

Mention "mental illness" and violence in a public forum, and most in the audience will think of the risk that "mentally ill" people pose to the public. There will be stories about how this or that mentally ill person committed a horrible act of violence, and the discussion will then focus on how society can protect itself from such acts. But as Brigit McWade notes in her chapter, this is a societal discourse belied by the facts, and such "persistently inaccurate media portrayals of mental illness" foster "community hostility to service-users." This is an example of how societal discourse can inflict "violence" on those labelled *Mad*. But McWade then goes further: Who benefits from this discourse? It arises, she observes, from psychiatrists and other mental health professionals, and serves to further secure their "dominance in common knowledge about madness and distress."

As the title of the collection states, this is a book about madness, violence, and *power*. If there is a root cause for the systemic violence explored in these pages, it can perhaps be found in this historical truth: whenever a society seeks to draw a line separating the "normal" from the "not normal," it leads the society to perceive the "not normal" group as the "Other." This is a categorization that is applied most readily to minorities, Indigenous people, poor people, LGBT folks, and other marginalized populations, and the reason it proves so harmful is that it calls upon a tribal instinct in the general population, as opposed to a sense of inclusion that is supposed to govern in modern democracies. With this instinct aroused, a society is prepared to treat the "other" in ways that violate all the usual norms. The Other, as Meghann O'Leary and Liat Ben-Moshe put it in their chapter, is no longer seen as capable of governing his or her own self: "Becoming psychiatrized does not just mean that you are labelled as 'crazy.' It also means that you are no longer seen … as capable of making decisions for yourself, your own insight and abilities are constantly questioned, and there is a definitive medical explanation for all your behaviours and feelings." This could be described as society inflicting a form of "existential violence." But it also provides a context for more overt violence, such as forced drug treatment, which leads to a provocative question: Is there something heroic in resisting such "treatment"? Will Aindow writes powerfully of his resistance:

> I was on a PICU [psychiatric intensive care unit] ward and got put on depot medication by the psychiatrist. I argued against this during the consultation and refused to have it. The following day a nurse asked me at breakfast when I wanted to have the depot. I continued to say I did not want it. Then, about two days later, six or maybe seven men came into my room, led by a male nurse I quite liked, charged with administering the depot. I backed into the corner of my room. I told them that I disagreed with the legislation that empowered them. I also told them that I understood the consequences of resistance to myself both criminal and psychiatric. I removed my watch and threw it on the bed. I told them that I would drop the first person that came near me with a needle and probably get a punch in on someone else. There was a momentary standoff and then the attempt was called off.

My favourite line in this powerful piece of prose is this: "I told them I disagreed with the legislation that empowered them."

The violence described in these pages, by the many thoughtful writers who have contributed to this volume, comes in many forms. Tobin LeBlanc Haley, writing as a "Mad woman," describes violence of a subtler kind, the "epistemic violence" she experienced while pregnant. She had to confront, in her own mind, the prevailing "knowledge claims" that, as a "mad person," she was "biologically and irrevocably broken," and thus was likely to give birth to a "sick child." As Haley notes, she does not come from a marginalized population, but rather, as a white, cisgender woman, from a place of relative privilege. Hers is an internal landscape of "violence," where one is encouraged to constantly monitor one's self for signs of abnormal thoughts and feelings, and it speaks to psychiatry's success, over the last 35 years, in prompting an ever-larger part of the population to think of themselves as depressed, anxious, or disordered in some way. In a sense, Haley is writing of "epistemic violence" that has been inflicted on our entire society.

It should be no surprise that such "violence," in its many forms, is occurring in our neoliberal societies. Neoliberalism places responsibility for unhappiness, disruptive behaviour, and emotional suffering on the individual, as though the individual's well-being arises solely from his or her chemical and genetic makeup, and not from unjust social environments. It takes Priya Raju and Nicole Penak, in their conversation about Indigenous communities, only one short sentence to reveal the bankruptcy of that neoliberal ideology: "Wellness or unwellness," they write, "is not an individual thing." Which brings readers to contemplate what can be done. Is it a matter of reforming psychiatry from within? Or is it, as O'Leary and Ben-Moshe write, that the institution of psychiatry is "beyond remediation and reform"?

While the immediate focus on psychiatry is understandable, the contributors to this book collectively tell of a broader, more pervasive problem. Much as Aindow "disagreed" with those who would forcibly drug him, perhaps we need to forcefully "disagree" with social systems that "psychiatrize" so many, designating them as the "other," and strive to create a society that understands that "wellness is not an individual thing."

Acknowledgments

We have many people to thank for making this book possible. First, we would like to thank members of our advisory group: Jaene F. Castrillon, Patricia Chambers, Ruby Dhand, Carole King, Brigit McWade, Jasna Russo, Tess Sheldon, and Lisa Walter. We greatly value the support and guidance this group gave us, helping us to move beyond our own ideas and assumptions. Sadly, we must also pay particular tribute to one of its members, Patricia Chambers who died in 2016.

We extend much thanks to our contributors. We want to thank all of them for their patience and for doing everything they could to make the best book we could.

To all the mental health service users/survivors and allies who have worked tirelessly in this field and whose efforts have provided the starting point for us writing this book and on this subject matter: we see you, we hear you, and we stand in solidarity. Thank you.

We are honoured by Robert Whitaker's enthusiasm for this collection of writings on madness, violence, and power, and feel much gratitude for his careful attention to the subtleties of the arguments made within and across its chapters.

We also want to thank Jaene F. Castrillon for generously contributing her art for the cover of the book. As editors committed to, and informed by, Mad Studies, it was important to us that the book's cover represent, in some way, a community voice or perspective. As such, we solicited book cover proposals from the community. We received submissions from seven artists, most of whom were mental health service user/survivors. Of those submissions, we selected Jaene Castrillion's *Still Life*, originally taken during 2015–16 while she was Workman Arts media artist in residence. The straitjacket serves as a metaphor for the key themes in this collection of writings, symbolizing the interrelationships and tensions between madness, power, and violence, and law, policy, discourses on mental health, and institutional practices. That is, the image of the straitjacket represents the various ways in which law, policy, discourses on mental health, and institutional practices coalesce into a web of power and violence – discipline and punishment – for mental health service user/survivors. Importantly, however, while we use the straitjacket image as a metaphor, we must not forget that although the straitjacket was invented by psychiatry and is no longer used by most psychiatric institutions, newer forms of restraints are being used, including seclusion rooms, chemical/medication restraints, and other devices, such as neck, wrist, waist, and leg restraints. The use of newer forms of restraint may come as a surprise to some readers, underscoring why we have brought together this collection of writings: to foster dialogue about, and engage a variety of audiences more deeply in, the ongoing issue of power and violence as emerging in the lives of mental health service user/survivors.

Appreciation must also go to the team at University of Toronto Press who helped get this volume into print: Eric Carlson, Stephen Shapiro, and Meg Patterson. And to our editor, Kerry Fast, and indexer, Judy Dunlop, we extend much appreciation for your careful attention to the details of this text. The manuscript was enriched by the detailed reading by and feedback from the external reviewers; we appreciate your interest in the collection of writings. We also recognize that all and any limitations the book has are our responsibility as editors and ours alone.

MADNESS, VIOLENCE, AND POWER
A Critical Collection

Introduction

ANDREA DALEY, LUCY COSTA, AND PETER BERESFORD

In preparing our book, we repeatedly considered issues of sensitivity relating to content and language used in the book. We realize that some people may find some of the words, language, themes, and ideas upsetting. As such, it is important to us to make clear that it is not our intention to cause any distress. We recognize that for some people the words and themes may be difficult to read about. We sincerely hope that readers will find that this book offers thoughtful insight despite this and feel encouraged to continue discussions within their own circles.

Violence is endemic in our world, commonplace in human and social relations, and legitimated and normalized in war and conflict. Nonetheless, unrelated and influential discourses have also developed that are narrowly concerned with the relations between violence, madness, and "mentally ill" people. This collection aims to disengage from the common forms of discussion about violence related to mental health service users/survivors, such as biomedical frameworks and statistical assertions that position them as more likely to enact violence or, alternatively, to be victims of violence compared to other people. This long-standing binary serves to keep mental health service users/survivors embedded within the predominant arguments of neuroscience while situating individualized violence as separate from social and structural forces. The purpose of the collection is instead twofold: first, we want to broaden understandings of the violence manifest in the lives of mental health service users/survivors and push current considerations to explore the impacts of systems and institutions that manage "abnormality," and second, we hope to allow for space to explore the role of our own communities in justice and accountability dialogues. Historically, reformers have defaulted to medicine or law to resolve problems, but what remedies might be available to us via our own experiential and written knowledges?

Violence takes many forms in our world. There is verbal, physical, emotional, sexual, and epistemic violence. There is personal, gender, state, civil, political, and military violence; individual and collective, legal and illegal, and consensual and non-consensual violence. There is media and cyber violence – intended to "Other," confuse, misrepresent, and divide. We talk of criminal violence as if it means only violence against a person, despite the sense of violation described by those who have been burgled, experienced identity theft, or felt their lives invaded in other ways. We have notions, rarely thought through, of violence as a continuum, from minor to major, from superficial to life-changing and life-ending.

Violence in its innumerable forms has affected global discussion across mental health service user/survivor organizations, such as the World Network of Users and Survivors of Psychiatry, Disability Rights International, and the UN Convention on the Rights of People with Disabilities (UNCRPD). These organizations (and others) highlight human rights issues and the legal protections required particularly for vulnerable mental health service users/survivors worldwide. In the last few years, the UNCRPD[1] has emphasized the need for further institutional accountability through Article 12's principle that all individuals with disabilities are equal before the law and Article 15's quest to ensure people with disabilities are not being subjected to torture or cruel, inhuman, or degrading treatment or punishment. As our book demonstrates, the law can be both empowering by giving voice to the voiceless and providing an opportunity for reporting extraordinary violence and persecution, and disempowering by becoming an instrument of violence itself, legitimating practices that are part of neo-liberal projects that are destructive to both citizens and political economies.

Our focus in this book is on the violence associated with madness or "mental health problems." This tends to be understood very narrowly in dominant debates as the propensity for violence by Mad and distressed people associated with their unpredictability and lack of reason. We have sought to open the discourse here to explore also the broader associations and meanings of violence in relation to Mad people and people identified as mental health service users/survivors. This includes violence in the personal, collective, psychiatric, spatial, and civil worlds that mental health service users/survivors and the rest of us inhabit. We want to bring new and different understandings to this from fresh perspectives and are very conscious that in doing this, we are opening up the boundaries of discussion. Yet at the same time, since we have a particular focus – madness, violence, and power – we know that our discussion has to be boundaried. There will inevitably be limitations and gaps in this collection of writings, but we expect and anticipate more conversation and future scholarly contribution to expand on themes started by the book's chapters.

Violence Past and Violence Present

Colonial violence is a global phenomenon – past and present – that is undeniably implicated in individual and community distress and trauma experienced by the world's Indigenous Peoples. Long-standing policies and practices of colonial governments have been used to enact violence against Indigenous Peoples, including the stealing of Indigenous children from their families and communities to erode Indigenous knowledges, cultures, and practices; the theft of land and related resources from Indigenous communities; the blatant failure of governments to honour treaties; and the lack of responsiveness to systematic violence against Indigenous girls and women, among other acts. However, colonial violence is not a product of governmental policies and practices only; it is also achieved through the application of psy-knowledge. Vaughan asserts that the "ambition of colonial psychiatry lay in elaborating and promoting a psychological language with which to discuss the dilemmas face by colonial administrators,"[2] including, among others, the legitimation of settler sovereignty over Indigenous land and people. Driven by capitalist interests, colonial governments obscure(d) the impact of state violence on Indigenous bodies and minds, drawing upon psychiatric theories to foreground pathologies of maladjustment to modernity and political resistance to colonial rule.

Notwithstanding ongoing colonial (state) violence, there have been some suggestions that violence, in a broad range of expressions and forms, has declined in modern life, from short to longer term, on personal and international scales (e.g., Pinker).[3] This has been widely challenged and is difficult to reconcile with what we know about the reach of violence resulting not only from colonial pasts and presents but also from modern methods of communication and weapons technology.[4] Thus the context of violence seems to be a worsening one where retaliation and revenge are celebrated as political acts of national patriotism. Since World War I (1914–1918), armed conflict has resulted in deaths and injury among civilians that increasingly outnumber those to the military. We know that violence has long been used as a weapon of war as well as being its inherent currency. We see it still in conflicts with organized rape, kidnapping, and amputation. We live in an age of tribal, sectarian, genocidal, terrorist, gender-based, national, supranational, and proxy conflicts. Even those of us lucky and privileged enough not to be directly affected by collective violence are increasingly affected by its omnipresence and increasingly brutal imagery in mass media – as both entertainment and "news." We are increasingly called upon to have complex views about violence, repudiating some while accepting the legitimacy of others.

Yet the violence associated with madness and distress, with mental health service users/survivors, still commands particular interest and visibility – compared, for example, with the violence of men against women or white against Black people, both of which tend to be underplayed in dominant discourses. The former, however, tends to be granted special attention, even if it is treated in a particular and partial way. Despite strategies to enlighten the mass media, among others, superficial tropes and cavalier and salacious fear-mongering are reproduced. Within the contemporary "war against terrorism" context, this is most notable in the ways in which madness is conflated with causal arguments about terrorism, being invoked to explain the actions of some (white) perpetrators of mass violence but not all (racialized).

We can certainly trace this focus on madness and violence back to the "enlightenment," the rise of the human sciences and interest in Mad people's behaviour as public entertainment.[5] The issue emerged again as a major public concern towards the end of the twentieth century following the running down and closure of psychiatric institutions and shift to *care in the community*. This was subsequently associated with increased violence by people in the psychiatric system, in high-profile cases like that of Christopher Clunis in England (a young man who had been failed by the mental health system and who killed Jonathan Zito in December 1992). In fact, the evidence did not support any increase in such violence,[6] although there was a hardening of policy and a further racializing of the issue. Mental health service users/survivors faced increasing stigma, hostility, and control.[7] Similarly in Canada, the high-profile case of Vince Li, who was found not criminally responsible for decapitating a passenger on an intercity transport bus in 2008, continues to stoke fears about extreme violence despite Li's story being a rare incident. Yet despite research that demonstrates that rates of recidivism for individuals found not criminally responsible are low,[8] fear endures not only with the public but also among mental health sector workers who can intentionally or unintentionally perpetuate discrimination and prejudice.

Why This Book?

This book looks to develop new terms of theoretical engagement in relation to madness, violence, and power. For too long this discourse has been prioritized as the domain of psychiatrists, lawyers, and judges. So much of the violence that impacts vulnerable people particularly, vis-à-vis powerful cultural narrative or hyper-surveillance, ironically makes invisible the ubiquity of violence and power. This book is also motivated by an increased discussion and coverage of violence in relation to mental illness within the public sphere, including the media, governments, community agencies, and psychiatric and penal institutions.

Within national and international contexts, such discussions and coverage often offer insubstantial or sensational accounts of the "mentally ill" in relation to criminalization, police interventions (gone wrong), and institutional trauma, as well as political and structural conditions that contribute to mental health vulnerabilities, including deportations of refugees, the impacts of colonization on First Nation and Indigenous communities, and chronic illness and early death by poverty as a result of neo-liberal economic policy. Such accounts are limited in their ability to critically question the relationship between power and the nuanced means by which violence is manifest in the lives of mental health service users/survivors. Rob Nixon has aptly captured this notion of nuanced violence or "slow violence" as social and structural forces "patiently dispense their devastation while remaining outside our flickering attention spans" to produce slow, long-lasting calamities.[9]

In this way, this collection of writings constitutes an integral contribution to critical scholarship on violence and mental illness. It makes visible and addresses a gap in the existing literature by broadening the violence lens while ensuring that the parameters of understandings remain in relation to mental health service users/survivors, by inviting an interdisciplinary conversation that is not narrowly biomedical and neuroscientific (i.e., reductionist). The collection offers robust and rich analyses by drawing from law, social science, history, critical disability studies, and critical race and Indigenous studies to introduce authors who are critically engaged and offer new perspectives, evidence, and calls for action to address violence as manifest in the lives of mental health service users/survivors and their chosen communities. In this regard, it will facilitate the advancement, solidification, and mobilization of knowledge required to make real the terms for self-determination and social justice, restorative justice, and reconciliation for those people impacted by the violence of systems and institutions. Thus, while the visibility of violence may remain elusive, the collection assists in the development of a number of theoretical frameworks and pedagogical tools for its illumination. Finally, the collection builds upon and extends the critical questions, themes, and advocacy work currently developed in the new and emergent field of Mad Studies by bringing together academic and non-academic community members and activists and allies within the consumer/survivor, ex-patient, and Mad movements thinking, researching, writing, and taking action about new considerations of power, violence, systems, and institutions in relation to mental health service users/survivors. As such, the collection's complex and nuanced approach to madness, violence, and power has the very strong potential to educate and challenge (conventional) practitioners, academics, students, and researchers in areas (e.g., psychology, social work, law, medicine, and public policy) that continue to be heavily reliant on psy-knowledge and related practices. This collection of writing encourages critical self-reflection on issues of violence and power as they operate in and through practices and policies that are too often assumed benevolent or neutral by those enacting them or teaching future practitioners to enact them. Relatedly, the book raises critical questions for practitioners, academics, students, and researchers about issues of perpetration, authority, and accountability.

Terminology

We had to grapple with issues of language and terminology in this book. All the terms that make up our title, *madness, violence,* and *power,* are problematic and contested. We have already touched on the normality of violence in our world and the need to problematize its meaning. The whole book is concerned with unpacking and exploring the nature and interrelationships of these three key concepts. They also demand some introduction themselves, if we are not to fall foul of the tendency in this field to rely on unstated assumptions and leave dominant discourses unquestioned.

There is no consensus about language in this field. Whatever terms we use and however we use them, we are inevitably likely to offend. We apologize for this and hope we cause the least possible offence. We know that many of the words that are regularly used can have unhelpful associations for some people. It is difficult enough trying to negotiate this ground with any one group of stakeholders, in any one society. But for a book like this, aimed at an international and diverse audience, it is perhaps an impossible task to attempt. We will use the term *mental health service user/survivor*, which hopefully will cause the least offence, although we did not impose our own preferences on contributors to the book.

Madness

We see this book as contributing to the evolving work of Mad Studies. Mad Studies, which have their origins in Canada, have come to prominence in recent years as a field of study and action. *Mad Matters*, the Canadian text that heralded increased international interest in Mad Studies, defined it as an umbrella term:

> Used to embrace the body of knowledge that has emerged from psychiatric survivors, Mad-identified people, anti-psychiatry academics and activists, critical psychiatrists and radical therapists. This body of knowledge is wide-ranging and includes scholarship that is critical of the mental health system as well as radical and Mad activist scholarship.[10]

While there is no agreed definition of Mad Studies, they are most closely associated with valuing the experiential knowledge, approaches, and practices of mental health service users/survivors, and questioning the prevailing biomedical model and psychiatric system while excavating more multifaceted, sophisticated, and fresh understandings that will support the emergence of new critical research and social action. Mad Studies can also be seen as part of a move on the part of mental health service users/survivors and others to reclaim the language of madness from its widespread pejorative use to ridicule, demean, and stigmatize people, alongside a growing thesaurus of abusive terms like *nutter*, *crazy*, *loony*, and *psychopath*. At the same time, user-led research suggests that views among mental health service users/survivors themselves are still divided. Some feel that the language of madness is now too compromised to be worth trying to salvage.[11] This is not a view we share, and we are happy to make use of the terms *madness* and (*mental/ emotional*) *distress* or the terms preferred by, useful to, and chosen by mental health service users/survivors themselves, across intersecting identities.

Perhaps the most contentious terms are those used to describe people experiencing madness and distress or coming within the orbit of the multifaceted and intersecting sites of mental health surveillance and regulation, including the psychiatric (health care), legal, and education systems. With the emergence of their organizations and movements, mental health service users/survivors challenged the passivity of the term *patient* and the medicalization of *mentally ill/disordered person*. A wide range of terms have developed internationally since. These include *consumer, customer, psychiatric system survivor,* and *people with psychiatric/psychosocial disabilities*. All have their advocates; all have their critics. Some are clearly underpinned by medicalized individual understandings, others by consumerist/free market ideology. In terms of the latter, evidence of this can be found in new trends to move health care dollars into the community and away from institutions. With this, there is urgent need to understand how narratives of violence (re)appear, for example, in new and varied tools of psychological and psychiatric assessment that are used to control where people live, supports they can or cannot receive, and ultimately how service user organizations fare in understanding these modernization strategies and immense data collection projects. Our hope is that future writing in the field will analyse new terms governing health care, resource allocation, and access to care for their utility.

Power

What is most conspicuous about power in the context of madness and distress is the inequalities that abound, the exclusion and disempowerment that go with being a mental health service user. This takes place at two obvious levels. The groups that are particularly likely to be caught up in the psychiatric, or coercive, systems are those that face structural inequalities, for example, on the basis of race, gender, sexuality, age, class, culture, disability, income, and life chances. Downwards social mobility, negative stereotyping, social isolation and poverty are all associated with becoming a long-term "revolving" or "chronic" mental health service user/survivor. Terms such as *bed blockers* (or *frequent flyers*), for example, have emerged to describe the ways in which long-term patients "block" beds for other (more deserving) patients. Systemic violence represents an additional expression of the imposition of power and disempowerment. For example, the number of police interactions across international regions with individuals in distress is alarming, to say the least. Inquests and other legal apparatus are deployed to make sense of suspicious deaths and make recommendations that are rarely implemented. This is further complicated as tensions increase through citizens becoming more conscious of the disparity between elites, the working class, and increasingly large middle class.

In light of this, mental health service users/survivors can expect to face both personal and political disempowerment. This is why the empowerment strategies that they, like other welfare service user groups, have developed to challenge unbearable situations, borrowing from the Black civil rights, feminist, and LGBTQ2S+ movements tend to be framed in terms of both. Changing the relations of madness and violence can be both an empowering and a disempowering process, according to what role mental health service users/survivors are able to play. Change raises issues about power, the location and distribution of power, and the relative power of different stakeholders in the process of change. This will be particularly apparent where change is imposed from the top down or externally. In this book we are particularly interested in participatory change, with mental health service users/survivors able to play an active role in it. When people have significant experiences of disempowerment, or of practice that is designed to blame, interpret, and accuse,[12] and have little understanding of their own capacity to exert power, even with a desire to increase their say and control, it may be difficult for them to use such opportunities for empowering change. It can be difficult for many of us actually to see ourselves as change makers.

Steven Lukes,[13] a political sociologist, developed the idea of three dimensions of power. The third dimension refers to the social construction of practices, ideologies, and institutions that secure people's consent to or at least acceptance of domination.[14] The community and developmental educationalist John Gaventa[15] drew on this to support approaches to social change rooted in the perspectives of marginalized communities. Instead of looking for the sources and the solutions of social problems in the theories and ideas of social science and social policy experts, he validated the narratives of the oppressed populations involved. In Gaventa's theory, such methodological subjectivity makes it possible for the framing of a social problem and its solution to arise from within the group. This both has an empowering effect on the group and provides a basis for it to take collective action to challenge dominant discourses and develop alternatives.[16]

Violence

The problem of violence, in its many forms, and its relationship to inequality, oppression, and domination has been differently conceptualized and theorized. Feminist, queer, critical race, critical disability, postcolonial, and intersectional scholars and activists have examined interpersonal, structural, and symbolic violence, often with attention to interlocking oppressions. In different and complex ways, gender, race, sexuality, class, and disability have been centred on analyses of structural formulations of violence that centre power as a relation that structures interactions between people. Most commonly, structural formulations of violence embed interpersonal violence in unjust social, political, and economic systems of inequality and associated social relations (e.g., sexist, racist, classist, and disablist) that permeate all social institutions. And unjust social, political, and economic systems of inequality are understood as being sustained by symbolic violence. That is, mechanisms of power and domination are considered to work through rather than on bodies as they are embedded in the routines of everyday life.[17] In this instance, consent, complicity, and misrecognition are implicated in symbolic violence as "the dominated apply categories constructed from the point of view of the dominant."[18] It is this imposition of categories of thought and perception by the dominant upon the dominated and the internalization of these by the latter that normalizes and naturalizes unjust social orders as legitimately just. In this regard, Dominquez and Menjivar[19] state:

> Every day, normalized familiarity with violence renders it invisible; power structures are misrecognized, and the mechanisms through which violence is exerted do not lie in conscious knowing but rather are entrenched in the "social order of things" (see Kleinman, 2000).

A critical understanding of familiarity as "noticing but being used to"[20] is integral to the formulation of symbolic violence as it is grounded and intertwined in the everyday practices of social exclusion and oppression. The interdisciplinary writings in this book work collectively to consider the interrelationship between interpersonal, structural, and symbolic violence as they collude to perpetuate social relations that serve the interests of the dominant.

It would also be a mistake to restrict our attention to the psychiatric system to understand systemic violence. Evidence from the United Kingdom, for example, highlights that the prison and penal systems increasingly now serve as places of last resort for people who may be failed by other services, as well as reflecting broader discriminations and exclusions in society. There is an over-representation of people with disabilities in the prison system. Thus, 49% of female prisoners in a British Ministry of Justice study were assessed as suffering from anxiety and depression, compared with 19% of the female population in the United Kingdom; 46% of women in prison have suffered a history of domestic abuse; 53% of women in prison reported having experienced emotional, physical, or sexual abuse as a child, compared to 27% of men. An estimated 36% of prisoners interviewed in a Ministry of Justice study were considered to have an impairment when survey answers about disability and health, including mental health, were screened. And 49% of women and 23% of male prisoners in a Ministry of Justice study were assessed as suffering from anxiety and depression compared with 16% of the general UK population (12% of men and 19% of women). A range of additional problems also emerged, including the increasing psychiatrization of crime, associating crime with "mental disorder" without independent evidence, further stigmatizing mental health service users.[21]

We have already touched on the numerous, complex, and contradictory understandings and meanings attached to violence across societies. As we have said, an underpinning reason for this book has been the narrow ways in which violence has been defined and discussed in dominant discourse. We hope to unpack this and explore other meanings and understandings, particularly from mental health service user/survivor perspectives.

Our Approach

Our early editorial discussions, across our respective personal and professional identities evolved slowly and carefully over a terrain of considerations and frameworks. To ensure we included a number of perspectives we invited eight people to help shape the deliberations that informed this collection. As such, the book emerged through a series of discussions with an international advisory group (AG) that included mental health service user/survivors, academics, and advocates from Canada, the United Kingdom, and Germany. Through our discussions (via Skype) it became particularly important to us that the collection of writings reflect diverse perspectives on madness, violence, and power, and that it serve as a useful resource for professional programs related to law, social science, social work, advocacy, and health (e.g., front-line practitioners and policy decision makers), as well as activists and allies of the consumer/survivor, ex-patient, and Mad movements, by offering theoretical frameworks and pedagogical tools. Guided by a terms of reference we initially drafted and then revised to incorporate the opinions and ideas of AG members, we collaborated over several months to explore and refine the focus of the book. More specifically, we sought the perspectives of the AG members on the preliminary themes we developed for the call for contributors, refining the focus of each theme and exploring distribution strategies to maximize the likelihood of reaching contributors internationally. The collection of writings offers perspectives on various international contexts, including Canada, the United States, and the United Kingdom, with the contributors writing for an international audience. However, future work could strengthen this area of scholarship by expanding contributions from other Western and non-Western regions. Having said this, we also recognize the contemporary context of globalized policymaking, and thus the relevancy and application of the contributions across international practice, research, and policy settings.

Organization of the Book

This collection of writings on violence in the lives of mental health service users/survivors is organized along four key themes, each of which constitutes a section of the book: Part I, Dispatches on Violence; Part II, Prevailing Problems; Part III, Law as Violence; and Part IV, Geographies of Violence. The themes traverse personal narratives of violence; institutional and institutionalized practices of knowledge production about mental health and mental illness informed by neo-liberal capitalist logic; legislated violence done to people through social policy and law; and the places and spaces in which violence happens. Notwithstanding the distinction that might be implied by the development of the discrete themes, we conceptualize violence as occurring simultaneously in complex and nuanced ways as it is depicted within and across the chapters included in the book.

Part I, Dispatches on Violence, foregrounds lived experiences in relation to the violence of institutions such as psychiatry, motherhood, risk assessment, and incarceration. In doing so, Part I not only serves the book's purpose of challenging "expert" "perpetrator" narratives of violence in relation to "mental illness" but also signals our desire to prioritize meanings of violence from mental health service user/survivor perspectives. Part II, Prevailing Problems, locates the collection of writings (and the problem of violence in the lives of mental health service users/survivors) within the particular socio-political-economic moment of neo-liberalism. The contributions underscore the hegemony of psy-knowledge in contemporary responses to mental illness through government policy, research processes, and cultural practices. They achieve this by implicitly and explicitly examining the issue of state violence against mental health service users/survivors and by implicating psy-knowledge in *slow violence* against, the *slow death* of, and *slow justice* for diversely situated mental health service users/survivors. Relatedly, Part III, Law as Violence, further articulates the book's interest in scrutinizing the relationship between madness and state-authorized power and violence, offering a collection of writings that raises questions about the ways in which law reinforces hierarchies and orders of patriarchal power in both local and international contexts. And finally, Part IV, Geographies of Violence, locates the book within the more immediate geographies of institutions and community that mental health service users/survivors traverse and in which they are subjected to the violence of "intervention."

In each section we provide a detailed introduction, outlining the overarching theme and key ideas presented by the contributors about the ways that violence occurs as people bump up against structures and systems that rely on psy-discourses and power.

Ultimately, as we have discussed, this collection of writings serves to expand the current parameters of violence narratives through a collection of writings that coalesce to push the boundaries of current acceptable practice and policy in the domain of madness, mental illness, and mental health service users/survivors. The book is a response to the dearth of literature and resources that hold systems and institutions accountable for the ways in which they participate in violence against mental health service users/survivors. While some existing literature does focus on broadly defined organizational violence within health care contexts, it is often setting and discipline specific (e.g., *(Re)Thinking Violence: in Health Care Settings: A Critical Approach*),[22] lacking an interdisciplinary focus on multiple systems and institutions experienced by mental health service users/survivors. This limitation has also become alarmingly evident to us through our respective work as academics, advocates, and activists. That is, our discussions with colleagues and students; community members; professionals within the mental health, legal, and criminal justice systems; and mental health researchers and consumer/survivor researchers suggest that the relevant bodies of research and theoretical literature fail to offer critical frameworks on power and violence as they are broadly experienced by mental health service users/survivors. Individualized narratives of power and violence fail to account for how various systems and institutions produce violence. In this regard, this book constitutes a remedy, of sorts, by offering accounts of modern/structural and postmodern/post-structural conceptualizations of power and violence within intersecting systems and institutions (i.e., "regimes of power"), such as psychiatric institutions, psychiatric discourses on mental disorders, economic policy, health and public policy, policing and criminal courts that impact mental health serviced users. We hope that this collection of writings spurs ongoing discussion and analysis about the creation of frameworks developed by services users themselves that look at restorative justice and positive models for communal intermediation.

NOTES

1 Office of the High Commission on Human Rights, "Convention on the Rights of Persons with Disabilities."
2 Vaughan, "Introduction," 7.
3 Pinker, *The Better Angels*.
4 Gray, "Why Pinker Is Wrong."
5 Scull, MacKenzie, and Hervey, *Masters of Bedlam*.
6 Taylor and Gunn, "Homicides by People With Mental Illness."
7 Suman, Ndegwa, and Wilson, *Forensic Psychiatry*.
8 Crocker et al., "The National Trajectory."
9 Nixon, *Slow Violence*, 6
10 Lefrançois, Menzies, and Reaume, *Mad Matters*.
11 Beresford, Nettle, and Perring, "Towards a Social Model"; Beresford et al., *From Mental Illness*.
12 Fleming et al. "Action Speaks Louder Than Words."

13 Lukes, *Power*.
14 Ibid.
15 Gaventa, *Power and Powerlessness*.
16 Ibid.
17 Morgan and Thapar Björkert, "'I'd Rather You'd Lay Me on the Floor.'"
18 Bourdieu, "Gender and Symbolic Violence," 339.
19 Dominquez and Menjivar, "Beyond Individual and Visible Acts of Violence," 187; Kleinman, "The Violences of Everyday Life."
20 Auyero and Burbano de Lara, "In Harm's Way at the Urban Margins."
21 Beresford, *All Our Welfare*.
22 Holmes, Perron, and Rudge, *(Re)Thinking Violence*.

BIBLIOGRAPHY

Auyero, Juvier, and Agustin Burbano de Lara. "In Harm's Way at the Urban Margins." *Ethnography* 13, no. 3 (2012): 531–57.
Beresford, Peter. *All Our Welfare: Towards Participatory Social Policy*. Bristol, UK: Policy Press, 2016.
Beresford, Peter, Rebecca Perring, Mary Nettle, and Jan Wallcraft. *From Mental Illness to a Social Model of Madness and Distress*. London, UK: Shaping Our Lives and National Survivor User Network (NSUN), 2016. https:// www.shapingourlives.org.uk/wp-content/uploads/2016/05 /FROM-MENTAL-ILLNESS-PDF-2.pdf.
Beresford, Peter, Nettle, Mary, and Perring, Rebecca. "Towards a Social Model of Madness and Distress? Exploring What Service Users Say." Joseph Rowntree Foundation. Accessed November 22, 2010. https://www.jrf.org .uk/report/towards-social-model-madness-and-distress-exploring-what -service-users-say.
Bourdieu, Pierre. "Gender and Symbolic Violence." In *Violence in War and Peace: An Anthology*, edited by Nancy Scheper-Hughes and Phillipe Bourgois, 339. Malden, MA: Blackwell, 2004.
Crocker, Ann, Tonia Nicholls, Michael Seto, and Gilles Côté. "The National Trajectory Project of Individuals Found Not Criminally Responsible on Account of Mental Disorder in Canada. Part 2: The People Behind the Label." *Canadian Journal of Psychiatry* 60, no. 3 (2015): 106–16.
Dominquez, Silvia, and Cecilia, Menjivar. "Beyond Individual and Visible Acts of Violence: A Framework to Examine the Lives of Women in Low-Income Neighborhoods." *Women's Studies International Forum* 44, no. 187 (2014): 184–95.

Fleming, Julie, Mark Harrison, Alan Perry, Dave Purdy, and Dave Ward. "Action Speaks Louder Than Words." *Youth and Policy* 2, no. 3 (Winter 1983–84): 16–19.

Gaventa, John. *Power and Powerlessness: Quiescence and Rebellion in an Appalachian Valley.* Chicago: University of Illinois Press, 1982.

Gray, John. "Why Pinker Is Wrong about Violence and War." *Guardian,* March 13, 2015. https://www.theguardian.com/books/2015/mar/13/john-gray-steven-pinker-wrong-violence-war-declining.

Holmes, Dave, Trudy Rudge, and Amelie Perron. *(Re)Thinking Violence in Health Care Settings: A Critical Approach.* Burlington, ON: Ashgate, 2012.

Kleinman, Arthur. "The Violences of Everyday Life: The Multiple Forms and Dynamics of Social Violence." In *Violence and Subjectivity,* edited by Veena Das, Arthur Kleinman, Mamphela Ramphele, and Pamela Reynolds, 226–41. Berkeley: University of California Press, 2000.

Lefrançois, Brenda, Robert Menzies, and Geoffrey Reaume, eds. *Mad Matters: A Critical Reader in Canadian Mad Studies.* Toronto, ON: Canadian Scholars' Press, 2013.

Lukes, Steven. *Power: A Radical View.* 2nd ed. Basingstoke, UK: Palgrave Macmillan, 2004.

Morgan, Karen, and Suruchi Thapar Björkert. "'I'd Rather You'd Lay Me on the Floor and Start Kicking Me': Understanding Symbolic Violence in Life." *Women's Studies International Forum* 29 (2006): 441–52.

Nixon, Rob. *Slow Violence and the Environmentalism of the Poor.* Cambridge, MA: Harvard University Press, 2011.

Office of the High Commission on Human Rights. "Convention on the Rights of Persons with Disabilities." Accessed November 12, 2017. https://www.ohchr.org/EN/HRBodies/CRPD/Pages/ConventionRightsPersonsWithDisabilities.aspx.

Pinker, Steven. *The Better Angels of Our Nature: Why Violence Has Declined.* New York: Viking Press, 2011.

Scull, Andrew, Charlotte MacKenzie, and Nicholas Hervey. *Masters of Bedlam: The Transformation of the Mad-Doctoring Trade.* Princeton, NJ: Princeton University Press, 1996.

Suman, Fernando, Ndegwa, David, and Wilson, Melba, *Forensic Psychiatry, Race and Culture.* London, UK: Routledge, 2005.

Taylor, Pamela, and John Gunn. "Homicides by People with Mental Illness: Myth and Reality." *British Journal of Psychiatry* 174 (1999): 9–14.

Vaughan, Megan. "Introduction." In *Psychiatry and Empire,* edited by Sloan Mahone and Megan Vaughan, 1–16. New York: Palgrave Macmillan, 2007.

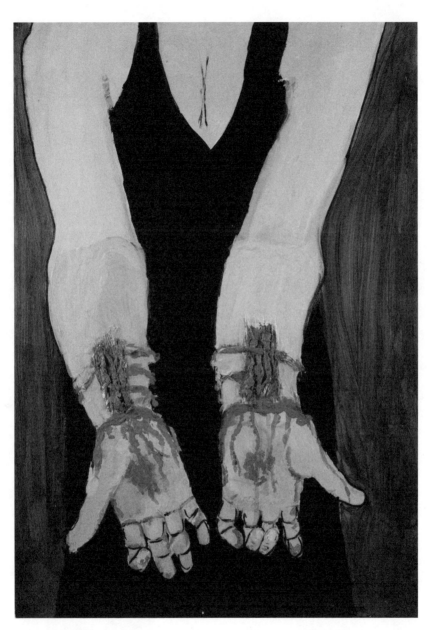

Untitled, by Ruth Beresford

PART I

Dispatches on Violence

Most texts about violence and mental illness tend to start and stop with accounts of violent behaviour and its perpetrators. In this book it has instead been our starting point for challenging the arbitrary and narrow boundaries of such conventional discourse. We have called this part *Dispatches on Violence* because we offer four very different first-hand accounts that relate directly to such experience to help make sense of its position and meanings in its much broader conceptual and material context. We have tried not to duck the pain and misery that such violence may bring, but we have also sought to improve understanding of it by not isolating or pathologizing it or those associated with it.

There are some general points to make about these contributions. All speak to people's lived experiences of violence in relation to institutions. This includes institutions of psychiatry, of motherhood, and of risk assessment, and the literal institutions of incarceration. Surprisingly, for us, these accounts are all by women. Surprisingly because women are most often associated with violence against *themselves* rather than others – notably in terms of self-harm. We don't know what this means. Are women more prepared to talk about violence in relation to themselves? Is it attributed to them arbitrarily and unreasonably or are such thoughts much more common than those accepting gender stereotypes feel comfortable believing? We do not know.

The first chapter, The Risk of Violence, by an anonymous female explores the lifelong consequences of being labelled as potentially violent without evidence or good cause. She speaks to the inherent violence of labelling someone as violent or having the potential for violence and the pain that comes from keeping this "secret." But she also cautions us as editors about the risks of producing a book like this about violence against mental health service users/survivors because of the potential that the book might exacerbate rather than ameliorate problematic associations between the two. This highlights the tension inherent in such a book – the risk of exacerbating dangerous associations between madness and violence by writing about it and the risk of exacerbating violence in the lives of Mad people by *not* talking about it. Her chapter also links with Tobin LeBlanc Haley's when she asks, How are you supposed to deal with that kind of knowledge about yourself?

Chapter 2, A Personal Account of Mental Distress in Motherhood, is also written anonymously. The author writes of wondering about her own potential for violence against her children. Again, she speaks of the experience of "secrecy" – not talking about it with others, not knowing whether other mothers have similar experiences. She speaks to the importance of not labelling mental distress, here associated with motherhood as a mental illness – not medicalizing the mental health of new mothers – and the need to acknowledge the impact of social factors such as loneliness, poverty, isolation, and adaption to parenthood. She highlights the importance of developing de-medicalized accounts of madness and mental distress.

In chapter 3, Sarah Markham speaks from her lived experience of engagement with a secure and forensic service (forensic inpatient) and the tensions created between patients' need to regain their personal freedom and clinicians' needs for clinical outcomes. There is no underplaying of the damage that violence can do in this critical first-hand account, which does not gloss over the issues that all involved can face and the challenge they present if we seek to do more than pathologize and punish.

In the last chapter, Carlyn Zwarenstein has explored what she calls "the opposite of violence" from her experience as a Mad person. She talks about the things that can make someone who is distressed feel safe and reassured, what she calls individual acts of kindness. She contrasts her image of the response to someone who has suffered physical trauma – "sitting near the scene of the incident, wrapped in a thermal or fuzzy blanket, head bent gratefully over a mug of hot tea or cocoa while someone – anyone – speaks to them kindly," with her experience of hospitals and other mental health settings. Here the emphasis is on minimizing expected hostility and risk rather than warmth and relationships of care. This is hardly calming or reassuring, and Carlyn reminds us of the need to reassess present "safety versus humanity trade-offs."

1 The Risk of Violence

ANONYMOUS FEMALE

Introduction

I have been finding it very difficult to write something for this book.
My life has taken a huge turn for the better recently and I want to keep
it that way; so, after careful consideration, I have decided to write this
chapter anonymously. I am also struggling with revealing information
that I have been unable to speak or write openly about for more than
three decades. So why would I want to write about it now, having kept
it to myself for so long? One reason is that I would have found it helpful
to read something like this when the "threat" of violence first appeared
in my own life. Another reason is that I am unsure whether this book
is a good idea. I want the editors, and readers, to think carefully about
ways in which the book itself might exacerbate rather than ameliorate
problematic associations between madness and violence; my hope is
that this chapter will help prompt such reflection.

I use the example of my own experience of the mental health system and its aftermath to illustrate my discussion of madness and violence. The chapter focuses on information I was given by medical and
psychiatric personnel when I came into contact with the mental health
system in the United Kingdom in the 1970s and 1980s. Every time I
was told something about my "mental illness," I was left wondering,
What am I supposed to do with this information? I found I had no way of
making sense of what I had been told, and each time I tried, I seemed
to dig myself deeper and deeper into a "mental illness" hole. One piece
of information I was given (about my own potential for violence) was
impossible to deal with, which is why I tried determinedly to push it
out of my mind for more than three decades. It could be argued (and in

general, I would agree), that it is always better to talk about things that worry you; but when it comes to madness and violence, that doesn't seem to apply.

I don't have a good view of psychiatry, but the concerns I have about the association of madness with violence are much greater than the concerns I have about psychiatry in general. The issue I have with psychiatry is that it individualizes problems. But what if you are one of those individuals in whom such problems are located? Being given a psychiatric diagnosis and realizing that psychiatry, the media, and indeed much of wider society view you as a "problem" can be very difficult; however, that difficulty is exacerbated and compounded when psychiatry locates in you the threat of violence. How are you supposed to deal with that kind of knowledge about yourself? This is what I want to discuss in this chapter. I begin by outlining my early experiences of psychiatry and then go on to discuss the weight of violence in my own life for the last 35 years before concluding with my concerns about this collection of writings.

I need to state at this point that I have never been violent towards another person. Nor have I ever threatened violence or incited anyone else to be violent. Throughout my life, I have held down responsible jobs, and my friends have frequently entrusted me with their babies and small children. I am not the sort of person you would expect to be violent.

My Experiences of Psychiatry

My contact with the psychiatric system started when I was a student in the 1970s. During my final year at university, I had a series of physical illnesses and was advised to take some time out from my studies and rest, but after six months I still had lots of aches and pains and was constantly tired. I also had a weird sense of being outside my body, like I was observing or looking in on my life taking place; and my head felt strange, like there was a force pushing against my forehead. After a series of medical tests, my GP told me that my aches and pains and exhaustion had no medical explanation and I was no longer physically unwell. I found it difficult to make sense of that information but concluded that if there was nothing wrong with me it would be fine to exert myself physically. I registered with a temporary work agency and for the next six months I was continually employed in a series of short-term factory jobs before obtaining a temporary contract as a nursing auxiliary at the local geriatric hospital. During this period, my life consisted of working, eating in the factory/hospital canteen, and returning home to sleep. I was so exhausted I could do nothing else, even on my days off.

Eventually my housemates persuaded me to go back to my GP as my joints were still painful, and I continued to feel weirdly distanced from my life, though I never once had a day off work for sickness. My GP prescribed chlorpromazine (which I'd never heard of), but when I looked closely at the tablets, I saw they had Largactil written on them. I knew what Largactil was, as this was given to some of the patients I worked with; the ones who were "mentally ill." I couldn't understand why my GP was giving me medication that was usually prescribed for "mental illness?" I didn't take any of the Largactil tablets and lay awake all night wondering what on earth was going on. When I queried the prescription with my GP the following day, I was told I needed to take the tablets as they would help me rest and not feel so tired. I felt very bewildered by this information. I didn't take the Largactil, nor did I return to my GP for some time.

The next time I received confusing information from my GP was about six months later when I was applying for a visa to travel and work temporarily at a children's summer camp in the United States. When I asked about the health section of the application, my GP said, "You've got what they would call a mental illness. I don't think there's any point in filling in this form. They won't let you work in America." The shock was enormous. I simply did not know what to do with that information. I couldn't even begin to understand myself as one of those problematic "mentally ill" people you see roaming the streets. I found myself unable to sleep for nights on end, as I could not take in this information. My housemates contacted my GP and told her I wasn't sleeping. After several weeks, she referred me to a psychiatrist. I agreed to the referral because I was utterly bewildered about what was happening to me.

The psychiatrist talked about dopamine imbalances in my brain and advised me to give up my temporary job, even though there were no complaints from my workplace. Indeed, the matron of the hospital asked to see me and praised my work; she also questioned why I needed to give up my job to receive psychiatric treatment, but I didn't take any notice of her concerns and chose instead to follow the psychiatrist's advice. The psychiatrist told me that I would recover more quickly if I stopped working and was admitted to hospital as a full-time voluntary patient. I agreed to treatment as an inpatient at the local psychiatric hospital but didn't realize I was being treated for "schizophrenia"; I discovered that several months later, when a new psychiatrist looked through my notes and said, "They think you've got schizophrenia." What was I supposed to do with that information? By then, I'd somehow accepted the role of mental patient and this diagnosis was just another facet of that role. As time went on, I found myself conforming to staff expectations of the role and even emulating aspects of other patients' behaviour.

The only "treatment" I received while in hospital was medication: Largactil, plus Kemadrin to counteract the side effects of the Largactil – these adverse effects were horrendous: feeling unable to control my tongue and trembling in my hands and arms. I thought they were caused by the Largactil, but the psychiatrist told me I was probably causing them myself because I'd read about "side effects" and I was imagining that I was experiencing them. By then I believed that I really was "mentally ill," so it was perfectly possible that I was imagining and causing the "side effects" myself. But when the psychiatrist eventually prescribed Kemadrin, it seemed to help. However, I then tortured myself thinking that I was perhaps imagining these improvements. I really didn't know what to think or feel by that stage and had completely lost any sense of my "self."

When I was discharged from hospital several months later, I didn't feel any better. In fact, I felt considerably worse; in addition to all my physical aches and pains and feelings of disconnectedness, I was also severely depressed and felt that my life was not worth living. Despite this, I registered again with the temporary work agency and got a short-term job in a department store, followed by a contract working as a receptionist, which I enjoyed. I went back to my GP to ask if I really needed to take the Largactil because it was making me feel very drowsy, but she suggested trying another brand of medication. I tried this for a while and then decided to take myself off medication altogether. I asked some medical students for advice about stopping medication and they suggested gradually reducing the dose. I did this, but it caused awful withdrawal effects – again, I wondered if I was causing these myself, but I was determined to be rid of medication, so I persevered and was eventually successful. I was, however, still exhausted all the time, ached from head to toe and felt like I wasn't real. I went back to my GP and told her that if my symptoms had a mental rather than a physical cause, I wanted to talk about any psychological problems I might have. I didn't know what these problems might be, but I wanted an opportunity to find out. My GP referred me to another hospital, which she told me was renowned for its residential program and psychotherapeutic approaches.

I spent half a day at the psychotherapeutic hospital undergoing an "assessment." The psychiatrist I saw (I'll call him Dr Green) interviewed me for less than an hour and wrote to my GP saying that I wouldn't benefit from the psychotherapy they offered as I had "schizophrenia." He also said there was a risk that I would kill my mother – my GP told me this the next time I saw her. I have never been violent in my life, ever. So how Dr Green could reach this conclusion I do not know, but his opinion clearly held a lot more weight than my own. I was devastated. That was 35 years ago. For three and a half decades I've had to live with that information, knowing that it's written in black and white in my medical records. When I was younger, I moved around the country quite a bit and each time I met a new GP it was an issue; it also restricted considerably my life opportunities for at least two decades as I was precluded from doing anything that required access to my medical records (medicals for employment or visas to work abroad, etc.). That sort of information also plays on your mind; when things are difficult it keeps popping up and won't go away.

For years I couldn't sleep at night. In my mind, I would go over and over my interactions with Dr Green and other staff at the hospital. I couldn't think of anything I'd said or done that would cause them to think I was potentially violent. And I certainly didn't make any reference to wanting to kill my mother or anyone else. I should mention here that when I attempted to get myself "undiagnosed" 15 years later, the psychiatrist I saw said that the hospital where Dr Green worked had a reputation for not accepting patients who had a "serious mental illness," and he wondered if the psychiatrists who worked there sometimes exaggerated patients' diagnoses as a reason for not accepting them; he thought this might have happened to me. When I'd been interviewed by Dr Green, I was successfully holding down a full-time job as a receptionist and wasn't taking any medication, so he needed some other sort of "evidence" of "mental illness" to justify his assessment that I was unsuitable for psychotherapy.

When writing about my experiences of psychiatry here, I have tried to present my thinking as it was at the time. But having since been in contact with many other people who have survived the psychiatric system, I now think very differently about my experiences. There are no physical tests for "mental illness," no blood tests, genetic profiles or X-rays that can *definitively* prove that a person has a particular "mental disorder," such as "schizophrenia," or indeed that there is a "risk" they will be violent. As a young person caught up in the psychiatric system, I didn't know this. I thought that being given a mental diagnosis was the same as being given a physical diagnosis. At that stage, I didn't know that there were any uncertainties or even ambiguities about diagnostic processes, and I thought that psychiatrists knew what they were doing. To make matters worse, I quite liked Dr Green when he interviewed me; he was friendly and humorous and I left the hospital feeling hopeful that he would take me on as a patient and my life might start to turn around. But his letter to my GP confirmed my status as a "schizophrenic" in need of medication; it also branded me as a potential murderer. I cannot tell you the number of nights I lay awake wondering if it really were possible that I would commit murder and if I should just kill myself as a precautionary measure.

Madness, Violence, and Empathy

Though this branding as a "potential murderer" was by far the worst thing that happened to me, psychiatry's other impacts on my life were also horrendous. Why then do I want to single out the association of madness with violence as particularly problematic? From a personal perspective, it was because I could not speak of this, as I explain below. But first, I want to say something about trying to make sense of my other experiences of psychiatry and the process of sharing and talking about those experiences before going on to discuss further the impacts of a "potential violence" diagnosis.

As a young woman in my twenties, I had little knowledge of "mental health" issues. I was a science student and to all intents and purposes I was unaware of social issues as I didn't read a newspaper regularly and rarely watched television or listened to the radio. I don't think I'd ever read any novels that explored issues of "mental health," and I'd never had any reason to think deeply about this sort of thing. I was dependent therefore on dominant mainstream understandings of "mental illness." For example, my childhood home was quite close to the local "lunatic asylum" and discussion of patients who lived there was almost always in derogatory terms. I had no desire to find out about the patients' lives or the psychiatric treatment they received, but when I came into contact with psychiatry myself, this suddenly became of interest to me. I started going to the public library to look up the "treatment" of "mental illnesses" in encyclopedias, and while I was there, I scoured the newspapers for anything related to "mental health."

The materials I accessed therefore reflected dominant understandings of "mental health and illness." This meant that these dominant understandings were the only framework I had for making sense of my own experiences. Even though I didn't want to understand the information I was being given in those terms, every time I tried to make sense of it, I pushed myself further and further into a "mental illness" hole – because I simply didn't have access to any other way of understanding or explaining my experiences. It wasn't until several years later, when I turned the pages of a book about feminist therapy in a radical book store, that I realized that there might be alternative ways of understanding madness and distress. I also made contact with other psychiatric system survivors, and since then I've been able to reframe my experiences and now understand them differently. In fact, writing the earlier part of this chapter was really difficult as I kept asking myself, *How could I have believed that?* and *Why on earth did I torture myself for years, thinking that I really was mentally ill?* I also found myself wondering if I would even have encountered the psychiatric system had the Internet been available at the time, with its wide range of alternative perspectives on madness and distress.

For several years after I left the hospital, I didn't talk about my encounters with psychiatry as it was fairly easy to hide my past, particularly when I moved to another part of the country; but after a while I started to talk to friends about some of my experiences. Sometimes they didn't take it too well, but generally people were very accepting and would often share their own experiences. Over time, I realized that being able to talk about my own experiences of mental and emotional distress meant that I often developed quite close friendships with people, quite quickly. I also found it liberating to be able to talk openly about my "psychiatric history" without having to censor everything I said for fear of people finding out. The same cannot be said, however, for talking about violence. My tentative attempts at sharing Dr Green's assessment of my potential to kill my mother were universally met with horror. One close friend (who had known me for many years, during which time I had never been violent in any way) responded by saying, "I'll call the police if you get violent," as he walked towards the telephone. Over time, I've come to realize that it is simply not possible to talk about this to anyone I am close to. I have had to keep it to myself.

My view therefore is that discussions of madness and discussions of violence are qualitatively different: whereas some, but not all, people can identify and empathize with another person's mental and emotional distress or madness; the same cannot be said of an assessment of "potential violence." No one has ever come close to empathizing with my experience of this; nor have I ever heard or read about anyone else's experience of being assessed in this way, which is partly why I decided to write this chapter. As I mentioned earlier, my understanding of psychiatry is that it locates problems in individuals. Its diagnostic processes are a means of stereotyping people as "Other." This Othering was particularly effective historically when people diagnosed as "mentally ill" were incarcerated in institutions and hidden from the rest of society. Now that people are less likely to be institutionalized, there are more possibilities for countering that Othering as mentally ill, as my own experience has shown. Branding an individual as potentially violent, however, is Othering of a different order, as it incites fear and the need for protection; it also positions an impassable gulf between that person and other human beings.

After an assessment of potential violence has been made, it is very difficult for that association with violence to be removed. I mentioned earlier that 15 years after my initial encounters with psychiatry, I attempted to get myself "undiagnosed." Despite a letter to my GP from a sympathetic psychiatrist, the "undiagnosis" didn't work because the original letter, with its assessment of "potential violence," remained on my medical records. For the most part, I have dealt with the assessment of my own "potential violence" by (a) keeping quiet about it; and (b) trying to push it to the back of my mind. Both of these approaches may be ill-advised, as it is generally better to talk about something that troubles us, rather than keep it to ourselves. As strategies for survival, however, they have served me well as my life has panned out with opportunities that I could never have imagined possible 35 years ago.

Social Climate

So far, I have talked about psychiatry's assessment of the potential for violence only in relation to me, and it could be argued that my experience is unusual. However, the American Psychiatric Association's resource document on violence risk assessment discusses the "social climate" in which psychiatry is now practised (deinstitutionalization, legal judgments against psychiatrists for failing to identify the risk of violence, increased claims for medical malpractice etc.), offering this as an explanation for the profession's increased focus on violence risk assessment and growing risk aversiveness.[1] The authors conclude that, "for the foreseeable future, no technique will be available to identify those who will act violently *that will not simultaneously identify a large number of people who would not*" (emphasis added).[2] This suggests that my experience is perhaps not unusual and increasing numbers of non-violent people could be living with the knowledge that they too have been assessed as "potentially violent." That's not to say however that psychiatrists always get it wrong. Clearly there are some individuals with "mental illness" diagnoses who do go on to commit unspeakable acts of violence; but so too do people without any kind of diagnosed "mental illness."

In addition to locating problems in individuals, psychiatrists also advise policymakers on problematic social issues, such as gun control and the "dangerousness" of people with "mental disorders." Gun control and "mental illness" has become a high-profile public debate in the United States, fuelled by media coverage and the agendas of lobby groups for both gun control and gun rights.[3] Similar high-profile discussions about "mental illness" and "dangerousness" are also evident internationally.[4] When debates about violence and "mental illness" are in the public domain, societal-level "dangerousness" cannot be hidden in the way in which I, as an individual, hid the issue of "potential violence" in my own life. The association between "mental illness" and violence is seared into public consciousness, and a generalized "fear of the mentally ill" is invoked and amplified; this has the potential, by association, to affect all mental health service users/survivors, even though the vast majority of people with "mental illness" diagnoses are never violent towards others. "Mental illness" is, however, strongly associated with suicide, and people with "mental illness" diagnoses are more likely to use firearms to take their own lives than to kill others.[5]

Over the years, several campaigns internationally have attempted to challenge mental health discrimination and stigma, but as Kate Holland notes, these campaigns "can themselves perpetuate stereotypes and assumptions that ultimately run counter to the original intent of challenging stigma."[6] For example, the recent UK Time to Change campaign reinforces the individualization of "mental illness" by locating "schizophrenia" in "parts of the brain."[7] Campaigns that challenge the association of "dangerousness" with "mental illness" by emphasizing that the vast majority of people diagnosed as "mentally ill" are never violent also, of course, serve to *reinforce* the location of violence in the small minority of mental health service users/survivors diagnosed as "potentially violent."

Conclusion

Although "mental illness" is founded on fear, deinstitutionalization policies and the increased numbers of people diagnosed as having "mental health problems" are removing some of this fear as diagnoses become normalized and experiences are shared through personal connections; but diagnosis as "potentially violent" is different. I found it impossible to share my experience of being branded as "potentially violent" in any kind of meaningful way. (To be fair, I too would have anxieties about being in the presence of someone who has been branded in this way and would want to think carefully about ensuring my personal safety.) There is no defence against an assessment of "potential violence." Just as there is no way of "proving" that you do not have a "mental illness," so too there is no way of proving that you do not pose a threat of violence. The process of sharing experiences of "Othering as mentally ill" may engender empathy and closeness; but when experiences of "Othering as potentially violent" are disclosed, empathy and closeness will likely be lost, with obvious impact on our "selves" and our humanity.

Psychiatrists' assessments of "potential violence" are individualized and dehumanizing. This individualization and dehumanization is further amplified by societal level fears of "the violent mentally ill." Psychiatrists are unable accurately to predict "potential violence" in individuals they identify as "mentally ill" and may also misdiagnose non-violent individuals as "potentially violent." The association of "potential violence" with "mental illness" is therefore profoundly problematic for the individuals in whom this association is located; it also (by association) impacts more widely on mental health service users/survivors in general. How then could the association of "mental illness" and "potential violence" be disrupted? Surely a book that explores madness, violence, and power would be a helpful contribution – or maybe not. My apprehension about this book is similar to my reticence about revealing my personal experience of assessment as "potentially violent"; just as there is no defence against a diagnosis of "mental illness" or assessment as "dangerous," so too is there no definitive way of demonstrating that the association between "mental illness" and "potential violence" is erroneous. Because psychiatric diagnosis as "potentially violent" is so deeply individualized and fears of "dangerous mentally ill patients" are seared into public consciousness, however critically this book is written there is a risk that it too may serve to reinforce this association.

NOTES

1 Buchanan et al., "Resource Document."
2 Ibid., 8.
3 Metzl and MacLeish, "Mental Illness."
4 Morse, "The Sun Newspaper's."
5 Swanson et al., "Mental Illness and Reduction of Gun Violence and Suicide"; Stuart and Arboleda-Flórez, "A Public Health Perspective."
6 Holland, "The Unintended Consequences," 217.
7 Time to Change, "Mental Health and Stigma."

BIBLIOGRAPHY

Buchanan, Alec, Renee Binder, Michael Norko, and Marvin Swartz. "Resource Document on Psychiatric Violence Risk Assessment." *American Journal of Psychiatry* 169, no. 3 (2012, Data supplement): 1–10.
Holland, Kate. "The Unintended Consequences of Campaigns Designed to Challenge Stigmatising Representations of Mental Illness in the Media." *Social Semiotics* 22, no. 3 (2012): 217–36.
Metzl, Jonathan M., and Kenneth T. MacLeish. "Mental Illness, Mass Shootings, and the Politics of American Firearms." *American Journal of Public Health* 105, no. 2 (2015): 240–9.
Morse, F. "The *Sun* Newspaper's '1,200 Killed by Mental Patients' Headline Labelled 'Irresponsible and Wrong,'" *Independent*, October 7, 2013. https://www.independent.co.uk/news/uk/the-sun-newspapers-1200-killed-by-mental-patients-headline-labelled-irresponsible-and-wrong-8863893.html.
Stuart, Heather L., and Julio E. Arboleda-Flórez. "A Public Health Perspective on Violent Offenses among Persons with Mental Illness." *Psychiatric Services* 52, no. 5 (2001): 654–9.
Swanson, Jeffrey W., E. Elizabeth McGinty, Seena Fazel, and Vickie M. Mays. "Mental Illness and Reduction of Gun Violence and Suicide: Bringing Epidemiologic Research to Policy." *Annals of Epidemiology* 25, no. 5 (2015): 366–76.
Time to Change. "Mental Health and Stigma." 2016. Accessed February 13, 2017. https://www.time-to-change.org.uk/mental-health-stigma.

2 A Personal Account of Mental Distress in Motherhood

ANONYMOUS

I am a 39-year-old mother of three children ages 10, 7, and 3. I have been with my partner for 18 years after we met at university, where I qualified to become a nurse. So far, my career has been interesting, varied, and successful. I am now a senior nurse and a specialist in my field, with an MSc in nursing. I receive good feedback and very rarely have time off sick – only one day off in the last six years. People I work with tell me I am organized, and I get the impression that I am perceived as a fairly calm person.

I mention all of this because it demonstrates that on paper I have a happy life and no obvious reason to have any mental health problems. Overall my childhood was happy: I have three siblings who I get on well with and my parents are still together after 40 years of marriage.

However, I have experienced mental distress. This was particularly after I became a mother, and it was characterized by anxiety and intrusive thoughts about harming my children.

I was desperate to have children starting in my mid-twenties. It took me some time to persuade my partner, who did not feel ready to become a father at that point. We almost broke up over it because I felt I could not wait until I was in my thirties. In the end he relented, and we had our first child when I was 29.

In truth, I would say that was when my mental health really began to break down. I had always been quite an anxious person and was aware that anxiety was a problem for me, but it was when I became a mum that this really began to impact on my life. Motherhood has lots of positive aspects – I loved my daughter and had lots of fun with her, but like many women I found the transition to motherhood difficult. It could be lonely, boring, upsetting, frightening, and isolating. Being the sort of person who felt it was important to do things "right," I would read lots of advice about how to bring up my daughter, which was often contradictory or difficult to follow. For example, the advice about waiting to wean until she was six months was impossible for me. I had to go back to work when she was five months old, and with her having been breast fed, she refused to take any milk from a bottle. Everyone had their own opinion and advice about the best way to child rear, but some of it just didn't fit with me and my child. It was all very stressful and I began to feel like a failure. My daughter had a lot of tantrums, which I found difficult to manage. I felt responsible for any negative behaviour and that I must be doing something wrong if she didn't behave well. I now realize that a lot of what she did was actually typical behaviour for a toddler, that she would grow out of it, and that I was learning how to manage it. Unfortunately, during this period instead of supporting each other, my partner and I did not get on very well and we both found our new life as parents difficult to adapt to. When my daughter was one, we almost broke up, but relationship counselling helped us through this difficult time, and we did go on to have our second child.

Although I then felt closer to my partner and I enjoyed my maternity leave with my second daughter, my feelings of anxiety and depression peaked around the time I went back to work part-time. I felt rather trapped in my job, where there was generally a bad atmosphere and morale was low. I was struggling to cope with the emotional demands of having two young children but felt I should be able to. I remember crying in the toilets at work and feeling like I couldn't cope with my life. I think that I had been used to being independent and even rather selfish before I had children, and it was difficult to get used to always being needed by someone else. I didn't see that I would be able to adapt to my life as a parent and be happy with it.

One incident stands out particularly. I was getting ready to go out with my children, and the eldest was playing-up about putting her coat on. I helped her to put her scarf on and as I did so, I felt so fed up with how she was behaving I imagined strangling her with the scarf. It was a sinister, dark feeling that affected me in the pit of my stomach. I felt really awful about it (although I now realize many parents must have similar feelings sometimes – it doesn't mean they would follow through with it). I know that this is when my anxiety began around my fear that I would harm my children. I would have intrusive thoughts about it, and it felt like a weight on my shoulders. I couldn't enjoy life because underneath it all was this belief that I might harm my daughters.

I became rather obsessive in some of my behaviour: I developed a fear of sharp knives, because I was afraid that I might stab the children in a moment of rage when they were being difficult. I couldn't leave sharp knives on the kitchen surface and would have to put them away as soon as they were washed. None of the knives were even sharp enough to cut food effectively, but I refused to buy any new ones because I didn't want to have access to knives that were any sharper. To be honest even now I haven't bought any new knives!

I remember feeling sick sometimes with anxiety. It was a horrible feeling, for which there was often no reason. Sitting in the cinema with my sister once I recall feeling terribly agitated and as if something bad was going to happen, but I couldn't work out what or why. I couldn't distract myself from how I felt. Occasionally, when I was in a social situation or on a rare evening out, I would find myself secretly wondering if I was going to stab my children one day. Sometimes I had this feeling that I wanted to put a plastic bag over my head and suffocate myself to block out the thoughts and the possibility of harming my children. Writing about it now is actually really difficult, because it felt very frightening and real. Although I do not experience those thoughts now and am having a positive experience of parenthood, I feel like that part of myself is hidden away in the background. I suppose I am still afraid that this could be triggered in me again, for example, if I have a difficult life event, such as bereavement.

One day that sticks out in my mind occurred when I went to meet a friend for a picnic with her young children. I parked at my parents' house because it was near the park. I unloaded the car and went in to see my dad first. I felt really miserable; I don't remember if it was anything in particular that had triggered it – perhaps the car journey had been stressful. My dad asked me how I was and it all came out. I cried and told him I was a bad mother, that I was a failure. On reflection I would say that although I continued to have difficulties for the next couple of years, that day was a turning point, because my dad didn't judge me about how I was feeling, and I began to realize that other people probably had similar experiences.

What Helped?

Thinking back to those years I have wondered what it was that helped me to get out of it. I never told any health professionals about my feelings – I didn't want to be labelled as "mentally ill." I didn't seek counselling about it (although I do think it could have been helpful). The following things definitely did help:

- SureStart, an accessible low cost service for parents and children. I used to attend the local SureStart Centre several times a week with my children, where there were activities, such as baby massage; play sessions; and other parents to talk to. This was an absolute lifeline, and I don't know how I would have coped without it. It seems to me to be incredibly important that places like this exist to bring people together and reduce the feelings of isolation and loneliness that parents can sometimes experience. I also made friends and we supported each other.
- Doing my masters degree and moving to a different place of work. It was helpful to focus on something other than being a mother.
- My family. Throughout my life they have always been a tremendous support. The main difficulty was that we live quite spread out across the county. My parents and sisters also work, so we cannot be there for each other as much as we would like to.
- Time. Some of what I went through I just had to go through. It gradually improved over time, as I became more confident and experienced in being a mother. Also, my children's behaviour became easier to manage as they got older and went to school. By the time I had my third child, I was much calmer and have so far found it much easier to cope.
- Moving house. We lived in a two bedroom flat until the two eldest were five and two. I did find it easier when we moved to a bigger home with a garden which I enjoy doing.
- An online cognitive behavioural therapy program. I did this sometimes and found it a useful way of challenging my negative thoughts.

These factors demonstrate that I am in a very fortunate position to be able to have a career, get an education, and have a nice home. Many people do not have these. I definitely believe that my mental health would be worse without the opportunities and support that I have had. The mental health of women when they become mothers has been a topic in the media recently, and there is more of an openness about it than when I had my first daughter. It is positive that mothers are being encouraged to be more honest about their feelings, and it would have helped me to know that other women may have similar experiences.

However, it bothers me that there is a tendency to medicalize the mental health of new mothers. I do not accept that postnatal depression is always an illness. I do not think what I experienced was exactly an illness, and therefore I did not want a medical intervention, such as medication or labelling by a doctor. Medicalizing the experiences of women when they have mental distress associated with motherhood is to deny some of the social factors that may contribute, such as loneliness, poverty, isolation, and adaption to parenthood. It also ignores the impact that cuts in local services, such as SureStart, may have on the lives of women and their families.

3 Patient Engagement and the Process of Self-Empowerment in Secure and Forensic Psychiatric Settings in the United Kingdom

I am a graduate of the University of Cambridge in the United Kingdom, and have a PhD in an area of pure mathematics. I am currently a visiting researcher in the Department of Biostatistics, Institute of Psychiatry, Psychology and Neuroscience, King's College, London. My interest in and experiential knowledge of the subject matter of this chapter stems from nine years' experience as an inpatient in various secure and forensic psychiatric hospitals in the South East of England and my six years of working in patient and public involvement with health care and clinical research services.

In the United Kingdom, "mentally disordered" individuals who have committed a crime in the context of suffering from a mental disorder may on sentencing be assigned a hospital order instead of a custodial sentence. This means they will receive treatment for their mental disorder and offending behaviour in a secure and forensic psychiatric hospital instead of a custodial sentence. Similarly, individuals who have been given a custodial sentence may be transferred to a secure and forensic psychiatric hospital for part or all their time under sentence.

In secure and forensic psychiatric settings, a tension exists between the promotion of responsibility and autonomy and the need to protect patients from posing a risk to themselves and others through qualification of their human rights and the restriction and confinement this entails. For me the relevance and efficacy of care planning and risk assessment and management were optimized through the development of mutual understanding between me and the clinicians working in the unit. While I was a forensic patient, I noticed barriers to achieving this mutual understanding, perhaps at times because the priorities of patients differed from those of their clinicians. Patients may place a greater emphasis on their need to regain their personal freedom whereas a clinician places a higher premium on first achieving certain clinical outcomes. Patients may enter forensic psychiatric services with a low sense of self-esteem and a confused sense of their place in society, with perhaps the belief that their offending behaviour was justified because of life or society dealing them a bad hand. This belief may lead to the conviction that the disabling effects of their mental disorder mean they have little chance of advance by conventional, law-abiding means.

According to the recovery model, as pioneered from within the consumer/survivor/ex-patient movement – a grassroots self-help and advocacy initiative, particularly within the United States during the late 1980s and early 1990s – recovery can be achieved through developing hope, a secure base, sense of self, supportive relationships, empowerment, social inclusion, coping skills, and meaning. In secure and forensic settings this is usually facilitated through clinically determined paced increases in responsibility and autonomy. However, if a patient has committed a serious offence(s), then the very need to qualify the patient's human rights through containment and restriction can act against a patient's need to express a sense of self and purpose through the reinstating of autonomy and reintegration into the community.

As a former inpatient of secure and forensic services, I am deeply aware of the need for effective and meaningful engagement between patients and all members of the clinical team to build a mutual understanding and respect for each other's roles and responsibilities and to develop a shared view of how best to achieve self-identified patient goals. While I was a resident of forensic inpatient units, I felt my co-patients were highly sensitive to how they were viewed by different members of their care team, especially if they felt misunderstood by their care team and similarly confused about what the care team expected from them. This has a direct impact on our ability to form the trusting relationships that lead us through therapeutic processes that are supposed to help us. It is valuable if the care team is responsive to people's perceptions during interactions and aims for the experience to be one that is constructive and empowering, rather than judgmental and restrictive.

No patient, however truculent or rebellious, wants to fail, although many may feel this is their lot in life and they may potentially never "succeed" in a sense that is meaningful to either them or those who place restrictions upon them. They may find it hard to own and take responsibility for their offending behaviour and say, "I know what I did, that it was wrong and that I shouldn't have done it," for fear of exposing themselves to a deluge of condemnation and chastisement from others, especially their own care team. I know from personal experience how much harder it is to talk about the guilt I felt after harming someone when the impression I received from my care team – and indeed what they said to me – was that they viewed me as being without remorse and devoid of empathy. This wasn't the case, I felt terrible for causing someone unnecessary injury and distress, yet no one seemed to believe me. I felt trapped; unable to talk about my experience and unpick the various reasons that had led me to making the choice I did. I was fortunate in that violence had been the tool I chose to deploy to catapult myself into the mental health system to get treatment after having exhausted conventional means and not an expression of anger or frustration. I knew I would never choose the same pathway again: it had led to such terrible consequences for both the victim and me and many other people. Not being able to talk about the guilt we feel at the harm we have caused while in the context of, say, raging against the desolation and unfairness of our situation, prevents us then from addressing the antecedents of the violent offending behaviour and can leave us predisposed to enacting further violence on ourselves or others within the confines of the ward or outside in the community.

Unfortunately, even the most dedicated and intelligent clinicians may fail to recognize what constitutes a good patient experience and the negative impact of the distress patients experience on their well-being as a consequence. Even if the clinician has a clear view of what would help the patient to recover and thrive, it may not be possible to construct the necessary care plan; it could conflict with accepted clinical, organizational, and legal protocols. Clinicians may also find their hands tied by the expectations of their colleagues and clinical peers. Similarly, clinical professionals may not understand what constitutes helpful and useful patient engagement, mistaking unquestioning receptivity and submission to their professional opinion as indicative of patient insight and compliance. In reality such seemingly meek and respectful affect may be indicative of little more than fear and a deep sense that their own opinion, as the "mentally disordered offender," will be discounted out of hand if it conflicts with the "professional" point of view. What the clinician believes to be a good example of patient engagement may be little more than a facade of submission and compliance.

Effective engagement of patients with their care team may only occur if both parties are aware of and appreciate each other's contribution. To discount the patient's point of view as indicative of a lack of insight if it counters the professional's view, especially if the patient has a poor educational background or lacks confidence in the ability to advocate for themselves, is not going to be helpful or build trust. However, patients can be acutely aware of their vulnerabilities and, independent of their care plan and care team, be learning how to manage their mental health through experiential learning and trial and error. This may be a natural consequence of developing the resilience necessary to survive the inpatient experience. In my opinion, patients will often not relinquish their more maladaptive behaviours (e.g., surreptitious substance misuse) until it seems more painful to stay as they are than to change and recover. Secure and forensic settings often seem like grotesque, stale, and barren kindergartens in which people are treated like children and yet are given little of meaning to do with their time. For those members of society whose failure to manage the disabling consequences of struggling with mental health problems has led them into conflict with the criminal justice system, the immediate outcome is a significant removal of their rights and restrictions, which severely limits their quality of life. No matter the severity of distress experienced before being detained, detention itself may feel so much worse, with those who are paid to care seeming to exhibit an inadequate degree of empathy, kindness, or even civility. Healing and recovering in secure settings can be an arduous process. Patients may need to develop a significant degree of resilience and pragmatic ability to adapt, heal ourselves, and regain freedom.

I found it most helpful when I actually received support that felt like real support and not punishment or degradation. We patients want services to help us to move forward in positive directions, preferably of our own choice. These are very human and understandable desires. For patient engagement with clinicians to be genuine and lead to recovery, we need to feel that we *are* at the centre of the entire process and that it is our well-being and human worth that are being prioritized. Again, conflicts between the priorities of the parties involved; the patients, their clinicians, front-line staff, managers, commissioners, and external agencies will often frustrate the delivery of even the most adaptive care and treatment package. However, on being given the opportunity to express our views and ideas in a constructive context and on a consistently regular basis, such as through pre-scheduled patient councils and service user involvement forums, it can be amazing how much rich and insightful innovation and capacity for positive change we forensic inpatients can exhibit.

In terms of my personal recovery, it was the consultant forensic psychologist in a medium secure setting where I was an inpatient who invested such trust in me in my first patient involvement role that he made a sustained significant positive impact on my recovery. When you feel you are a terrible, pathetic failure as both a human being and a member of society, being treated positively and respected for your abilities by someone who you hold in esteem can make a huge difference to your sense of self and potential for recovery.

Many other specific factors can influence the success of a person's inpatient experience. For example, indeterminacy of length of stay (an invariably negative factor) and the associated sense of powerlessness in determining one's own future and not being able to take advantage of the positive opportunities that present in society are significant barriers to recovery. Patients need to be informed of what the service has in store for them, the criteria that must be met for them to be allowed more freedom, access to the outdoors or to other parts of the unit, self-medicating, self-catering, transfer to less secure settings, and of course discharge. Ideally, we patients need to be involved right from the start in the care planning process and the determination of specific goals and how our progress is to be measured and achieved.

Traditionally, forensic psychiatry places significant weight on the association between past violence committed by a patient and their potential for future violence. Accordingly, minimization of a patient's perceived risk with regard to others and themselves is viewed as the overarching aim of a patient's treatment in secure hospital settings. Unfortunately, the various actuarial and clinical judgment-based violence risk assessment tools have yet to be shown to exhibit significant positive predictive power and may be described as being, at best, heuristic. Furthermore, according to James Livingston, "defining success in one-dimensional, negative terms can create a distorted view of the diverse objectives of the FMH [forensic mental health] system."[1] I believe this point cannot be emphasized enough and to be specific, in risk assessment this means taking into account positive factors such as secure attachment in childhood, educational achievement, and history of long-term employment. As sensitive, sentient beings, inpatients do respond to kindness and humane treatment which seeks to optimize their quality of life. For a patient to experience their care team as respectful and positively concerned for their well-being can have a significant positive effect on the sincerity and efficacy of therapeutic relationships and thereby facilitate transparency and recovery. All too often the forensic patient experience is that the purpose of *everything* (detention, restriction, medication, therapy, etc.) is to protect everyone else from the patient themselves regardless of the levels of distress it may cause a patient. There are also long-standing concerns that patients are subject to institutional violence that has become embedded in the system. For a patient to report an instance of what they perceive to be institutional violence and for their claims to not be dismissed or invalidated by an invocation of the statement that they are mentally disordered and the implicit or explicit assumption that this means their account or concern isn't to be trusted may unfortunately be a quite infrequent occurrence. For a patient to be treated by services in such a manner that they feel valued and safe optimizes responsiveness to care and treatment and ultimately self-empowerment.

On a positive note, collaborative risk assessment with patients being involved with all clinical team discussions that occur as part of the risk assessment process is now becoming part of the contract of many UK National Health Services secure and forensic mental health providers. It is a part of the 2014/2015 CQUIN commissioning framework in keeping with the UK Department of Health best practice regarding managing risk. It seeks to ensure a collaborative approach to risk assessment and management, aiming at delivering a holistic approach to risk by focusing on incorporating the patient's strengths. Providers are required to deliver an education package jointly to staff and patients around risk assessment and risk management. Recently, I have been involved in developing a web-based decision support for mental health risk, safety, and well-being called GRiST,[2] which allows patients to formulate their own risk assessment and management and support plans. Patients can share this, should they want to, with their care teams and enable up-to-date and real-time communication of risk concern and support requests. GRiST provides a structured and systematic approach to risk assessment and one which is based on a consensual and holistic model of risk shared by multidisciplinary mental health experts and service users. However, little literature is available concerning patients' views and experiences of risk assessment and management. In one observational study it was found that patients "attempted to understand the system of assessment and sought to affect and reduce their risk status by engaging in overt, compliant behaviours."[3] The study claimed that the "risk assessment process is subverted by the restriction of the flow of information, and patients are left with frustrations that they must contain and manage."[4] Another study of patient involvement in risk assessment found that practices were variable and depended upon individual professional initiative.[5] Some patients influenced the support they received, but generally, patients' main role was to accept or reject what was offered. After an audit of patient involvement in risk assessment on low secure wards, several recommendations were made including that "all patients should be informed that a [risk assessment] has been undertaken and, if clinically appropriate, they should be actively involved in the process; assessors must document reasons if this is inappropriate."[6] In another study, it was reported that some professionals lacked confidence or experience in openly discussing risk with patients.[7] This indicates a need for more robust training in this area for clinicians. Research is required to determine the extent and efficacy of collaborative risk assessment, including what constitutes an adequate formulation, how it translates into a treatment plan, and how it can be evaluated. It is, of course important in hospitals not to place too much emphasis on negative risk at the expense of other aspects of patient well-being. Patients do have free will and are able to learn from bad (and good) experiences and move on to lead fulfilling lives.

Multiple barriers to self-empowerment exist within forensic psychiatric services: the enduring culture and practice of risk averse restrictions, conflation of risk prediction with risk assessment, and paternalistic notions of preventive detention. The upcoming revision of the FMH system may or may not address these long-standing issues. In the interim patients may help themselves by using and developing their communicative and collaborative skills to make their voices better heard. Engagement, involvement, and other forms of working together can help patients to begin to actualize their own identities and in the process aid staff to come to recognize the human individuals behind the *mentally disordered offender* label.

In short, to effectively counter stigma and negative bias within forensic psychiatric services (I think this is referred to as *clinical bias*) there needs to be more focus on improving the quality of hospital treatments as experienced by patients. I think that in general, the more an individual believes their concerns and experience have been taken into account, the more likely they are to be open to working with their clinical teams. No one genuinely wants to be ill or to hurt themselves or others. We all, in our various ways, want to succeed and live good lives. The people that I have met, either as a fellow inpatient or as a peer support worker, who have been given the *mentally disordered offender* label have expressed a need to feel that they are seen as so much more than mere walking, talking units of potential harm; objects to be contained and controlled. They long to be appreciated for their positive human qualities, for their relationships and their individuality, and the support they provide for each other. We are human, we want to recover, and we need the positive support and faith of our clinical care teams and community to help us to do this.

NOTES

1 Livingston, "What Does Success Look Like," 1.
2 GRiST, "The Grist Solution."
3 Reynolds et al., "Playing the Game," 3.
4 Ibid., 3.
5 Langan, "Involving Mental Health Service Users."
6 Gough, Richardson, and Weeks, "An Audit of Service-User Involvement," 7.
7 Askola et al., "The Therapeutic Approach," 1.

BIBLIOGRAPHY

Askola, R., Nikkonen, M., Putkonen, H., Kylmä, J., and Louheranta, O. "The Therapeutic Approach to a Patient's Criminal Offense in a Forensic Mental Health Nurse-Patient Relationship – The Nurses' Perspectives." *Perspectives in Psychiatric Care* 53, no. 3 (2017): 164–74. https://doi.org/10.1111/ppc.12148.
Gough, K., Richardson, C., and Weeks, H. "An Audit of Service-User Involvement and Quality of HCR-20 Version 2 risk Assessments on Rehabilitation and Low Secure Wards." *Journal of Psychiatric Intensive Care* 11, no. S1 (2015): e2, 1–8. https://doi.org/10.1017/S1742646415000084.
GRiST: Galatean Risk and Safety Tool. "The GRiST Solution." Accessed February 19, 2017. https://www.egrist.org/content/grist-solution.
Langan, J. "Involving Mental Health Service Users Considered to Pose a Risk to Other People in Risk Assessment." *Journal of Mental Health* 17, no. 5 (2008): 471–81.
Livingston, James D. "What Does Success Look Like in the Forensic Mental Health System? Perspectives of Service Users and Service Providers." *International Journal of Offender Therapy and Comparative Criminology* (March 2016): 1–21. https://doi.org/10.1177/0306624X16639973.
Reynolds, L. M., Jones, J. C., Davies, J., Freeth, D., and Heyman, B. "Playing the Game: Service Users' Management of Risk Status in a UK Medium Secure Forensic Mental Health Service." *Health, Risk and Society* 16, no. 3 (2014): 199–209.

4 The Opposite of Violence

CARLYN ZWARENSTEIN

As a teenager, I had the idea that I might one day become a lawyer. A family friend who often works on civil rights and police brutality cases kindly offered me a student job as his occasional assistant. In this role, I poured over the transcripts of inquests into the deaths of Raymond Lawrence and Lester Donaldson, reading the actual words spoken on the stand by people who had loved, or those who had shot and killed, each of these two Toronto Black men with mental health issues, neither of whom represented serious threats to the officers who shot them in the belief or under the pretext that they did. As a well-off, white kid raised in the Toronto suburbs, this was my first exposure to violence ending in death; to police brutality; and to people who could be variously described as being in emotional distress, having psychological or psychiatric issues, or Mad. It was my first exposure, too, to the way racism and sanism (or the presumed association of both Blackness and madness with violence) result in police pulling the trigger too quickly.

Only a few years after that, an episode of what was diagnosed as major depressive disorder launched my career as a Mad person subject to an endless series of relatively non-invasive cures. I did not at first draw a connection between Lawrence's and Donaldson's fatal experiences and my own experience of depression. Still, after I diagnosed myself using a friend's psychology textbook and found my way to University Psychiatric Services, I was treated in a dismissive and brusque way that left me feeling shame and further distress. I am not saying that I experienced violence. I did not. However, the ways in which people are treated when they are emotionally distressed often reflect societal discomfort with madness and a lack of demonstrated empathy. There are many reasons for this discomfort, which magnifies existing prejudices based on class, age, sex, sexual orientation, gender, ability, race, and other differences. Regardless of the reason, though, I believe that the lack of incorporation of kindness (the human expression of one-on-one compassion) as a fundamental goal for provider interactions within the psychiatric system opens the door to the Othering experience that, magnified by racism, classism, and other biases that confer further Otherness, allow for people to be mistreated within the psychiatric system that is supposed to help us. Unkind (or worse) treatment in the psychiatric and mental health systems is one branch on the same tree that also allows Mad people to be inaccurately judged to be a threat and as such more liable to be mistreated or killed in a confrontation with the law, which is so often a waystation or endpoint for a person voluntarily or involuntarily in the mental health world. Addressing lack of kindness – the establishment of individual relationships of thoughtfulness and compassion – within the mental health system is a complicated question. I will look at the issue, and possible ways of addressing it, from four angles.

The Hospital as a Place of Healing

A hospital is meant to be a place of healing. That is the premise and the point: you are sick, and you go in to get well. It is the premise that draws people to work in these places, and it is the premise that draws people to seek help there when the symptoms of mental illness are too confusing, too distressing, too unfamiliar, or just too much to bear. And yet, hospitals are just as much sites of trauma as they are sites of healing. My friend Kate Robson, a parent coordinator in a neonatal intensive care unit (NICU), makes this point in an article about the NICU. The trauma in an NICU is partly to do with the circumstances – in the NICU, the lives, deaths and previously unanticipated futures of tiny premature newborns – but also partly to do with the way personnel and practices may reinforce a sense of helplessness, of despair, of emergency, or of insignificance in the parents who spend time there. Robson and her co-authors argue that while NICU parents did not plan to be there, and despite the circumstantial trauma of the situation, policies and practices can reduce the disempowerment or further trauma associated with an NICU stay, and even bring out another aspect that ought to be part of the experience: celebration. They emphasize that careful design of practices and care taken to reduce sensory impact within the unit can facilitate a reframing for families of the tiny patients so that time spent there is understood as an ultimately positive experience, as well as an educational one, preparing parents and their children for the rest of their lives together. These practices would include what they call "psychosocial support," family presence and reunification, and social connection.[1]

Indeed, the person – not yet self-identified, perhaps, as a consumer, a survivor, a proud Mad person, a chronic depressive/bipolar/schizophrenic, or a patient – who presents voluntarily at any site for mental health intake (a phone helpline, say, or a mental health or regular hospital emergency room, a private therapy waiting room, or a first appointment in a hospital or clinic) – is not that different in important ways from the NICU patient. We are in a state of acute distress, mental and sometimes physical as well. We are in urgent need of help. We are fragile, easily crushed emotionally, and yet we have gotten this far, which shows the strongest of desires and the most vital of strengths: the drive for survival. We are in a moment of transformation: the person who leaves this place will be either better or worse for their experience, on a rocky but upward path of healing or bruised and scarred by being there. We may come out with a new identity based on a first or new diagnosis, which in turn may be the beginning of a long series of diagnoses and psychiatric experiments. Or we may then carry with us the beginnings of rebellion, of a personal and eventually political critique of our experience and of the causes and values of being mad.

Now, a premature infant has very specific physical needs – a certain percentage of oxygen, a particular temperature. And while these needs must be met, perhaps the most vital thing for future physical, cerebral, emotional, and cognitive development is actually kindness, at least, the way an infant recognizes kindness, which is through skin-to-skin contact. So too a person in psychiatric or emotional distress suffers from symptoms that may be explained and addressed in a number of specific ways (psychopharmaceutic, psychotherapeutic, social, behavioural, or electrochemical for example) – but all, universally, need kindness to set us on a path out of the hospital or emergency room or clinic: stabilizing our sense of self and self-esteem, refraining from creating extra trauma from a confusing, over-stimulating, infantilizing (despite my analogy with premature infants in other respects) or unfeeling environment. For adults who do not know each other, kindness involves individual interactions reflective of thoughtfulness, which is why it seems like a fuzzy concept, hard to implement in the concrete terms of practices, policies, and training. Hard does not mean impossible, though.

Teaching Kindness

There is relatively little research relating to mental health care on what is described as *patient experience* and little that is quantitative. A few studies, though, reflect the importance of individual relationships – between the person experiencing psychological distress and anyone they encounter within institutions in which they seek or are referred for help.[2] Likewise, an image that comes to me again and again is that of the survivor of a fire or a car accident who we see so often in movies, sitting near the scene of the incident, wrapped in a thermal or fuzzy blanket, head bent gratefully over a mug of hot tea or cocoa while someone – anyone – speaks to them kindly. Not better, but safe, comforted, in a holding situation from which healing can arise. For me, mental distress most often takes the form of depression, or hopelessness, or extreme low mood, and when I have felt at my worst, it is to that comforting image that I cling.

Google *kindness* and *mental health* and you will find many, many online links to information about how being kind can improve your mental health. It is far more difficult to find anything relating to how we can be treated with kindness by the structures and people we encounter when experiencing emotional distress. And yet, as a counterpoint to the experience of violence that, to varying degrees, is all too common among those involved with the mental health system, and as one aspect of working towards a trauma-informed (and trauma-preventing) system, kindness is a vital concept. Further, kindness is an expression of empathy in settings invariably freighted with power imbalances and so represents a first step towards solidarity and the potential for individual acts, as well as collective political action, to equalize relationships that are unequal in our current world. And yet, kindness is nearly absent in the psychiatric literature (although the creation of environments and actions that facilitate the establishment of therapeutic relationships is a major preoccupation of most psychotherapeutic literature, as well as of architects and others interested in hospital environments). Meanwhile the word – describing the longing for it – emerges repeatedly in the often-heartbreaking stories related in *Mad Matters*, the seminal text for Mad Studies in Canada.[3]

Even more – the failure of empathy is persistent within mental health care system interactions in cases of both "mild" and "severe" mental illness, in the sense that patients repeatedly express their distress at personal interactions with health care personnel in which they experienced a lack of kindness.

Mad activist and researcher Erick Fabris describes cycles of power that generally inform psychiatric practices and interventions, focusing his analysis on Community Treatment Orders in Toronto, Canada, which "break trust and erode the supposed therapeutic aims of both worker and inmate."[4] These cycles include the use of psychiatric drugs that may in fact provoke diagnosable psychiatric conditions – what he calls a cycling of chemistry; cycling of evidence, where any behaviour is further evidence to validate a diagnosis; and cycling of biology, where diagnoses and treatments alike may change frequently and suddenly, and everything is reducible to a presumed biological cause. These cycles are not exclusive to psychiatry.

Despite the substantial literature devoted to various forms of person-centred, humanistic, holistic, empowering psychotherapy, the most basic modelling of empathy – not skills, like rote reflective listening, but genuine recognition that as humans we all possess the same needs and the same essential value – seems largely absent from both undergraduate medical and psychiatric specialist education, and so that moment of seeking the comfort and the peaceful place to rebuild remain largely absent from the mental health emergency rooms, psychiatrist offices, group meeting rooms, and psychiatric wards they inhabit.[5] A major step that could be taken to address this would be getting psychiatric survivors into medical education classrooms to speak directly to residents and medical students about their experience, and having the Mad Studies' perspective inform compulsory courses in psychiatric medicine and nursing.

Relationships of Care

In a way, and despite the process of systemic deinstitutionalization of psychiatric inpatients over the past few decades, we have given to professionals – because of their training, their understanding of the human mind and brain chemicals, their encyclopedic knowledge of the latest *Diagnostic and Statistical Manual of Mental* – a role that used to fall, for better and for worse, to families. And so the person in distress is still looking for the sort of care that comes because of mutual obligation and bonds of friendship or kinship, a compassion that is less hierarchical than the patient–health care provider relationship. I think that this need remains unfulfilled in most people seeking help for emotional distress, and it remains a vital one.

I can offer my recent experience as an example. Last year, I experienced a several-months-long episode of intense depression. The cause was not at all mysterious: low moods have been common, recurrent, and tolerable for many years. In this case there was a clear inciting factor: I had been suddenly struck by dramatically worse symptoms of my previously tolerable degenerative spine disease.

For a long time, I relied on the support of friends who I could text or meet for coffee and a consoling chat to get me through the moment-to-moment struggle with pain and stiffness. But the more desperate I felt, the darker my outlook, the more these friends felt inadequate to the task. Depending on their own experiences and personalities, some suggested antidepressants and others suggested a professional psychotherapist. The advice to lean on professionals instead of (carefully and with restraint) depending on friends to support me as I managed emotions of hopelessness did not feel right: it seemed to me that the key to this problem lay not in my thinking (suggesting a need for cognitive behavioural or other brief psychotherapy), my understanding (maybe some psychoanalysis or deep psychotherapy), or my biochemistry (a psychiatrist and antidepressants). But I didn't want to wear out my welcome, or stress out my friends, or put them in situations they felt inadequate to deal with. On the other hand, my depression was caused by a situation that was by no means unfamiliar to me. What I needed, I felt, was someone to hold my hand and give me moral support to survive an experience that seemed to be pushing the limits of my capacity to endure, to strengthen my own resources rather than to provide a solution. However, although all psychiatrists will have had a certain amount of training in psychotherapeutic methods that universally stress the importance of the therapist-patient relationship, the professionalization of mental health care into a system in which emotional distance is thought to be vital fails to consider the way in which the expression of being personally touched by the suffering of the other is integral to healing, and the observed absence of the same can be wounding. I felt fragile, and so all interactions were easily measured as either harsh or kind.

After first requesting a referral from my rheumatologist to Toronto's Centre for Addiction and Mental Health, a major mental health centre located in my neighbourhood, my first contact with the organization came in the form of an automated message reminding me of my evaluation appointment. The message warned that if I did not call back to confirm my already-confirmed appointment within a certain time, it would be cancelled. The tone of voice was hard and punitive, upsetting to a person already on an emotional edge, and wholly unnecessary. By contrast, when I arrived for my evaluation, the intake secretary spoke to me gently. I told her how much I appreciated this. While there is no research that I know of specifically into whether feeling like you've been wrapped in a fuzzy blanket upon intake in a mental health facility translates into quantifiable and sustained improvements in mental health, I can think of few practices that would be more likely to translate into therapeutic gains. Of course it's not just the little things – addressing social determinants of health would be the most important set of policy changes that could improve mental health. However, small practices reflective of kindness should be a natural outcome of a system based more on solidarity and the state's responsibility to care for its members. And meanwhile, kindness can be an important counterweight, establishing one-on-one compassion and equality even in a world where some people are unfairly privileged while others are burdened by unfair obstacles.

The Safety versus Humanity Trade-Off

One day, in great distress, I asked a friend with a long history of psychiatric in- and outpatient treatment whether she thought I should try emergency psychiatric services. She told me that in her experience, one goes to emergency voluntarily only because one is in great distress, looking to feel better. Instead of wrapping the distressed person in a metaphorical fuzzy blanket, "they" take away your keys (for your own safety, but the emotional effect is punitive), making you wait a long and uncertain time with little information and no comfort, in a room with lots of other disturbed people.[6] This image has stayed with me and haunted me. Surely the emergency room atmosphere of a psychiatric hospital is designed primarily for expediency and physical safety – rather than for the creation of an environment that sets patients at ease, instils them with hope and provides a sense of both personal efficacy and trust. Indeed, having worked as a writer with an architect on descriptions of his projects that included emergency mental health services, I now know that discrete safety measures (to prevent suicide, to prevent assaults on staff, to ensure vigilance) are key. Here we get back to the question of violence. Fear of violence means that, given the necessity of ensuring patient safety and safe work conditions, psychiatric facilities tend to give precedence to utility and safety over comfort and kindness in design. This is not always the case, and designers and architects certainly have tried to instil tranquility and thoughtfulness in their designs. But the assumption of violence perpetrated by psychiatric patients trumps consideration of the violence ultimately inflicted *upon* patients by degrees as the sense of shared health care provider–patient humanity is leached away in a cold and bureaucratic process of intake, diagnosis, and treatment.

Because of the almost-spontaneous nature of true kindness on an individual basis, it seems contradictory to call for systemic implementation of kindness. But numerous small and large decisions about framing, resource allocation and time form the substrate upon which a thoughtful, compassionate, gentle culture, a culture of kindness, can be built. Whether the health care system is a largely publicly-funded one as in Canada, or largely private and corporate, as in the United States, there are challenges. To address them with any success, kindness needs to be identified as a value at the highest level of mission-setting, and then for this value to be enacted, not just blandly expressed, it must inform every decision, making sure that staff have the emotional resources and are sensitized to the sensory and emotional strains that mental health system interactions can cause, and that they are taught and supported with adequate resources (such as time, adequate pay, safe working conditions, and relevant education) to mitigate them. Psychiatric patients need to be involved at the highest level of planning to ensure that representative concerns of this diverse population are addressed in all aspects of planning, from physical design to staff training to communications.

It might (might) be too much to ask for a mental health hospital or intake clinic, any more than a regular or paediatric emergency ward, to be a site of celebration. But reducing unnecessary trauma? Building a sense of compassion, of kindness, of thoughtfulness and care into the experience? Beginning the work of re-creating a fractured identity, a new life, and an autonomous future? Why on earth not? That work, of imagining how the process of seeking help for emotional distress might itself be made less distressing, is to me the work of imagining a small piece of a more caring and cohesive society. It is the opposite of violence.

NOTES

1 Robson, MacMillan-York, and Dunn, "Celebration in the Face of Trauma."
2 Gilburt, Rose, and Slade, "The Importance of Relationships in Mental Health Care."
3 Lefrançois, Menzies, and Reaume, *Mad Matters*.
4 Fabris, *Identity, Inmates, Insight, Capacity, Consent, Coercion*, 6.
5 Everything from the eponymous person-centred psychotherapy and Gestalt to cognitive-behavioural or psychoanalytic approaches spotlight the individual and their developmental or other needs, with little consideration of the systemic and political or environmental issues that are more often the province of philosophers and social scientists than psychotherapists, let alone psychiatrists (by contrast to those individual need-focused approaches, systemic or group psychotherapy does focus more on social system issues). Addictions expert Gabor Maté has recently written about the impact of capitalism and associated structures on individual mental health (as cited, for example, in Meili, 2014). Most recently, psychotherapist and former community organizer Roger Brouillette's article "Why Therapists Should Talk Politics" garnered considerable attention. By and large, though, mental health services fail to incorporate corrective responses to mental health-challenging political and social needs or lacks.
6 Therapeutic solidarity may emerge via individual acts of kindness and shared internal and externally-imposed suffering on psychiatric wards between institutionalized patients. Among my usually outpatient friends with ongoing or recurrent experience of mental distress I've developed a similar rapport of "checking in" and mutual support. Perhaps more "peers" should be available to provide comfort in emergency settings?

BIBLIOGRAPHY

Brouillette, Roger. "Why Therapists Should Talk Politics." *New York Times*, March 15, 2016. https://opinionator.blogs.nytimes.com/2016/03/15/why-therapists-should-talk-politics/?_r=0.

Fabris, Erick. *Identity, Inmates, Insight, Capacity, Consent, Coercion: Chemical Incarceration in Psychiatric Survivor Experiences of Community Treatment Orders*. Toronto, ON: OISE, 2006.

Gilburt, Helen, Diana Rose, and Mike Slade. "The Importance of Relationships in Mental Health Care: A Qualitative Study of Service Users'

Experiences of Psychiatric Hospital Admission in the UK." *BMC Health Services Research* 8, no. 92 (2008). https://bmchealthservres.biomedcentral .com/articles/10.1186/1472-6963-8-92.

Lefrançois, Brenda, Robert Menzies, and Geoffrey Reaume, eds. *Mad Matters: A Critical Reader in Canadian Mad Studies.* Toronto, ON: Canadian Scholars' Press, 2013.

Meili, Ryan. "Gabor Maté: How Capitalism Makes Us Sick." *Briarpatch Magazine*, November 13, 2014.

Robson, K., MacMillan-York, E., and Dunn, M. S. "Celebration in the Face of Trauma: Supporting NICU Families through Compassionate Facility Design." *Newborn and Infant Nursing Reviews* 16, no. 4 (2016): 225–9. http:// www.sciencedirect.com/science/article/pii/S1527336916300058.

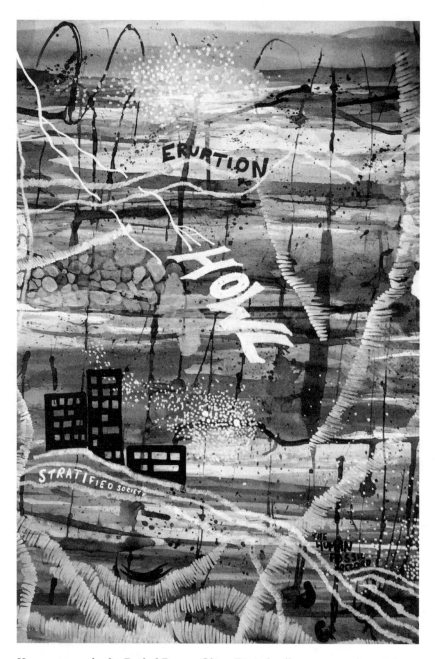

Human geography, by Rachel Rowan Olive. Digital collage: watercolour, ink, paint marker, and digital image work.

PART II

Prevailing Problems

Part II contains six chapters that, in different ways, associate neo-liberal discourse and practice related to *mental illness* as violent or associated with violence in the lives of mental health service users/survivors. Collectively, the authors' analyses showcase and integrate various violence-related concepts to interrogate knowledge production processes related to mental illness, mental health crisis, and madness. Each contribution uniquely details the relationship between the ways in which mental health service users/survivors and mental health crisis become known through psy-knowledge informed by neo-liberal logic, and how psychiatric power is reified through associated government policy, research processes, and cultural practices.

Christopher Van Veen, Katherine Teghtsoonian, and Marina Morrow centre a mayor's task force on mental health and addictions (Vancouver, Canada) to reveal "ways in which violence, care, and neo-liberalism are intertwined" in the text's "problematization" of "mental health crisis." Conceptualizing neo-liberalism as a set of practices that translate justice and equity concerns "into an economic register," they identify practices of violence that are visible within the text. In doing so, the productive power of neo-liberal rationality to shape "crisis" and related solutions that privilege cost efficiency or that introduce coercive practices into existing mental health programs are offered as instances of violence. Their textual analysis integrates the concepts of responsibilization, slow violence, and epistemic violence, and considers the notion of *slow justice* in relation to resistance strategies that emerge from an understanding of problems as constituted rather than given. The authors invite readers to engage with their analysis beyond its local relevance to consider the implications of neo-liberal political rationality across geographies.

The ideas of slow violence and slow death are taken up by Jijian Voronka in an exploration of how randomized controlled trials (RCT) are implicated in structural violence vis-à-vis approaches by the state to solve the "crisis of the chronically homeless mentally ill" through research. Jijian locates the RCT within the "tight governance of neo-liberal biopolitical logics" underscoring its use as a knowledge production process that serves the modern state's propensity for "techniques which try to make known, order, and manage whole populations." Her ethnographically informed case study of the At Home/Chez Soi interrogates the RCT specifically, and evidence-based research generally, for its role in configuring "social problems and troubled bodies" as economic opportunities in neo-liberal improvement projects. In doing so, Jijian implicates research in the reconceptualization of homelessness as a health condition rather than a social injustice produced by neo-liberal capitalism and troubles the changing configurations of housing and mental health services as they are administered through research projects. She concludes with a consideration of how both prolong precariousness for homeless people within the context of scientific rationalism and economic austerity.

Chapter 7 offers a textual analysis of Canada's first national mental health strategy, *Changing Directions, Changing Lives: The Mental Health Strategy for Canada*. Merrick Pilling takes the strategy to task for its reliance on a neo-liberal individualizing framework that fails to advance a strong structural analysis of homophobia, transphobia, and other forms of violence in shaping experiences of mental distress and recovery for sexual and gender minority people (e.g., lesbian, gay, bisexual, queer, gender-queer, trans, Two Spirit). Configuring conditions that cause distress as individual risk factors inherently associated with gender and sexuality, Merrick argues that the strategy does not address state accountability for alleviating the impacts of systemic violence (i.e., transphobia and homophobia). Underscoring historical and contemporary harms to sexual and gender minority people subjected to biopsychiatric approaches to "treat" dissent genders and sexualities, as well as the mental health impacts of discrimination, Merrick asks critical questions about the implications of the strategy's promotion of recovery that further integrates "LGBQT people into mental health systems through increasing accessibility" – in the absence of recognizing their potential for violence in these spaces. His analysis concludes by considering how returning to the concept of recovery as originally defined by psychiatric survivors and engaging critical theoretical frameworks (e.g., critical race, queer, and trans theories) may be more useful responses for articulating understanding and reactions to the impacts of systemic violence in the lives of gender and sexual minority communities.

Meghann O'Leary and Liat Ben-Moshe weave narrative and analysis in "recounting the psychiatrized life and eventual death" of Spencer. A young man of 23 years, Spencer committed suicide having lived through several years of psychiatric commitment and attempts to rebuild his life after being given a diagnosis of bipolar psychosis. The authors bring to light important ideas about the ways that "neo-liberal models of choice create a regime of violence that is not necessarily coercive," but that pulls individuals into harm's way through projects of self-improvement that rely upon discourses of "personal responsibility," "betterment," and "recovery" and ignore the ways in which structural oppression restricts lives. The authors unequivocally locate the violence of psychiatry in its embeddedness in the discourses of neo-liberalism and capitalism. Similar to Christopher Van Veen, Katherine Teghtsoonian, and Marina Morrow's use of "responsibilization" and Merrick Pilling's attention to "individualizing" accounts of distress, the authors' hold these discourses to account as they operate to absolve society of any responsibility for Spencer's distress and death. It is this absolving of responsibility that perpetuates violence. Meghann and Liat offer important insight into the ways in which neo-liberal psy-discourse on "choice" and related practices maintain a racial capitalist regime as they are applied to surveil and control marginalized communities, including trans people of colour.

In chapter 9, through an Indigenous storytelling approach, Priya Raju and Nicole Penak invite readers to understand their perspectives on how the authoring of mental health experiences occur for Indigenous Peoples applying for Ontario government disability supports. As a racialized psychiatrist and an Indigenous social worker, the authors describe the tensions in the work they do at an Indigenous health centre, exploring the ways in which day-to-day practices serve to (re)entrench intersecting relationships between neo-liberalism, capitalism, colonialism, racism, and classism. In doing so, they shine light on invisible and yet dangerous practices. Their discussion outlines the violence inherent in a social welfare system that requires the social construction of the deficient Other through "expert" psy-knowledge to determine eligibility for social support. Yet, it is a layered story as they examine their relationships and the relationships of their professions to colonialism. As importantly, the authors' approach to the chapter offers an example of what might be done about the violence of reducing marginalized communities mental health service users/survivors to deficit or deviant categories through process of categorization. Priya and Nicole model storytelling as a practice of collectivization within the contemporary context of neo-liberal social service delivery as this chapter centres relationship building as a path towards change.

Brigit McWade brings us into the realm of madness and violence in the media, examining their representations and how their relationship to each other is "imagined, produced, circulated and resisted." Through a critical analysis of existing research literature, Brigit begins by considering that ways in which people's beliefs about and stigmatization of Mad people have been understood as an effect of the media. She raises the important issue of the limitations of research that uses narrow conceptualizations of both madness and violence based on the individualizing deficit model of biomedical psychiatry. Importantly, Brigit asks that we conceptualize the relationship between madness and the media more broadly to explore how the media works with psy-discourse to reproduce psy-power through medicalized representations of madness. In doing so, she reveals psychiatry's dependency on the media for its constant promotion to "maintain and increase its market share of the mental health industry." In concluding, Brigit presses us to think even more broadly about psychiatry as culture and our self-understanding is "mediated through psychiatrized media cultures."

5 Enacting Violence and Care: Neo-liberalism, Knowledge Claims, and Resistance

CHRISTOPHER VAN VEEN, KATHERINE TEGHTSOONIAN, AND MARINA MORROW

Violence is customarily conceived as an event or action that is immediate in time, explosive and spectacular in space, and as erupting into instant sensational visibility. We need ... to engage a different kind of violence, a violence that is neither spectacular nor instantaneous, but rather incremental and accretive.[1]

Introduction

In 2013 the Vancouver municipal government declared that this large city located in the Canadian province of British Columbia (BC) was in the midst of a "mental health crisis." This crisis was said to be evident in worrying trends identified by the local police department, including growing threats to public safety resulting from violent incidents perpetrated by individuals characterized as "mentally ill," without access to proper treatment, and responsible for excessive demands on emergency room and police services.[2] The mayor announced the establishment of a task force on mental health and addictions charged with considering this urgent problem and developing strategies for responding to it. In this chapter we engage critically with the final report produced by the task force – *Caring for All: Priority Actions to Address Mental Health and Addictions* – and the policy – and service-oriented reforms it supports.[3] Our analysis excavates the practices of violence that are visible within this document, even as it describes and seeks to move forward initiatives that are presented as caring, inclusive, respectful, supportive, and culturally sensitive. We also highlight ways in which violence, care, and neo-liberalism are intertwined in the city's efforts to address the "mental health crisis." Using Carol Bacchi's discussion of *problematization*, we aim to destabilize established understandings of how violence is implicated in the "crisis" and to suggest that while neo-liberalism may dominate the city's response to it there is nevertheless room for – and evidence of – resistive practices.[4]

In trying to think more broadly about violence we draw on Rob Nixon's discussion of "slow violence." Arguing that conventional notions of violence are too narrow, Nixon suggests slow violence as an alternative that also extends our understanding of structural violence by adding a temporal dimension. Thus, he defines it as "a violence that occurs gradually and out of sight, a violence of delayed destruction that is dispersed across time and space, an attritional violence that is typically not viewed as violence at all."[5] Rather than the "explosive and spectacular" versions of violence that drive concerns about Vancouver's mental health "crisis," Nixon's concept foregrounds practices of violence that are reproduced through a broad time frame within which marginalization, discrimination, and impoverishment are enacted through government policies, economic systems, and colonial exercises of power. Such thinking recasts the violence that unfolds around mental health reform in Vancouver as historically endemic and multifaceted, rather than as a temporally contained "crisis." We supplement slow violence with the concept of epistemic violence that has been so useful in illuminating the erasure of Mad people's understandings of their own experience. Maria Liegghio, for example, argues that fundamental to epistemic violence is "the denial of the person as a legitimate knower" and suggests that "being constructed as dangerous is a powerful mechanism that sets the stage for epistemic violence."[6]

In examining *Caring for All* we start from the premise that any set of circumstances can be represented as a "problem" – problematized[7] – in many ways and that different problematizations will have different effects, including what they draw our attention to and the solutions that they invite. We explore how current circumstances in Vancouver are being problematized in ways that make some forms of violence – but not others – visible and that make particular types of interventions – those that privilege cost efficiency or that introduce coercive practices into Assertive Community Treatment (ACT) models[8] – appear to be sensible and effective rather than, themselves, instances of violence. As we will see, problematizations that are developed and promoted by authoritative actors are presented as accurate and true so that the solutions they imply are privileged while others are left out of the discussion. The idea of "problems" as *constituted* rather than *given* opens up space for considering critically the knowledge claims through which a particular problematization and solutions to it are generated, as well as alternatives to these. This is a key goal of our analysis. We argue that just as there are multiple forms of violence at work in constructing the problem of the "mental health crisis" and its solutions, so are there multiple forms of resistance. This possibility is our central concern in the concluding section of the chapter, in which we consider the "spaces of power"[9] that *Caring for All* signals and the opportunities for resistive practices these might offer. We also consider the possibilities and potential pitfalls of "slow justice" as a basis for responses that arise from problematizing the present in terms of slow and epistemic violence rather than as a "mental health crisis."

We write this piece as individuals who live the tensions that we write about directly in our work and in our lives. One of us (Chris) has navigated spaces of care and control as a manager of Vancouver-based mental health and addictions supportive housing programs for eight years. Another (Marina) has been a researcher in the field of mental health reform for 20 years with a focus on intersecting and overlapping forms of structural and systemic oppression and has sat at policy tables where decisions are made about mental health policy directions, including discussions related to the projects we critique in this chapter. And a third (Kathy) has wrestled with questions of whether and how to engage critically with problematic public and organizational policies alongside practitioners, activists, and colleagues in her courses and in other diverse settings over the past two decades. We constantly grapple with the ethical tensions that arise as we strive to make a difference in policy and practice; our experiences – as critical policy analysts, educators, practitioners, and social activist scholars who live in the spaces of power that we analyse – inform our writing.

Vancouver's History of "Crisis" and Resistance

Visibly marked by extreme disparities in wealth, Vancouver has a past and present characterized by practices of colonization, significant homelessness, and well-researched rates of morbidity and mortality for its most disenfranchised residents. During their long tenure as the governing party in the province (2001–2017), the BC Liberals enacted deep cuts to social programs that radically reshaped policies and practices related to housing, employment, and income security in directions that undermined the well-being of people living in marginalized circumstances, including those with diagnoses of "mental illness."[10]

The effects of these policy shifts have been starkly apparent in Vancouver's Downtown East Side (DTES). Located to the east of the city's business centre, the DTES is conventionally referred to as "Canada's poorest postal code" although the life circumstances of its residents are mirrored in urban centres across the country. While area residents are poorly served by current policies, they nevertheless often attract attention from various levels of government, researchers, and community non-profits who exercise countless interventions and practices of health care surveillance. Indeed, it might be said that a disproportionate amount of the BC evidence base as it relates to poverty, homelessness, mental health, and addictions arises from studies done on people and programs in the relatively small neighbourhood.

Despite these and other problematic features of local policies and practices, Vancouver nevertheless enjoys a progressive reputation when it comes to its health care and support services, and the city's health research community is touted internationally.[11] At the same time the DTES neighbourhood has been constructed by media, police, and epidemiologists as a pathological community populated by "sick" individuals. For example, a decade ago a local newspaper dubbed the core of the neighbourhood "four blocks of hell," where it "is so filthy and hazardous that sanitation workers have asked for police protection when they go in on routine duties."[12] And during the 1990s the public's attention was repeatedly drawn to the proliferation of HIV cases and drug-related overdose deaths in this part of the city. While each set of circumstances, like the present moment,[13] has been constituted as a "crisis," we suggest that the chronology of the neighbourhood reveals not a series of "crises," but rather a monotonous and continuous history of slow violence experienced by the population that inhabits its streets and single-room occupancy hotels.

Absent from these crisis-oriented representations of the DTES are local activities and initiatives through which this area of the city emerges as a lively site of community building and anti-poverty activism. Many of the organizations operating in the DTES have been strong advocates for improved policy and services. Community leaders have also worked to protect the area and its residents from encroaching gentrification and other challenges.[14] These efforts have included successful appeals to the Supreme Court of Canada leading to landmark decisions establishing the rights of drug users to access supervised injection sites and the movement towards the decriminalization of sex trade work. Community-based action research has also played a positive role in highlighting the voices, needs, and contributions of people on the DTES, including survival sex trade workers and those living with HIV/AIDS.[15] These achievements, and the practices of community involvement that they are built on, have not gone unnoticed by Vancouver's municipal government. Indeed, the mayor's task force made significant efforts to incorporate inclusive practices into its consultation and policy development processes. It thus drew together 140 "leaders in government, police, the health sector, academia, non-profit agencies and people with lived experience" to participate in workshops that were held over a 10-month period in 2013.[16]

These multiple and contradictory practices of engagement with the DTES and its residents are visible in the *Caring for All* document produced by the taskforce, which is why it is of interest to us. Although our analysis is focused on this locally situated document, we see it as having a broader relevance because *Caring for All* makes visible practices and problematizations that extend far beyond Vancouver. For example, the Housing First and ACT strategies that it posits as central to solving the "problem" of the "crisis" take as their evidence base research from the Mental Health Commission of Canada's At Home study, which was conducted across five major Canadian cities between 2010 and 2013.[17] Similar interventions are currently being implemented across Canada and the United States.[18] In addition we anticipate readers will recognize many of the processes (establishing a consultative task force), practices (tracking and measuring success), and knowledge claims ("evidence-based") in their own backyards. Thus, although our research is focused empirically on one urban location and text, our intent is to offer a critical lens that may be useful in other sites where similar conversations and initiatives are unfolding.

Neo-liberalism and Violence

Neo-liberalism is a concept often used to refer to government policies that sustain inequalities in wealth, privatization of public goods and services, and the privileging of business interests by government. Such policies have had wide-reaching material effects that have significantly reduced access to income security and government services, resulting in increased poverty and homelessness.[19] A vast literature explores the origins of such policies and their harmful effects on people's lives. We extend these findings by considering neo-liberalism not just in terms of government policies but also as a set of practices that enact a particular rationality or way of conceptualizing the political, the economic, and the social and the relationships among them. In doing so, we suggest linkages between these practices and forms of slow and epistemic violence visible in dominant problematizations of Vancouver's "mental health crisis."

A key element of neo-liberalism as a political rationality is the practice of translating concerns about justice or equity into an economic register, so that all issues must be addressed in terms of fiscal sensibility rather than social or political necessity. This thinking is reflected in the prominence of cost arguments in *Caring for All* where recommended interventions are viewed as effective only insofar as they provide a net economic benefit.[20] New funding or initiatives are not referred to as *social spending* but rather as *investments*, conjuring the promise (and requirement) of fiscal return and prudence. When individuals caught in the "crisis" use what the report deems inefficient emergency services (such as first responders or temporary shelters) this is constituted as a problem of capital expenditure rather than of suffering or slow violence. And when individuals are successfully targeted by programs viewed to be more fiscally efficient their lives are understood to be improved, even if what they are actually experiencing is violence in the form of the increased surveillance and coercive psychiatric treatment that ACT involves.

Neo-liberalism is also often enacted through efforts to "responsibilize" individuals, that is, to minimize direct government involvement by encouraging people to carve a personal path to recovery rather than addressing the structural conditions in which they live.[21] *Caring for All* thus proposes directing individuals to recovery through early preventive interventions, cultural connection, the arts, and other medical and non-medical interventions. These "responsibilizing" impulses sit somewhat awkwardly alongside practice recommendations that reveal a more directly disciplinary form of power, forms of care and support such as the locally implemented version of ACT that uncharacteristically brings police and health authorities together to "aggressively" target individuals constructed as sick and dangerous for treatment and monitoring in the community. Thinking about neo-liberalism as a political rationality and set of practices allows us to see it as uneven rather than monolithic, with its various elements open to reconfiguration in specific spatial and temporal environments, such as the activities of the mayor's task force. It also opens up particular kinds of questions about *Caring for All* and the "crisis" it seeks to address: Where and how are neo-liberal rationalities and practices visible? What forms of knowledge are evident and are some privileged over others in presenting the problem of the "crisis" and its solutions?

Competing Problematizations

The discussions and recommendations of the mayor's task force were preceded by a sequence of previously-released, highly publicized reports written by the Vancouver Police Department that argued vigorously that officers are increasingly being called upon to respond to violent situations involving untreated "mentally ill persons," a problematization that is visible at the heart of the way in which the Task Force characterizes the current "crisis."[22] Thus, the first paragraph of *Caring for All* indicates that the work of the Task Force is necessitated by a "surge in people with severe, untreated mental illness and addictions at St Paul's Hospital, a dramatic increase in people taken into police custody under the Mental Health Act, and several violent episodes that indicated a major crisis in the health care system."[23] Right up front, the "crisis" is defined in a manner that forges a seemingly-obvious connection between "people with severe mental illness and addictions" and threats to public safety. Not only is this focus on "ill" individuals and their (violent) behaviours congruent with neo-liberalism, but it also opens the door to policy responses that intertwine violence with care by establishing a significant role for the police in enforcing the delivery of services to those deemed incapable of "self-managing."

We can see significant traces of this in *Caring for All*, which notes that "[the At Home study] demonstrated that a 'housing first approach' aggressively supported by appropriate community based treatment and other key supports can address homelessness and is a sound investment."[24] The police are explicitly identified as one of these "key supports" and a "joint treatment model" involving collaboration between law enforcement and a local health authority is noted as a successful step towards solving the problem of the crisis.[25] Resonating with a neo-liberal interest in cost-effectiveness, this discussion in *Caring for All* draws together problematizations advanced by the municipal police force with those generated by the BC Liberal government and suggests that they have been validated through scholarly research. It is worth noting, however, that police participation in ACT was not locally researched, nor is it included in conventional best practices associated with the model. Nevertheless, police are now members of some

Vancouver ACT teams, a development that is unintelligible without mental health first having been constituted as a public safety problem. Foregrounding the potential violence of persons with untreated "mental illness" makes the involvement of police on care teams possible and, as Liegghio has argued, lays the groundwork for epistemic violence. At the same time, it decentres an alternative problematization: someone who has been traumatized by psychiatry or the criminal justice system may be concerned about very different forms of violence when receiving a joint home visit from a police officer and psychiatric nurse. Troubling dominant problematizations and the knowledge claims they rely on could thus have significant practice implications as well.

This is not an impossible task; in fact, we can see traces of alternative problematizations of the violence associated with the "crisis" already present in *Caring for All*, which notes that individuals apprehended under the provincial Mental Health Act (BCMHA) between 2010 and 2013 were significantly more likely to be the victims of violence than those in the general population.[26] As another example, we know that people with diagnoses of "mental illness" are subject to forms of coercion not sanctioned for any other health related issue; that is, the BCMHA permits forcible confinement or treatment. Moreover, and importantly, notions of "mental illness" as dangerousness can be challenged by drawing attentions to alternative understandings of the problem of violence along the lines suggested by Nixon. Instead of characterizing existing circumstances as a "mental health crisis," they could be problematized as resulting from the practices of slow violence enacted through a lack of a federal housing strategy, an economy that structurally prevents many from accessing basic social goods, colonization and its legacies, and the psy-disciplines. Competing problematizations such as these allow us to avoid "[misrepresenting] the duration and scale of the situation by calling a crisis that which is a fact of life and has been a defining fact of life for a given population that lives it as a fact in ordinary time";[27] it also opens space for considering a wider range of responses.

Competing Knowledge Practices

In *Caring for All* and the task force processes that it describes, the local research community sits atop an epistemological hierarchy of knowledge producers and is tasked with creating and monitoring evidence-based responses to the problem presented by "the crisis." For example, the report notes the Task Force's intention to partner with local universities to develop a data sharing model that will support "an integrated and evidence-based collaborative system," with the purpose of developing "a common vision" and "shared measurement across a service system."[28] The report also makes clear that "best practices" can only be such if validated through "rigorous research."[29] These knowledge practices establish that researchers and trained health administrators ultimately define success with indicators based on what they view to be "evidence." Setting parameters around what counts as data and who gets to collect and measure, they summon neo-liberalism's favourite hall monitor: "expertise." In so doing, epistemic violence is enacted, as locally grounded understandings of problems and solutions are subordinated to knowledge arising from practices deemed more authoritative.

Nevertheless, conventional notions of expertise – seen to reside in university-trained researchers – were contested as other forms of knowledge found space in politically important ways. For example, *Caring for All* recommends Aboriginal leaders join an "advisory group" to "create concepts/models for Aboriginal Healing and Wellness in Vancouver" in keeping with the task force's principle that "outcome measures and indicators are culturally relevant and demonstrate the value of lived experience."[30] A "peer leadership table" was also recommended to review current practices in care and support services, and several peer-based organizations were similarly asked to partner in generating self-defined needs and models of support. These acknowledgments make visible in the text the contributions by task force members who refused the notion that "expertise" is the sole property of psy-science. On the other hand, the involvement of people with lived experience comes with a disclaimer that suggests that they are in need of validation by researchers: "Although more evidence-based research on the topic of peer roles in health care is needed, local examples of peer practice show positive results."[31] Just as lived experience is evoked, it is also marginalized. A similar tension is visible in the way that *Caring for All* summons the importance of peer involvement at a time when many local community-based supports led autonomously by people with lived experience have had their funding withdrawn.[32] Epistemic violence is also evident where the document lists health authorities, government ministries, non-profit agencies, police, and researchers as *partners* in the task force, while Aboriginal leaders and people with lived experience are there to provide *input*.[33] Those with lived experience are thus engaged with in contradictory ways: subtly demoted even as they are allocated space to challenge dominant constructions of their lives.

The Opening and Closing of Democratic Space

As the discussion above suggests, the Task Force process that led to, and is described in, *Caring for All* was deliberately constructed to be inclusive and to that end ensured a place for the voices of those with lived experience, youth, and Aboriginal groups. While this is to be welcomed, it is notable that the report does not address the circumstances or views of members of other marginalized groups, nor were their representatives invited to participate in the task force process. This stands as a significant omission in a city that is home to many different racialized communities and constitutes a problematic limit to the "inclusion" on offer. Wendy Brown alerts us to an additional difficulty, arguing that when inclusion and participation are enacted in spaces and places where neo-liberal rationalities dominate, the scope for democratic practice is significantly constrained. As she suggests, a strong emphasis on consensus building (among other things) means that civic participation is reduced "to problem solving and program implementation, a casting that brackets or eliminates politics, conflict and deliberation about common values or ends."[34]

Several features of *Caring for All* provide examples of things that Brown is worried about. For example, the existence of "strong consensus on 23 key priority actions" is presented as a positive outcome indicative of substantial progress, and yet such consensus also signals that the space for advancing alternative problematizations of "the crisis" and responses to it has been closed down.[35] The text also indicates that evaluating future successes will be assisted by various measures including "agreement on shared principles, metrics and indicators of success" and "tracking of key metrics and data sharing."[36] Success thus requires consensus about what counts as evidence and what can be defined as improvements in relation to the "crisis." While some initiatives resonate with claims that have been advanced by members of disenfranchised communities (practices of peer support, incorporating Aboriginal and youth understandings of positive outcomes), the emphasis is on a series of technical solutions (i.e., more training for community workers, more research on "best practice," "tracking progress in the number of specialized addictions practitioners"), including the translating of Aboriginal, peer, and youth views into "outcome measures and indicators," rather than on initiatives aimed at creating a more just and equitable economy and distribution of social goods.[37] In this way, the slow violence that has been long endured by communities and individuals – deemed only just now to be "in crisis" – goes unrepresented and unaddressed. Instead, the space for naming and responding to this problematization is populated by quantitative measures that contain the parameters of "the crisis," both substantively and temporally.

Knowledge Practices and Slow Justice

The mayor's task force demonstrates how the "problem" of "mental illness" in the city is cast as one to be solved by normative agreement on the "evidence-based best practices" that ought to guide system responses to problems understood to reside in episodic crises. What escapes scrutiny in this process are the structural conditions that produce poverty, racism, sexism, and homelessness, and the slow violence that these visit upon those whose lives *Caring for All* addresses. We wonder, then, whether *slow justice* might be a way of thinking about practices that challenge those arising from the convergence of dominant biomedical, police and neo-liberal problematizations. Slow justice emerges from the seams where consensus might *not* have been achieved, where the efforts to problematize the crisis differently have shined through, opening up spaces for problems and solutions to be enacted in alternative ways. We see evidence of slow justice in the attention to the lived experience of psychiatrized people and drug users, and to Aboriginal knowledges, in the recommendations outlined in *Caring for All* and in the participation by members of these communities in the task force's process. The spaces afforded to these knowledges and communities are constrained, to be sure, but they have been created and occupied through slow but steady efforts that are instructive and can be built on.

While research remains a strong force in determining what counts as evidence in the "truth games"[38] surrounding the crisis, other groups historically excluded from policy processes in the city have been able to resist through practices that emerge from problematizations that are different from those that dominate *Caring for All*. For example, activist groups continue to host forums that showcase alternatives to biomedical treatment for people experiencing mental distress and to provide peer support and advocacy to people experiencing poverty and homelessness.[39] Workers in the mental health care system devise ways to defy government funding mandates that restrict advocacy activities by helping people obtain state benefits. Scholar activists speak out in public forums to question the ethics of research on homelessness and Mad activists hold Mad Pride events that celebrate rather than pathologize their "difference."[40] In response to the fear of being detained under the BCMHA after reaching out to medical professionals in moments of distress, a peer-to-peer helpline was set up by activists wanting to offer care and compassion without threat of hospitalization.

We see these resistive strategies and the alternative ways of thinking about mental health that they enact as elements of what we imagine slow justice to include. They work to expand the social and political space(s) within which people whose views/experiences have been marginalized, yet who bear the burden of decisions made, can engage through processes that foster participatory democracy and respect the epistemic value of lived experience. On this view, justice accrues not just in major policy and political shifts but also slowly accumulates in day-to-day resistive activities which contribute over time to significant social and cultural change.

Such practices could be understood cynically as "neo-liberal cooptation," as could participation in the consultative processes organized by the mayor's task force. Others might dismiss our temporal optimism, evoking the adages "slow justice is no justice" or "justice delayed is justice denied."[41] We agree that for individuals suffering the material repercussions of slow violence, psychiatrization, and colonization in their day-to-day lives, the absence of "fast justice" – and the presence of slow violence – is indeed unjust. However, we see local strategies of resistance as part of a process of reconfiguration taking place slowly, over time, through the actions of resistive subjects working in the "spaces of power."

Brown notes that as critical thinkers our democratic task is to puncture the neo-liberal common-sense rationalities that pervade the local spaces in which we work and live. A good place to start is to question practices of inclusion that close off democratic possibility, enact structural violence, and ignore the historical endemics of slow and epistemic violence. Just as there are many forms of violence, there must also be many forms of resistance. Some might resist by advancing competing problematizations within official processes – what Foucault calls "playing the same game differently"[42] – others by refusing to play the game at all. Both are part of a process of slow justice, the nimble exercises of resistance practised in non-ideal situations over time. Thus, even though slow and epistemological violence march on, eroding people's access to basic care, dignity, and voice, discursive struggles continue around Vancouver's "mental health crisis." Here and elsewhere, slow justice is at work when activists bring critical practices to bear on problematizations that enable harm to occur in the first place.

NOTES

1 Nixon, *Slow Violence*, 2.
2 Vancouver Police Department, *Vancouver's Mental Health Crisis*.
3 City of Vancouver, *Caring for All*.
4 Bacchi, *Analysing Policy*.
5 Nixon, *Slow Violence*, 2.
6 Liegghio, "A Denial of Being," 126.
7 Bacchi, *Analysing Policy*.
8 ACT is a recent and widely implemented interdisciplinary care team treatment model for individuals identified as "mentally ill" and homelessness. For a complete description of the model as promoted by researchers in the Mayor's Taskforce see Sommers et al. "Vancouver at Home."
9 Newman, "Spaces of Power."
10 See Morrow, Frischmuth, and Alicia Johnson, *Community-Based Mental Health Services in BC;* Caledon Institute of Social Policy, *A New Era in British Columbia*.
11 Elliot, "Debating Safe Injection Sites in Vancouver's Inner City."
12 Shore, "Welcome to Hell."
13 After this chapter was substantively complete yet another "crisis" was declared, this one focusing on opioid-related deaths. In June 2017, Vancouver Mayor Gregor Robertson proclaimed that "the near record number of overdose deaths in the fentanyl crisis is a bloodbath in all corners of the Vancouver with no end in sight" (see Kearney, "Fentanyl Crisis").
14 See Blomley, "The Right to Not Be Excluded."
15 Teréz, "Investigating the Geographies"; Kate Shannon et al., "Social and Structural Violence and Power Relations"; Boyd and the NAOMI Patients Association, "Yet They Failed to Do So."
16 City of Vancouver, *Caring for All*, 11.
17 For the Vancouver arm's final report see Currie et al., *At Home/Chez Soi Project: Vancouver Site Final Report*.

18 See for example Employment and Social Development Canada, "Harper Government Invests"; Lowery, "'Housing First.'"

19 See for example Morrow et al., *Community-Based Mental Health Service*; Teghtsoonian, "Social Policy in Neo-liberal Times."

20 City of Vancouver, *Caring for All*.

21 Morrow, "Recovery: Progressive Paradigm or Neo-liberal Smokescreen?"

22 Vancouver Police Department, *Vancouver's Mental Health Crisis*; Wilson-Bates, *Lost in Translation*.

23 City of Vancouver, *Caring for All*, 4.

24 Ibid., 8.

25 Ibid., 15.

26 Ibid., 7.

27 Berlant, "Slow Death Sovereignty, Obesity, Lateral Agency."

28 City of Vancouver, *Caring for All*, 20, 14.

29 Ibid., 14.

30 Ibid., 31, 30.

31 Ibid., 22.

32 For example, the West Coast Mental Health Association, Gastown Art Studios, Drug Users Resource Centre, and the Gallery Gachet have all had their government funding discontinued in 2014–2016.

33 City of Vancouver, *Caring for All*, 11.

34 Brown, *Undoing the Demos*.

35 City of Vancouver, *Caring for All*, 38.

36 Ibid., 38.

37 Ibid., 38.

38 Foucault, "The Ethics of the Concern."

39 For example, the regular forums held by the West Coast Mental Health Network.

40 See Patton, "Can a Research Question Violate a Human Right?" (unpublished manuscript) for a discussion of ethics and research on homelessness. See the Mad Pride events hosted by Gallery Gachet in Vancouver, http://gachet.org/2015/06/07/mad-pridedevelop -madness/ and http://www.spotlightonmentalhealth.com/mad-pride -2014-gallery-gachet/.

41 The phrase "justice delayed is justice denied" was used by Martin Luther King Jr. in "Letter from Birmingham jail," in which King expressed frustration with a "tragic misconception of time'. Some moderate activists believed that a more fulsome citizenship for African Americans would inevitably come with cultural change over time. For King, change required direct action and pressure from oppressed groups. See Martin Luther King Jr, *Why We Can't Wait*. New York: Signet Classic, 2000.

42 Foucault, "The Ethics of the Concern."

BIBLIOGRAPHY

Bacchi, Carol. *Analysing Policy: What's the Problem Represented to Be?* Frenchs Forest, Australia: Pearson, 2009.

Berlant, Lauren. "Slow Death Sovereignty, Obesity, Lateral Agency." *Critical Inquiry* 33, no. 4 (2007): 754–80.

Blomley, Nick. "The Right to Not Be Excluded: Common Property and the Struggle to Stay Put." Accessed February 27, 2017. https://sfu.academia .edu/NickBlomley.

Boyd, Susan, and the NAOMI Patients Association. "Yet They Failed to Do So: Recommendations Based on the Experiences of NAOMI Research Survivors and a Call for Action." *Harm Reduction Journal* 10, no. 6 (2013). http://harmreductionjournal.biomedcentral.com/articles/ 10.1186/1477-7517-10-6.

Brown, Wendy. *Undoing the Demos: Neo-liberalism's Stealth Revolution.* New York: Zone Books, 2015.

Caledon Institute of Social Policy. *A New Era in British Columbia: A Profile of Budget Cuts across Social Programs.* Ottawa, ON: Caledon Institute of Social Policy, 2002.

City of Vancouver. *Caring for All: Priority Actions to Address Mental Health and Addictions.* Vancouver, BC: City of Vancouver, 2014. https://vancouver.ca/ files/cov/mayors-task-force-mental-health-addictions-priority-actions .pdf.

Currie, Lauren, Akm Moniruzzaman, Michelle Patterson, and Julian Somers. *At Home/Chez Soi Project: Vancouver Site Final Report.* Calgary, AB: Mental Health Commission of Canada, 2014. http://homelesshub.ca/resource/ homechez-soi-project-vancouver-site-final-report.

Elliot, Denielle. "Debating Safe Injection Sites in Vancouver's Inner City: Advocacy, Conservatism, and Neo-liberalism." *Contemporary Drug Problems* 41 (2014): 5–32.

Employment and Social Development Canada. "Harper Government Invests in Housing First Homelessness Initiatives in Toronto." News release, February 13, 2015. Accessed September 1, 2018. http:// www.mhchs.ca/articles/harper-government-invests-in-housing -first-homelessness-initiatives-in-toronto-61/.

Foucault, Michel. "The Ethics of the Concern of the Self as a Practice of Freedom." In *Ethics, Subjectivity and Truth: The Essential Works of Foucault 1954–1984*, edited by Paul Rabinow, 281–301. New York: New Press, 1998.

Kearney, Cathy. "Fentanyl Crisis 'a Bloodbath,' Says Vancouver Mayor." *CBC News*, June 2, 2017, http://www.cbc.ca/news/canada/british-columbia/ new-numbers-robertson-opioid-crisis-feds-bloodbath-1.4144404.

Liegghio, Maria. "A Denial of Being: Psychiatrization as Epistemic Violence." In *Mad Matters: A Critical Reader in Canadian Mad Studies*, edited by Brenda Lefrançois, Robert Menzies, and Geoffrey Reaume, 122–30. Toronto, ON: Canadian Scholars' Press, 2013.

Lowery, Mollie. "'Housing First': What L.A. can learn from Utah on Homelessness." *LA Times*, June 3, 2015. http://www.latimes.com/nation/la-oe-0603-lowery-homeless-utah-la-20150603-story.html.

Morrow, Marina. "Recovery: Progressive Paradigm or Neo-liberal Smokescreen?" In *Mad Matters: A Critical Reader in Canadian Mad Studies*, edited by Brenda Lefrançois, Robert Menzies, and Geoffrey Reaume, 122–30. Toronto, ON: Canadian Scholars' Press, 2013.

Morrow, Marina, with Silke Frischmuth, and Alicia Johnson. *Community Based Mental Health Services in BC: Changes to Income, Employment and Housing Supports*. Vancouver, BC: Canadian Centre for Policy Alternatives, 2006.

Newman, Janet. "Spaces of Power: Feminism, Neoliberalism and Gendered Labor." *Social Politics* 20, no. 2 (2013): 200–21.

Nixon, Rob. *Slow Violence and the Environmentalism of the Poor*. Cambridge, MA: Presidents and Fellows of Harvard College, 2011.

Patton, Cindy. "Can a Research Question Violate a Human Right? Randomized Controlled Trials of Social-structural Conditions." Paper presented at Centre for the Study of Gender Social Inequities and Mental Health, Critical Inquiries in Mental Health Inequities: Exploring Methodologies for Social Justice. Vancouver, BC, 2012.

Sadler, Ian. "Press Release: Exhibition: Mad Cartographies: Wilderness of the Soul." *Spotlight on Mental Health*. Accessed February 27, 2017. http://www.spotlightonmentalhealth.com/mad-pride-2014-gallery-gachet/.

Shannon, Kate, Thomas Kerr, Shari Allinott, Jill Chettiar, Jean Shoveller, and Mark Tyndall. "Social and Structural Violence and Power Relations in Mitigating HIV Risk of Drug-Using Women in Survival Sex Work." *Social Science and Medicine* 66 (2008): 911–21.

Shore, Randy. "Welcome to Hell: Enter at Your Own Risk," *Late Nights in Lotusland: Reblog about Lives and Times in Vancouver* (blog). December 8, 2006. http://wig2.blogspot.com/2006/12/four-blocks-of-hell-on-earth.html.

Somers, Julian M., Michelle L. Patterson, Akm Moniruzzamam, Lauren Currie, Stefanie N. Rezansoff, Anita Palepu, and Karen Fryer. "Vancouver at Home: Pragmatic Randomized Trials Investigating Housing First for Homeless and Mentally Ill Adults." *Trials* 14 (2013): 1–20. https://www.biomedcentral.com/content/pdf/1745-6215-14-365.pdf.

Sylwia. "Mad Pride: Develop Madness." Gallery Gachet. June 7, 2015. http://gachet.org/2015/06/07/mad-pride-develop-madness/.

Teghtsoonian, Katherine. "Social Policy in Neo-liberal Times." In *British Columbia Politics and Government*, edited by Michael Howlett, Dennis Pilon and Tracy Summerville, 309–29. Toronto, ON: Emond Montgomery Publications, 2010.

Teréz, Szöke. "Investigating the Geographies of Community-Based Public Art and Gentrification in Downtown Eastside." MA thesis, University of Guelph, 2015.

Vancouver Police Department. *Vancouver's Mental Health Crisis: An Updated Report*. Vancouver, BC: Vancouver Police Department, 2013. https://vancouver.ca/police/assets/pdf/reports-policies/mental-health-crisis.pdf.

Wilson-Bates, Fiona. *Lost in Translation: How a Lack of Capacity in the Mental Health System Is Failing Vancouver's Mentally Ill and Draining Police Resources*. Vancouver, BC: Vancouver Police Department, 2008. Accessed April 7, 2017. https://vancouver.ca/police/assets/pdf/reports-policies/vpd-lost-in-transition.pdf.

6 Slow Death through Evidence-Based Research

Introduction

This chapter explores how the "gold standard" research norm of randomized controlled trials (RCT) is implicated in structural violence, contributing to the slow death of subjugated peoples. Understanding research as a key technology of neo-liberal biopolitical governance, I map how changing configurations of housing and mental health services administered through research projects sustain research subjects as precarious life. Drawing on an ethnographicallyinformed case study of the At Home/Chez Soi research demonstration project (2009–2013), I consider the direct connection between research as a practice that allows for the continued administration of state violence. Addressing how Mad people are managed as populations through research, I show how violence and power are tethered through what is often conceived as the benevolent quest for evidence-based research (EBR).

The At Home/Chez Soi project was a $110 million research demonstration project that studied how to best house "the chronically homeless mentally ill" in five cities across Canada.[1] A RCT, the project was funded by Health Canada through the Mental Health Commission of Canada, exemplifying how homelessness is increasingly functionally understood as a health condition rather than a consequence of neo-liberal capitalism.[2] Over 2000 homeless people across five sites in Canada were screened for "mental illness" and randomized into the intervention group or control group. The intervention group received Housing First programming, while the control group was left to access whatever pre-existing services were in their communities. The project was meant to provide the state with EBR that Housing First programs are the best model to solve the "crisis of the chronically homeless mentally ill" in Canada. Having experiences of homelessness/distress, I was hired as a consumer research consultant for the project. My work included advocating for and supporting service user involvement throughout the course of the study.[3] As service user involvement solidifies as a best practice in health and social service research and delivery, this chapter implicitly raises questions about the structures within which peer workers are included.

The consequences of normalizing RCTs (and EBR more broadly) as key to addressing homelessness/mental illness raises a number of ethical issues that this chapter considers. In Part One I explore the contexts through which EBR on social and structural inequities has emerged as best practice. I unsettle the idea that research is foundational to solving social problems. Instead, I unpack how through neo-liberal biopolitical management tactics, research works in conjunction with a wide array of neo-liberal tactics to sustain rather than solve structural violence. Part Two of this chapter explores consequences of the deployment of EBR as it aligns with neo-liberal biopolitical investments. I consider the constraints that RCT's place on research, researchers, service provisions, and especially those subjectified as research participants. By demanding EBR on the clinical and cost-effectiveness of housing homeless people before committing to affordable housing infrastructure, I understand EBR as a technology of rule that contributes to the prolonged subjugation of homeless people, emphasizing that systemic violence lands in very material ways on very real bodies. Studying imperilled bodies rather than acting to resolve housing insecurity inevitably prolongs precariousness in the lives of homeless individuals. In this way, marginalized research participants become material embodiments of the structural violence that austerity economics and the scientific rationality of EBR secures.

This chapter is also about intimate violence, despite its structural focus. Specifically, it involves the story of how researchers can become embedded in studies that, while couched as "benevolent projects" meant to offer help, are bound to a history of Western "improvement projects" that organize and manage subjugated peoples.[4] Currently, research intervention projects target subjects that are constituted by structural violence (racism, ongoing colonization, ableism, global capitalism) and enjoin them into social experiments, whereby subjects or their environments are altered and manipulated and the effects studied. Research endeavours are now part of an assemblage of tactics that are harnessed to implement neo-liberal technologies of governance. In this way, the implementation of EBR in the social and mental health sectors produces and sustains structural violence.

Part One: Evidence-Based Research in Context

Currently, knowledge production emerges within the tight governance of neo-liberal biopolitical logics. Foucault marked the nineteenth century emergence of biopolitics as modern states moved to manage populations through strategies of fostering respectable and productive bodies while divesting in degenerate abject bodies, a process of "making live and letting die."[5] Biopolitics harnesses both techniques that discipline and regulate individual bodies, as well as techniques that try to make known, order, and manage whole populations.[6] Through biopolitics, what Foucault termed state racism is used to stratify the population, making distinctions between productive and regressive bodies and determinations about who should live and who should be left to die.[7] Thus, "biopolitics deals with the population as a political problem. As a problem that is at once scientific and political, as a biological problem and as power's problem."[8]

With neo-liberalism, strategies of population management have changed, relying upon techniques that permeate economic, ideological, governance, and policy directives.[9] This includes managing the social welfare state though neo-liberal tactics that manage public assets and expenditures through private corporate means. Neo-liberalism works to reduce or "nullify all forms of social protections, welfare and transfer programs while promoting minimalist taxation and negligible business regulation," fosters precarious work, and positions "individualism, competitiveness, and economic self-sufficiency as fundamental virtues."[10] This means that for disabled people our interdependency as humans is negated, and those that fail to live up to neo-liberal tenets inevitably become subjects that need to be managed through it.[11] Paradoxically, disabled people are largely excluded from employment because of the cultural and material aversion towards impairment and difference while at the same time their economic disenfranchisement has generated "the multi-billion dollar industry that houses and 'cares' for the disabled population."[12]

Slow Death and Neo-liberal Biopolitics

Conjoining biopolitics to current neo-liberal management offers new ways of thinking about improvement projects.[13] Willse's work on the administration of homeless populations under neo-liberal management explores how social problems and troubled bodies are now reconfigured through neo-liberal biopolitics as economic opportunities. Willse shows how marginalized bodies that hitherto under Fordist-Keynesian social welfare models had been disinvested and left to die are renewed through neo-liberal biopolitical projects as economically generative. Marginalized populations as "surplus life" offer opportunities for capital growth. Through the privatization of social problem management, investing in the administration of marginality allows for the growth of professional management industries, including "the development of new service and knowledge industries directed towards managing surplus populations."[14] In the case study of the At Home/Chez Soi project private landlords, public health and housing agencies, government officials, researchers, and peer workers all become key professionals in administrative, provider, and knowledge industries enjoined to best manage (not solve) the "crisis of the chronically homeless mentally ill."

Berlant uses the concept of "slow death" to elaborate how populations rendered deficit to productivity are managed through biopolitics. As a process, "*slow death* refers to the physical wearing out of a population and the deterioration of people in that population that is very nearly a defining condition of their experience and historical existence. ... the phenomenon of mass physical attenuation under global/national regimes of capitalist structural subordination and governmentality."[15] It is the result of long processes of intertwined violence (environmental, spatial, racial, sexual and gendered, disabling and debilitating) imbued with long histories of privation. Yet crucially, by marrying concepts of slow death to the economic life generated through the management of such subjugated populations, we see how populations regulated into slow death under neo-liberal biopolitics now offer economic opportunities for professionals to grow research, knowledge, and service industries based on their abjection.

Attention turned to those living out slow deaths is often couched in the language of "crisis." Yet the rhetoric of crisis belies the long-standing subordination of abjected populations, misrepresenting "the duration and scale of the situation by calling a *crisis* that which is a fact of life and has been a defining fact of life for a given population that lives it as a fact in ordinary time."[16] The ordinary living of populations regulated to slow death is often deemed *crises* when posing problems to state management and economic profit – for example, the problem that the *crisis in mental health* poses to health insurance companies, the loss in profits for companies through absenteeism, the increase in disability-related state benefits, or the costs associated with accommodating workers and students in public and private sectors.[17]

While both homelessness and mental illness are often referred to as crises, a combined subset of both populations allow for action based on the crisis management of the "chronically homeless mentally ill." The *chronically homeless mentally ill* is an emerging population category, requiring interventions distinct from the management of the "chronically homeless."[18] Distinct, because mental illness is prioritized as causing and sustaining homelessness. This process marks what Morrow calls the "healthification" of social problems, which reconfigures socio-economic inequities as health issues.[19] Often, intervention projects are justified not only to help those in crisis but as a response to the problems that they pose to white civil society. To sustain ongoing colonial nation-building projects of a nativist white and English Canada, those that pose trouble to white civility – good polity, conformity to the principles of social order, polite or liberal education – must be oriented towards acquiring such civilizing mores.[20] The chronically homeless mentally ill are construed as a population that threatens not only white civil society but also neo-liberal capitalism. The problem that the chronically homeless mentally ill pose to us as a nation is primarily that of cost. Improperly managed and let loose they are positioned as costing the state more than they contribute to it. Yet importantly, they are also positioned as harbingers of violence that must be dealt with to keep citizens safe. For example, research that ties divestments in housing and mental health care to increasing crime rates speaks to how such crises are not only about managing the slow death of subjugated peoples but also about protecting the lives of those who are deemed worth living.[21]

Research through Neo-liberal Biopolitics

Critiques that speak to the ways in which social problems are organized through neo-liberal biopolitical economies have emerged, including how non-governmental organizations as "non-profit industrial complexes" sustain subjugation.[22] Under "new managerialism," corporate model logics manage social issues by "importing ideas and practices from the private world of business into the world of public service, on the assumption that the latter are superior to the former."[23] This means that new kinds of external accountability, performance, and audit cultures, and prioritizing cost efficiency and program efficacy have become the rule.[24] Public services are run through corporate models: for example, social and health service sectors now use and promote evidence-based practices based on EBR. As a neo-liberal management strategy EBR is used to "engage the authority of 'hard science' to give weight to their propositions," and thus the growth of EBR projects investigating social problems, to be transformed into evidence-based practice.[25] In this way, EBR is a key technology used to investigate "how to do things best" based on "objective evidence about their effectiveness, and then measuring outcomes in order to assess their degree of success."[26] While my analysis interrogates RCTs as one research design used to investigate social inequities, many research methods can be put to work within particular discursive frames to solidify logics that align with neo-liberal management strategies.

One of the consequences of current neo-liberal management tactics is increasing demand for pilot research demonstration projects to provide the state with EBR to plan future policy and program directions. Motivated primarily to ensure cost and program efficiency, the call for EBR through RCTs has proliferated in recent years.[27] RCTs now extends beyond clinical health and drug trials to social policy and programs.[28] This means that temporary fragmented pilot project programs are increasingly moving in to supplant fully funded health and social service programs. Not only Band-Aid solutions, these are sites where research data is collected and being a research participant becomes a condition of receiving help. This raises questions of informed consent, limited choice, and consent under duress. In the case of the At Home/ Chez Soi project, few people were in the position to turn down an opportunity to become a research participant, leading to questions of undue inducements for those seeking basic necessities for life.

Part Two: Research as Violence

By using the At Home/Chez Soi project as a case study, in this section I explore four consequences of this move towards relying on RCTs to help know and manage populations living through slow death. I start by exploring what now counts as research in research and performance cultures, and how that binds us as researchers to state violence. Using Housing First as an example, I show how projects that are couched in benevolence work to sustain structural inequities through the privatization of social problems. I engage with the risks of tying human rights to positive research outcomes and end by considering the lives that are left when research studies end.

The Politics of Research

Research is political. As Beresford notes, "powerful hierarchies for the production of knowledge still operate in research, not least in mental health research."[29] This project was funded and framed as a health intervention, and it structurally proceeded as a registered clinical trial approved by 11 hospital and university research ethics boards.[30] Positioned as a clinical intervention, project methods thus fit into the norms of drug and other clinical RCTs that research ethics boards are used to reviewing. While RCTs have long been valorized as the "gold standard of evidence" that favour "drug trials over all other types of research" in the medical realm, shifting this method of evidence-based medicine and applying RCTs to broader social realms and the study of structural violence is concerning.[31] In this example of the At Home Project/Chez Soi, research ethics boards are thus implicated in condoning the medicalization of social issues through their active approval of research projects that position social policy issues as medical problems. For this to change, those that hold purview at the ethics review stage of medical research would have to resist such conceptualizations, which would likely require a shift in board compositions to include scholars critical of health and drug trial logics when applied to issues of social justice.

For researchers trying to unsettle dominant logics, chances of accessing funding for social justice research is significantly undermined. Social science research under neo-liberal biopolitical logics is understood as a technology that should benefit governance by directly serving state strategic priorities and directives and not social justice. State-sponsored research granting bodies are subject to the governing rules of new managerialism. To secure their own funding dollars, they face pressure to reward research grants to projects that directly align with state interests. Further, special calls for research that tap into municipal, provincial or territorial, or federal strategic priorities are now regularly issued, and researchers become responsible for crafting research grants that correspond to what governments want done (but often no longer funds directly). In this way, researchers are bound to the terms of working within state interests.

This applies to the At Home/Chez Soi project. The motivation for this RCT was aligned with state interests given the federal government's

2009 endorsement of the Housing First model based on research in other countries. Patton argues that the primary motivation of the project was "to assess the 'cost/benefit' and 'cost/effectiveness' of 'Housing First in comparison to care as usual' in the Canadian context."[32] Patton contends that conducting a RCT to provide cost-benefit data to a government that is already interested in Housing First as an intervention for the problem of the chronically homeless mentally ill is unethical research practice. She notes that an "RCT is not the only, indeed, it is not even the best way to answer costing questions, which are usually addressed using historical data and service utilization models."[33] Yet through the valorization of RCTs as the benchmark research method, it is now normalized to use in social experiments to provide "objective science" for social policy change.

One desired outcome of the project was for the research data to show that it is cheaper to house people than to leave them homeless. Thus, research data needed to demonstrate significant cost offsets to the state. This meant providing data that showed a decreased use of costly emergency, police, and criminal justice contact, as well as a reduction in housing people in prison, hospital, transition, and shelter systems. Here, the goal was to show overall that public service costs would be reduced through "assertive community care." In fact, not only reduced but also re-directed: one key component of Housing First models is the move away from public housing/institutional settings and towards reliance on private housing units to solve affordable housing shortages.

Housing First: Privatizing Social Problems

The intervention under study in the At Home/Chez Soi project was the Housing First model. Housing First models work to rapidly house a homeless individual, and then provide services and support through ACT or intensive case management teams. An eligibility screening assessment included MINI International Neuropsychiatric Interview 6.0, a standardized instrument used to first ensure that the participant is mentally ill. They are then signed up for welfare or disability benefits. The rental portion of their benefits is put towards their housing, and the project tops up the remaining portion through a capped rent supplement. Crucially, participants are predominantly housed in private units, and thus rent paid goes directly to private landlords.

Housing First programs are a prime example of how public-private partnerships grow financial opportunity through neo-liberal biopolitical economies. One of the critiques of the Housing First model is that it divests government of the responsibility of supporting more affordable housing units. Further, since it requires no investment in building housing infrastructure, there is a temporality to commitment – funding for Housing First programs can fluctuate more easily than the commitment of bricks and mortar. A reliance on pre-existing private dwellings offsets state responsibility in building and maintaining affordable housing units. It does not solve the housing crisis caused by the shortage of affordable housing units, instead finding a solution within capitalism and privatizing the social problem of affordable housing. However, the tenancy problems of capitalism are sustained, including allowing for landlord discrimination and rental refusals based on participants' status as the chronically homeless mentally ill; racism, especially against Indigenous Peoples; drug use; gender and sexual variance, and so forth. In cities where unoccupied market rental units are low, this is especially so. Consequently, participants are often spatially relegated to undesirable rental units that those who are living well won't consider.

Researching a Human Right

How we seek to solve the problem of lack of affordable, accessible, and accommodating housing matters. Housing is a basic human right as declared in Article 25 of the United Nations Universal Declaration of Human Rights (1948), the UN Convention on the Rights of Persons with Disabilities (2008), and the Canadian Charter of Rights and Freedoms (1982). Because housing is a human right, there is no need to generate an evidence base to justify it.

Patton's rights-based analysis critiques the At Home/Chez Soi project by addressing the consequences of studying homelessness through an RCT, raising a number of ethical risks that come with studying a human right. Specifically, how such research positions human rights as contingent on outcomes – the right to housing becomes conditional to cost, health, and safety benefits. Patton argues that market and commodity rationales undercut the purpose of human rights:

> One of the main purposes of defining human rights is to set a floor underneath what a society is permitted to do to its most vulnerable members – but research of this kind moves housing from the domain of rights and into the marketplace of goods ... In this way, the study design expresses social responsibility in actuarial rather than human rights

terms. Essentially, the costing aspect of the housing study puts a price on a human right. To ask disempowered individuals to consent to participating in a study which diminishes their value as persons by actuarializing their right is, in itself, a violation of the human right implicitly under scrutiny.[34]

Patton goes on to outline risks associated with project findings, asking what happens if study results show that housing is ineffective at cost savings, improving health outcomes, or otherwise managing the problems that populations living out slow deaths cause the state. In this way, "agreeing to be in this study amounts to [participants] agreeing to the possibility of losing the *right* to housing."[35] Further, because Housing First is funded as a mental health intervention and not a housing intervention, the project works to solidify housing as connected to improved health results. This works to reinforce "the significance of housing as a 'treatment,' [and] it undermines the *status* of housing as a right by making its value contingent" on improved health outcomes.[36]

Patton ends her critique by noting that the concepts "and the research designs that we assent to – RCT and no doubt others – are part of the actuarialization of human rights. Simply couching this as 'science' does not absolve our responsibility for the violations we commit in the name of 'producing evidence' that does not speak to fundamental problems, and does not help the ever receding human beings that we now call 'research subject.'"[37] Through such research, we offer conditional aid to populations that are sustained as marginal, further subjecting bodies to slow death under new terms. This shows how neo-liberal biopolitical projects as economic opportunity offers state and knowledge professionals opportunities for growth. Yet those made marginal are offered the limited choice of commodifying their marginality anew: as research participants that at once generate for the state yet places them in further precarious situations.

Bodies of Research

The history of commodifying imperilled subjects – racialized, disabled, mad, queer, and other nexuses of endangered bodies – through research is extensive.[38] As objects of study, we have long been subject to experiments because our lives are deemed worthless. Productivity can be made from those deemed unproductive; using our lives and bodies as objects of study works to reduce us, prevent us, and cure us. To step back into how intimate structural violence is, I want to end this chapter by attending to the research subjects of the At Home/Chez Soi project. Ample research products have been generated through study findings.[39] Lost in the "success" narrative of this research project are the post-study intimate material lives of participants.

Those captured by the study are "hard bodies": hard to house, hard to treat, hard to handle through mainstream measures. Unruled bodies disrupt public space, they create spectacle, cause trouble, are often met with police intervention (and police violence), and cost money and lives. Cast out from civil society, many of the potential participants who made contact with the project were living at the extremities of life. The project offered potential access to basic living needs that could move them back from the realm of imminent death to the space of slow death. By way of this project, such imperilled bodies were offered the chance to reintegrate back into services and systems that would offer them little more than rejoining the realm of slow death. The project (temporarily) worked to regroup unruly bodies back into the management of neo-liberal biopolitical industries.

When the At Home/Chez Soi project began, critiques from community activists, advocates, service providers, and other researchers were met with the tenets of hope, optimism, and promise for the future. Proponents argued that it was better than nothing. The state now demands EBR to inform evidence-based policy and practice, and that this is what researchers now have to work with. Hands are tied, we do what we can, and we have to act: people are homeless and dying. Further, there was the promise of what this RCT could produce. If the research outcomes showed program efficacy and cost savings, this would improve the landscape of housing policy.

However, there was no promise of housing and service sustainability. Those in the intervention group risked losing their rent supplements and services at the end of the pilot project. At the beginning of the project, housing and mental health activists and advocates were met with the promise that hard work would not only be put into sustaining the housing and services of the intervention group but also be expanded to those in the control group and beyond. Further, with evidence, the state would expand investments in Housing First initiatives across Canada. The promise of a future groundswell of housing and support for the chronically homeless mentally ill allowed for project implementation.

As the project wore on, such promises wore thin. This is not to say that project leads didn't work extremely hard at trying to secure sustainability of housing and services for participants. But the promise of, for example, expanding housing and services to the control group or that positive early findings would lead to immediate federal funding to sustain project participants ceased. In practice, the focus was on trying to secure the housing and services of the thousand participants who risked losing their place at project end. Thus, these early promises were tactical responses to critique, public speech acts that allowed research initiatives to proceed.

For those in the business of neo-liberal biopolitical investments, the project was a success. Housing First as a program model was affirmed, research careers advanced, and the federal government explicitly and repeatedly cited the project as an evidence base, leading to federal policy change. While EBR has led to policy change supporting Housing First programs, in practice this has largely entailed a shifting of funds from pre-existing services (not a significant increase) towards Housing First models for local municipalities who apply for (time-limited contractual) Federal Homelessness Partnering Strategy funding. While the Housing First model in theory has now been legitimized through EBR, the financial investments required to fully implement this program model across Canada remain limited.[40]

The promise of EBR has not extended as well to those under study. In the end, those harnessed as the intervention group through the RCT landed on uneven ground. Because housing and mental health services are predominantly administered municipally and provincially, a patchwork of negotiations with a variety of governments was required to advocate for housing and service sustainability. Toronto was the most successful site as intervention group participants were promised sustained housing and services, indefinitely. Other sites were mixed: housing alternatives were found for many intervention group participants requiring moves, new housing, and service providers.[41] Yet much of what was found were the same transitional and rooming housing solutions that created housing insecurity for them in the first place. While the large assemblage of professional players that drove the project splintered back out into the safety of their respective research, service, policy, and administrative fields, in the end, participants were largely left behind.

For those who have been regulated to and through slow death, we are no longer surprised by what bad outcomes wait for us as precarious clients, users, and objects of research. Through the entanglements of neo-liberal capitalism, we are expected to hustle like those who live well – we are reminded that there are no free meals, no guaranteed income benefits, no social safety nets left for anyone. Yet as hustlers working within the spaces of slow death, our choices are limited. This abrupt end for participants to the promises of EBR shows the violence of research on subjugated populations.

Yet the cyclical game of research isn't over. A number of former At Home/Chez Soi sites have received research grants to follow and study what happens to project participants as they emerge back out of the project, with some, no doubt, landing back where they started. As Fine notes, as researchers in austere times, we are recruited "to create a *science of banal dispossession* – to engage in the systematic collection of evidence that demonstrates (usually) that state programs don't make up for historic and cumulative oppression, legitimating the slashing of the safety net."[42] Quick fixes to clean up the problems of systemic violence through regimes of capital always fail. As researchers, we are directly tied to the violence of EBR and practice, and thus tethered to systems that relegate study participants to slow death.

NOTES

1 Goering et al., *The At Home/Chez Soi Trail Protocol.*
2 Kotz, *The Rise and Fall of Neo-liberal Capitalism.*
3 Nelson et al., "Collaboration and Involvement of Persons"; Voronka et al., "Un/helpful Help and its Discontents."
4 Razack, *Dying from Improvement.*
5 Foucault, *Society Must Be Defended*, 247.
6 Ibid., 249.
7 Ibid., 254–5.
8 Ibid., 245.
9 Larner, "Neo-liberalism."
10 Springer, "Neo-liberalising Violence," 137.
11 Mingus, "Changing the Framework."
12 Taylor, "The Right Not to Work," 12.
13 Razack, *Dying from Improvement.*
14 Willse, *The Value of Homelessness*, 47.
15 Berlant, "Slow Death," 754.
16 Ibid., 760.
17 Reid, "The University as the Next Mental Health Treatment Facility."
18 Willse, "Neo-liberal Biopolitics."
19 Morrow, "Recovery: Progressive Paradigm," 329.
20 Coleman, *White Civility.*

21 See Torrey, *American Psychosis*.
22 INCITE! Women of Color against Violence, *The Revolution Will Not be Funded*; Manazala and Spade, "The Nonprofit Industrial Complex"; Munshi and Willse, "Introduction."
23 Deem and Brehony, "Management as Ideology," 220.
24 Power, *The Audit Society*.
25 Davies, "Death to Critique and Dissent?", 100.
26 Hammersley, "Some Questions about Evidence-Based Practice in Education," 8.
27 Mykhalovskiy and Weir, "The Problem of Evidence-Based Medicine."
28 Kerr, Leve, and Chamberlain, "Pregnancy Rates among Juvenile Justice Girl"; Herman et al., "Randomized Trial of Critical Time Intervention."
29 Beresford, "Control: User-Controlled Research," 192.
30 Goering et al., *The At Home/Chez Soi Trail Protocol*, 1.
31 Fischer, "Politics," 231.
32 Patton, "Can a Research Question Violate a Human Right?", 8.
33 Ibid., 8.
34 Ibid., 11.
35 Ibid., 11.
36 Ibid., 12.
37 Ibid., 12–13.
38 Duster, *Backdoor to Eugenics*.
39 Aubry, Nelson, and Tsemberis, "Housing First."
40 Government of Canada, "Housing First: Types of Support."
41 Aubry, "Housing First Strategy."
42 Fine, "Troubling Calls for Evidence," 4.

BIBLIOGRAPHY

Aubry, Tim. "Housing First Strategy." *CBC Radio*, November 30, 2016. http://www.cbc.ca/news/canada/new-brunswick/programs/informationmorningmoncton/tim-aubry-housing-first-strategy-1.3874274.
Aubry, Tim, Geoffrey Nelson, and Sam Tsemberis. "Housing First for People with Severe Mental Illness Who Are Homeless: A Review of the Research and Findings from the At Home-Chez Soi Demonstration Project." *Canadian Journal of Psychiatry* 60, no. 11 (2015): 467–74.
Beresford, Peter. "Control: User-Controlled Research." In *Handbook of Service User Involvement in Mental Health Research*, edited by Jan Wallcraft, Beate Schrank, and Michaela Amering, 227–43. West Sussex, UK: Wiley-Blackwell, 2009.

Berlant, Lauren. "Slow Death: Sovereignty, Obesity, Lateral Agency." *Critical Inquiry* 33, no. 4 (2007): 754–80.

Coleman, Daniel. *White Civility: The Literary Project of English Canada.* Toronto, ON: University of Toronto Press, 2008.

Davies, Bronwyn. "Death to Critique and Dissent? The Policies and Practices of New Managerialism and of 'Evidence-Based Practice.'" *Gender and Education* 15, no. 4 (2003): 91–103.

Deem, Rosemary, and Kevin J. Brehony. "Management as Ideology: The Case of 'New Managerialism' in Higher Education." *Oxford Review of Education* 31, no. 2 (2005): 217–35.

Duster, Troy. *Backdoor to Eugenics.* 2nd ed. New York: Routledge, 2003.

Fine, Michelle. "Troubling Calls for Evidence: A Critical Race, Class and Gender Analysis of Whose Evidence Counts." *Feminism and Psychology* 22, no. 3 (2012): 3–19.

Fischer, Daniel B. "Politics of Research in Mental Health." In *Handbook of Service User Involvement in Mental Health Research,* edited by Jan Wallcraft, Beate Schrank, and Michaela Amering, 227–43. West Sussex, UK: Wiley-Blackwell, 2009.

Foucault, Michel. *Society Must Be Defended: Lectures at the Collège de France, 1975–76.* New York: Picador, 1997.

Goering, Paula N., David L Streiner, Crol Adair, Tim Aubry, Jayne Barker, Jino Distasio, Stephen W. Hwang, Janina Kamaroff, Eric Latimer, Julian Somers, and Denise M. Zabkiewicz. "The At Home/Chez Soi Protocol: A Pragmatic, Multi-site, Randomized Controlled Trial of a Housing First Intervention for Homeless Individuals with Mental Illness in Five Canadian Cities." *BMJ Open* 1, no. 2 (2011): 1–18.

Government of Canada. "Housing First: Types of Support." Accessed January 1, 2017. https://www.canada.ca/en/employment-social-development/programs/communities/homelessness/housing-first/supports.html.

Hammersley, Martyn. "Some Questions about Evidence-Based Practice in Education." Paper presented at the Annual Conference of the British Educational Research Association, University of Leeds, England, September 13–15, 2001.

Herman, Daniel, Sarah Conover, Prakash Gorroochurn, Kinjia Hinterland, Lorie Hoepner, and Ezra Susser. "Randomized Trial of Critical Time Intervention to Prevent Homelessness after Hospital Discharge." *Psychiatric Services* 62, no. 7 (2011): 713–19.

INCITE! Women of Color against Violence. *The Revolution Will Not Be Funded: Beyond the Non-profit Industrial Complex.* Cambridge, MA: South End Press, 2007.

Kerr, David C. R., Leslie D. Leve, and Patricia Chamberlain. "Pregnancy Rates among Juvenile Justice Girls in Two Randomized Controlled Trials of Multidimensional Treatment Foster Care." *Journal of Consulting and Clinical Psychology* 77, no. 3 (2009): 588–93.

Kotz, David M. *The Rise and Fall of Neo-liberal Capitalism.* Cambridge, MA: Harvard University Press, 2015.

Larner, Wendy. "Neo-liberalism: Policy, Ideology, Governmentality." *Studies in Political Economy* 63 (2000): 5–25.

Manazala, Rickke, and Dean Spade. "The Nonprofit Industrial Complex and Trans Resistance." *Sexuality Research and Social Policy* 5, no. 1 (2008): 53–71.

Mingus, Mia. "Changing the Framework: Disability Justice." *RESIST Newsletter,* November 2010. Reprinted on Leaving Evidence (blog). https://leavingevidence.wordpress.com/2011/02/12/changing-the-framework-disability-justice/.

Morrow, Marina. "Recovery: Progressive Paradigm or Neo-liberal Smokescreen?" In *Mad Matters: A Critical Reader in Canadian Mad Studies,* edited by Brenda Lefrançois, Robert Menzies, and Geoffrey Reaume, 323–33. Toronto, ON: Canadian Scholars' Press, 2013.

Munshi, Soniya, and Craig Willse. "Introduction: Navigating Neo-liberalism in the Academy, Nonprofits, and Beyond." *Scholar and Feminist Online* 13, no. 2 (2015). http://sfonline.barnard.edu/navigating-neo-liberalism-in-the-academy-nonprofits-and-beyond/soniya-munshi-craig-willse-introduction/.

Mykhalovskiy, Eric, and Lorna Weir. "The Problem of Evidence-based Medicine: Directions for Social Science." *Social Science and Medicine* 59 (2004): 1059–69.

Nelson, Geoffrey, Eric Macnaughton, Susan Eckerle Curwood, Nathalie Egalité, Jijian Voronka, Marie-Josée Fleaury, Maritt Kirst, Linsay Flowers, Michelle Patterson, Michael Dudley, Myra Piat, and Paula Goering. "Collaboration and Involvement of Persons with Lived Experience in Planning Canada's At Home/Chez Soi Project." *Health and Social Care in the Community* 24, no. 2 (2016): 184–93.

Patton, Cindy. "Can a Research Question Violate a Human Right? Randomized Controlled Trials of Socio-Structural Conditions." Paper presented at Critical Inquiries in Mental Health Inequities: Exploring Methodologies for Social Justice. Centre for the Study of Gender Social Inequities and Mental Health, Vancouver, BC, 2012. http://www.socialinequities.ca/knowledge/can-a-research-question-violate-a-human-right-randomized-controlled-trials-of-social-structural-conditions/.

Power, Michael. *The Audit Society: Rituals of Verification.* Oxford, UK: Oxford University Press, 1999.

Razack, Sherene H. *Dying from Improvement: Inquests and Inquiries into Indigenous Deaths in Custody.* Toronto, ON: University of Toronto Press, 2015.

Reid, Jenna. "The University as the Next Mental Health Treatment Facility: Fixing the #brokengeneration." Paper presented at the American Educational Studies Association Conference, Toronto, ON, November 1, 2014.

Springer, Simon. "Neoliberalising Violence: Of the Exceptional and the Exemplary in Coalescing Moments." *Area* 44, no. 2 (2012): 136–43.

Taylor, Sunny. "The Right Not to Work: Disability and Power." *Monthly Review: An Independent Socialist Magazine* 55, no. 10 (2004). https://monthlyreview.org/2004/03/01/the-right-not-to-work-power-and-disability/.

Torrey, E. Fuller. *American Psychosis: How the Federal Government Destroyed the Mental Illness Treatment System.* New York: Oxford University Press, 2014.

Voronka, Jijian, Deborah Wise Harris, Jill Grant, Janina Komaroff, Dawn Boyle, and Arianna Kennedy. "Un/helpful Help and Its Discontents: Peer Researchers Paying Attention to Street Life Narratives to Inform Social Work Policy and Practice." *Social Work in Mental Health* 12, no. 3 (2014): 249–79.

Willse, Craig. "Neo-liberal Biopolitics and the Invention of Chronic Homelessness." *Economy and Society* 39, no. 2 (2010): 155–84.

Willse, Craig. *The Value of Homelessness: Managing Surplus Life in the United States.* Minneapolis: University of Minnesota Press, 2015.

7 Changing Directions or Staying the Course? Recovery, Gender, and Sexuality in Canada's Mental Health Strategy

MERRICK PILLING

Canada's first national mental health strategy, *Changing Directions, Changing Lives: The Mental Health Strategy for Canada* mobilizes recovery as a key concept in "changing directions" in the mental health system. In this chapter I examine sections of *Changing Directions* to critically analyse the strategy's understanding of gender, sexuality, and recovery as it pertains to lesbian, gay, bisexual, queer, and trans (LGBQT) people. I argue that despite the acknowledgment of some of the social factors related to mental distress, the strategy relies on a neo-liberal individualizing framework that fails to advance a strong structural analysis of homophobic violence and transphobic violence in shaping experiences of mental distress and recovery. *Changing Directions* individualizes social problems by positioning the conditions that can cause distress as "risk factors" inherently associated with gender and sexuality, rather than partially created and perpetuated by the state. This erases state violence and accountability and has troubling implications for recovery for LGBQT people who experience mental distress. Recovery is envisioned as further integrating LGBQT people into mental health systems through increasing accessibility without acknowledging or changing the ways in which such systems can be violent.

Changing Directions is the work of the Mental Health Commission of Canada (MHCC), which was established by the Conservative-led federal government in 2007 with a 10-year mandate, recently renewed for an additional 10 years. *Changing Directions* is a 113-page document outlining six strategic directions for implementing change in the system, published in 2012. This national strategy is the first of its kind in Canada, standing in contrast to most countries in the global north where such documents were developed in the 1990s following deinstitutionalization. The committee responsible for background research in preparation for *Changing Directions* (Standing Senate Committee on Social Affairs, Science And Technology) attributes this late development to issues related to federalism and refers to this lack of national planning as "relative backwardness."[1] As the first national strategy, *Changing Directions* is a significant document that provides the theoretical foundation for the future of Canadian mental health care.

Changing Directions is comparatively unique in that it includes an explicit discussion of issues related to gender and sexuality. Of the countries studied in preparation for the development of *Changing Directions*, only England has a national plan that makes mention of gender, "sexual orientation," and "gender dysphoria," and only superficially.[2] With the advent of the legalization of same-sex marriage in Canada in 2004, some gays and lesbians (viz. white, middle-class, monogamously coupled gays and lesbians) enjoyed more rights and have become increasingly normalized within mainstream society. Correspondingly, there is increased recognition of these groups in legislation and policy documents, such as *Changing Directions*. While this could be perceived as a positive development legitimizing the existence of some gay and lesbian ways of being, it is important to think critically about what is accomplished by such inclusions. LGBQT people have not been well served by mental health systems and the biomedical model of "mental illness" more generally.

Indeed, dissident genders and sexualities have been, and continue to be, positioned as psychopathologies. The *Diagnostic and Statistical Manual of Mental Disorders* has been key in this process, with historical and current diagnoses that pathologize LGBQT people.[3] Likewise, LGBQT people continue to experience discrimination and erasure within mental health care systems and organizations.[4] What does recovery mean within this larger context of pathologization and discrimination? As will be seen, *Changing Directions* interprets the effects of this context as "risk factors" inherently linked to gender and sexuality, an individualizing approach that erases systemic violence, with troubling implications for recovery.

What Is Mental Health Recovery?

The concept of recovery originated within the psychiatric survivor movement in the 1980s as a way of challenging biomedical prognoses of lifelong "illness" and reduced capacity for self-determination.[5]

Psychiatric survivors developed an understanding of recovery in contradistinction to the biomedical view of recovery as the lessening or elimination of "symptoms."[6] In this view, recovery refers to (re)creating a meaningful life with or without experiences of mental distress and recovering from the harmful effects of the psychiatric system.[7] The initial conceptualization of recovery focused on psychiatric survivor agency, exploring means of addressing distress outside of medical systems, and addressing the social factors that can cause or exacerbate mental distress, including the effects of psychiatrization and biomedical "treatment."

Recovery has since been taken up as a concept informing policy change and mental health service provision in the global north. The use of *recovery* in such contexts has changed its meaning, and some argue that it has been reconfigured in the service of neo-liberal state agendas.[8] Social-justice-oriented scholars have critiqued this reconfiguration of recovery for failing to address structural inequities.[9] Indeed, some contend that recovery is now used to "incorporate psychiatric survivors into medical systems" and reinforce "medical authority," as mental health professionals become "experts" in recovery.[10]

This reconfiguration of recovery is evident in *Changing Directions*. The document defines recovery as "living a satisfying, hopeful, and contributing life, even when there are ongoing limitations caused by mental health problems and illnesses."[11] This definition sounds similar to the way the psychiatric survivor movement defined recovery, in that it does not require the elimination of symptoms. However, it differs in that there is no acknowledgment of the fact that people may need to recover from the effects of psychiatrization. The definition also suggests that both mental distress and the resulting "limitations" placed on those experiencing it are caused by "problems" and "illnesses," leaving no room for those who do not see mental distress as a deficit or who see it as a social issue rather than a medical one.[12] In this way, the MHCC uses the positive sounding message of hope while jettisoning the critical repositioning of the origins of mental distress and the resulting limitations as social and structural, thereby side-stepping state responsibility for structuring and addressing those conditions. This fundamentally neo-liberal approach turns recovery into an individualized "personal journey."[13] Further, state-produced conceptualizations of recovery as being able to "contribute" are telling; if one can contribute one is not perceived as a "burden" on the state or society. This positioning of "recovery" as an individualized process ideally resulting in the ability to contribute puts the focus on making personal change rather than social and structural change. The section following looks more closely at sections of the strategy to examine the implications of this for how the MHCC envisions facilitating recovery for LGBQT people.

Recovery in the Context of *Diversity* and *Disparity*: Strategic Direction 4

Strategic direction four describes five priorities, which are named in the executive summary as 4.1: social determinants, 4.2: immigrants, refugees, ethno-cultural, racialized, 4.3: northern and remote, 4.4: minority official language, and 4.5 gender, sexuality. I briefly discuss the introduction before focusing on priority 4.5, which is the only section of the document that examines the specific concerns of "lesbian, gay, bisexual, two-spirited, trans-gendered, and trans-sexual" (though notably not queer) people. While not always speaking directly to recovery, this section illuminates the MHCC's understanding of the relationship between gender, sexuality, and mental health, and the conditions that lead to mental distress. It therefore has implications for recovery and how such distress will be addressed.[14]

The introduction sets the stage for the strategy's approach to analysing "disparities" in mental health. The MHCC uses the language of the social determinants of health to explain how certain groups are both "at greater risk" of developing "mental health problems and illnesses" and experiencing "disparities in access" to services.[15] For example, the MHCC explains that those with "better incomes, more education, and stronger social networks" are often healthier. This acknowledgment of social factors seems like a clear departure from the individualizing logic of the medical model of mental illness, which locates the primary cause of distress within the biological characteristics of the individual. However, with the exception of "experiences of racism and … discrimination," the "risk factors" listed focus on characteristics of the individual rather than the environment (e.g. "socio-economic status" as opposed to "class oppression," and "living in a remote/northern community" as opposed to "lack of services in northern/remote communities").[16] The list does include racism, but this is the only place in Strategic Direction 4 where this word appears, and opportunities to include structural analyses of racism are ignored.[17]

Theorizing the "risk factors" as individual characteristics rather than environmental ones has consequences for perceived responsibility and intervention. If the *risk* is gender or sexuality rather than transphobia, sexism, and homophobia, then there is no reason to look for external conditions that create these risks, and the state cannot be held responsible for perpetuating or alleviating these conditions. Any intervention is less likely to target structural causes and can also be framed as "charitable" and "humanitarian" efforts to "help" marginalized groups rather than a necessary responsibility of the state. For the most part, Strategic Direction 4 stays focused on this individualistic level, though at times it does make mention of structural conditions. As will be seen, even when structural conditions are described, the MHCC does not recognize state violence by including a strong structural analysis that holds the state responsible for creating, promoting, enabling, and accepting these conditions.

Priority 4.5: Gender and Sexuality in *Changing Directions*

Priority 4.5 lists several ways in which gender makes a difference in mental health problems and illnesses. These include the following: "Women are more likely than men to experience anxiety and depression, including depression following the birth of a child. Men are more likely to develop schizophrenia at a younger age. Girls and women attempt suicide at higher rates, but men and boys … die by suicide more often."[18] It is clear from this quotation that the MHCC espouses a binary, cisnormative understanding of gender, referencing studies using cisgender participants only and making no mention of trans and intersex people in its discussion of gender. This is further evidenced by cissexist assumptions such as the one that only women give birth to children.

Furthermore, the MHCC reinforces a biomedical view of mental distress by presenting these differential rates of various illnesses as medical facts. For example, the document states that women are more likely to experience anxiety and depression, rather than stating that women are more likely than men to be *diagnosed* with depression and anxiety and have their experiences medicalized. Moreover, the role of race and racism goes unexamined in the discussion concerning gender. For example, Suman Fernando argues that there is a "racist tendency to designate black people as schizophrenic" because of the ascription of "violence, suspiciousness and dangerousness to black clients."[19] The MHCC ignores the racialized character of this diagnosis, stating only that men "develop" (as opposed to saying they are diagnosed with) schizophrenia at a younger age. Indeed, the MHCC uses "women" and "men" as universal categories, without acknowledging differences based on any form of social difference.

The MHCC then goes on to state that "gender makes a person vulnerable to mental health problems and illnesses" and this means that "the impact of gender needs to be considered in prevention and early intervention efforts."[20] Despite the fact that this declaration is followed by lists of risk factors for cisgender women and men that are clearly created by inequity and sexism it is *gender* that is blamed for this "vulnerability," rather than structural inequity and expectations associated with hegemonic gender norms.

For example, the risk factors listed for women are "caregiving responsibilities, higher rates of poverty," "domestic violence and abuse," and higher likelihood of experiencing "childhood sexual abuse." It is positive that the MHCC acknowledges the existence of such experiences in the lives of many women. However, the expectation that women will perform the majority of caregiving, the feminization of poverty, and violence against women and girls can be seen as effects of sexism. Furthermore, it has been argued that poverty and violence affect racialized women in even higher numbers, indicating the interlocking effects of racism and sexism.[21] If these facts can be ignored and the blame placed on gender, the state can sidestep responsibility for addressing these conditions through, for example, funding or creating social services for low-income racialized women.

Likewise, the risk factors for men are listed as those that "threaten their sense of success and achievement, such as job loss," men's inability to recognize having an "emotional problem" and their desire to "handle it alone," and the fact that men "do not always present signs and symptoms in ways that are easily recognized by service providers."[22] It is positive that the MHCC recognizes that men also experience mental distress. However, the MHCC presents these risk factors as facts about men, as opposed to contextualizing them as part of hegemonic masculinity. The expectation that men will be "breadwinners," non-emotional, independent, and "strong" is part of the same problematic belief system that positions women as dependent, emotional, and weak.[23] By presenting this neutrally as "gender difference" as opposed to the result of social processes that (re)enforce and discipline gendered behaviour, the MHCC arguably becomes part of the social processes that recreate this world view and naturalize hegemonic gender ideals and behaviours.

This approach individualizes the problem and thus also the potential solutions. For example, if the problem is the way men present signs and symptoms, one logical way to facilitate recovery would be to educate men on recognizing the signs of mental illness. This strategy treats men as a homogenous, monolithic group, which runs the risk of perpetuating binary, cisnormative, heterosexist (and likely white-centric) gender expectations. It also encourages men to pathologize any evidence of distress as mental illness. Another logical solution would be to train providers in recognizing the ways that men apparently present symptoms, thus homogenizing and essentializing men's behaviour based on hegemonic gender ideals.[24] Again, this also keeps the biomedical model intact, placing the problem on the inability to recognize symptoms of an underlying illness, rather than examining how diagnostic criteria and the way they are applied are enculturated and subjective. An alternative would be to explore how men's experiences are less likely to be medicalized because the diagnostic criterion for many mental illnesses have been feminized and used as tools of social control of women. Does it follow that men who are perceived as *feminine* are more likely to be diagnosed as mentally ill? Another alternative would be to examine how race and racism inform gendered expectations and diagnostic processes. For example, how does the racist cultural association linking Black men with violence and danger inform how they are perceived and diagnosed with mental illness?[25]

While it is encouraging to see the MHCC consider gender at all, the way in which it is considered is limited. The total of the strategy's gender analysis is 217 words. The words *sexism* and *transphobia* are nowhere to be found; nor are a whole set of related words and concepts. While it is not essential to use these specific terms, the strategy does not in any way discuss violence and discrimination based on gender within the mental health care system, whether against trans people, those who are perceived as non-normatively gendered, or cisgender women. The strategy is based on a normative understanding of gender that does not allow for female masculinities, male femininities, and non-binary genders. It also does not consider how race, sexuality, class, disability, or any other factors may inform experience. It is refreshing to see the recognition of "social determinants" of mental health such as poverty and violence, rather than a rigid biomedical explanation based solely on brain chemicals and genetic factors. However, without a structural analysis of oppression both within and outside of the mental health care system, the strategy falls short of addressing the salience of gender in mental health needs and recovery.

The next 240 words address LGBT people, which the MHCC lists as "lesbian, gay, bisexual, two-spirited, trans-gendered, and trans-sexual people."[26] The use of "two-spirited, trans-gendered, and trans-sexual" suggests that the MHCC either disregards or is unaware that the latter two terms are not generally spelled with a hyphen and that the use of -ed at the end of *transgender* is contested.[27] Even more problematic is the fact that this section includes trans people in name only. The section discusses "sexual orientation" and there is no mention of gender identity, gender expression, transphobia, violence against trans people, or any of the issues facing trans people, indicating that the MHCC conflates *sexual orientation* with *gender identity* and *gender expression*, a problem that is also widespread in health care education and protocols.[28] Despite the use of the term "two-spirited," the MHCC makes no mention of this group either, whether in this section or in Strategic Direction 5, which is devoted to First Nations, Inuit, and Metis people. Notably, despite its increased popularity and use, the term *queer* is also not included, indicating that it is perhaps viewed as too radical or controversial and it possibly is seen as equivalent to lesbian, gay, and bisexual, which is a notion that many reject.[29] This approach erases a large group of people who identify as queer rather than as lesbian, gay, or bisexual.

The MHCC then goes on to state that "stigma and discrimination on the basis of sexual orientation have an impact on the mental health of ... LGBT people."[30] This is an important acknowledgment. Similar to the paragraph about gender, the risk factors affecting mental health are then listed, which are "sexual and physical assault" and "bullying for youth."[31] According to the MHCC, these risks can be mitigated by an "accepting family" and "connection with other LGBT youth."[32] Furthermore, the MHCC states that "older people may be particularly reluctant to access mental health services because of past negative experiences with the service system, including prejudice, discrimination and lack of knowledge."[33]

The acknowledgment of the impact of assault and bullying is crucial. The suggested method of addressing these problems, however, is limited. While an "accepting family" and peer support are important, these are both suggestions that download the responsibility onto the individual, the family, and the community and that sidesteps state responsibility for addressing very serious issues of abuse, assault, discrimination, homelessness, poverty, and violence. Framing these problems as primarily affecting youth does not acknowledge that abuse, assault, discrimination, and violence against LGBQT people is widespread and affects those of all age groups. Likewise, suggesting that "older people" are the ones affected by "past negative experiences" minimizes the issue by erasing the fact that this affects all LGBQT people, regardless of age. Moreover, framing the experiences as being in the past suggests that discrimination within the system is largely historical, which is inaccurate.[34]

The MHCC then goes on to explain that "stereotypes of all kinds" affect the treatment of LGBT people "within the mental health system and within the LGBT community."[35] The report states that

> on the one hand, mental health service providers must be mindful not to stereotype or discriminate against LGBT people because of their sexual orientation, and also to recognize the impact that discrimination and stigma can have on an LGBT person's mental health … On the other hand, LGBT organizations should seek to strengthen their understanding of stigma and other issues related to mental health and mental illness and be ready to provide support.[36]

This acknowledgment of discrimination is positive and stands out in comparison to the section concerning gender, which does not mention discrimination. However, by suggesting that stereotyping can be addressed by being "mindful" not to discriminate suggests that it is a simple matter of reminding service providers as opposed to an issue that requires more systematic and structural forms of intervention. It also reduces the issue to a problem with individual service providers, as opposed to acknowledging that homophobic violence and transphobic violence are structural and deeply embedded in the mental health system in myriad ways. For example, simply being "mindful" does not address administrative systems that classify people according to name and gender given at birth, causing problems for trans people who have not changed their identification, and often even for those who have, as these systems and those operating them are often not amenable to such changes. This kind of institutional erasure of trans people is endemic.[37]

Further, the contrast between mental health service providers being mindful and LGBT organizations learning more about stigma is problematic. The phrase that begins the sentence about LGBT organizations, "On the other hand," suggests that it is a commensurate problem to the one regarding mental health service providers. Presenting the shortcomings of LGBT organizations as commensurate with those of the mental health system is inappropriate, given that LGBQT organizations do not even exist in many areas of the country and where they do, are often underfunded by the government. Furthermore, the citation given at the end of this claim is to an article written about the public mental health system in the United States, based on data collected in 1998 and published in 2004 (though incorrectly cited as being published in 2008). This 17-page article devotes six sentences to the lack of attention paid to "LGBT people with serious mental illness" by LGBT community organizations. This seems like a dubious basis on which to make claims about Canadian LGBT organizations.

The MHCC also states that "people who provide mental health services ... to the LGBT community need to have a positive attitude and to be knowledgeable about the needs of people from these communities, while at the same time not making global assumptions that can obscure differences among ... individual[s]."[38] Like the recommendation to be "mindful," the recommendation to have a "positive attitude" makes it a matter of service providers' disposition rather than a process of challenging deeply held homophobic and transphobic beliefs about LGBQT people. Given the widespread and structural nature of homophobia and transphobia in the mental health system, the emphasis should be on changing this institutional violence. Instead, the section includes only one sentence about how providers need to be knowledgeable while resisting "global assumptions." Yet the MHCC does not say how providers will become more knowledgeable or explain the state's role in making this happen.

Priority 4.5 ends with four "recommendations for action," which replicate the approach and attending problems outlined above. With a few exceptions, Strategic Direction 4 focuses on increasing access to services, making existing services more "welcoming" to marginalized groups, and challenging stigma associated with mental illness. In addition to the erasure of state accountability regarding the creation of conditions that can lead to distress, there is a lack of examination of power relations embedded within the biomedical model. There is no questioning of who is considered in need of psychiatric services and why, nor the ways in which oppressive beliefs are entrenched in diagnostic processes and interactions between service providers and those experiencing mental distress. There is, therefore, no examination of the ways in which recovery may in some cases be hindered by the dominance of the biomedical model. For these reasons, *Changing Directions* does not adequately address what needs to change within the existing system as it stands or the possibility of alternative ways of understanding and addressing mental distress and recovery. As a guiding strategy for changing Canadian mental health policy and practice, it will further entrench individualist approaches that leave intact or perpetuate the structural conditions that create distress and hinder recovery.

The work of the MHCC has created "an important political moment in Canadian history for discussing and debating how best to meet the diverse mental health needs of the population."[39] With more attention being paid to the mental health of Canadians, there may be opportunities to influence the ways in which LGBQT people are understood in relation to concepts of *mental health and illness*. It is therefore necessary to think critically about the implications of the MHCC's approach for LGBQT people. Positioning gender and sexuality as *risk factors* may be more palatable than the overt pathologizing involved in the listing of *homosexuality* and *gender dysphoria* in the *Diagnostic and Statistical Manual of Mental Disorders*. However, it accomplishes similar work in that it reproduces individualist ideologies that problematize marginalized genders and sexualities rather than structural violence and oppression.

A growing body of literature argues that discrimination causes mental illness and calls for better access to mental health services for LGBQT people are increasing.[40] This is a well-intentioned yet potentially worrisome trend. These arguments can easily be made compatible with the approach espoused by the MHCC in that they do not question the concept of mental illness and advocate further integration into mental health care systems as a means of facilitating recovery. This approach may also appeal to the contemporary mainstream LGBQT rights-based movement, which is increasingly aligned with state interests. Given the power of the state to involuntarily institutionalize and enforce biomedical forms of treatment such as drugs and electroconvulsive therapy (ECT), the state cannot be seen as neutral or protective. Advocating for increased accessibility to mental health systems for LGBQT people may facilitate such punitive approaches to recovery, which elide agency and bodily autonomy.

There is no doubt that discrimination and oppression cause distress and that it is crucial to address the devastating effects of this violence. Yet biomedical approaches to treatment, psychiatry, and mental health care systems have long been instrumental in the social control of marginalized groups.[41] Given the simplistic, individualistic changes to existing mental health care systems proposed by the MHCC, will increasing access to such systems facilitate recovery for LGBQT people? Returning to the concept of recovery as originally defined by psychiatric survivors as recovering from the effects of psychiatrization is informative. If psychiatrization itself is potentially damaging and violent, will improving access to mental health systems create more oppressive experiences to recover from? What approaches are already in place outside of the system that could be adapted for LGBQT people? What new approaches could be imagined? The work of psychiatric survivors and Mad Studies scholars in rethinking the ideology of mental illness and how it informs mental health care could usefully be combined with critical race, queer, and trans theories of racialization, gender, and sexuality in answering these questions.

Community accountability models, for example, that centre on queer and trans people of colour and seek to address violence "without reproducing the technologies of individualization, pathology, penality, protection under the authority of heteropatriarchy and white supremacy, and criminalization" could be possible sources of inspiration for devising ways of preventing and recovering from experiences of mental distress.[42] Such approaches foreground systemic violence, including oppression perpetuated by the state.[43] This is compatible with the work of those who have challenged the damaging effects of mental health systems and state intervention into the lives of psychiatric survivors through mental health legislation.[44] A combination of such approaches would challenge intersectional structural violence; centre on people with lived experience of psychiatrization, homophobia, transphobia, racism, and other forms of oppression; emphasize agency; and offer alternatives to individualizing, biomedical strategies for recovery. The MHCC could usefully be informed by community accountability models and Mad Studies/psychiatric survivor efforts in terms of envisioning what changes could be made to address structural oppression and violence. Such considerations are foundational to truly "changing directions" in recovery from mental distress for LGBQT people.

NOTES

1 Mental Health Commission of Canada, *Changing Directions, Changing Lives*, 1.
2 The Standing Senate Committee on Social Affairs, Science and Technology studied the health care systems of Australia, New Zealand, the United States, and England.
3 Daley and Mulé, "LGBQTs and the DSM-5."

4 Bauer et al., "'I Don't Think This Is Theoretical; This Is Our Lives"; Daley and Mulé, "LGBQTs"; Lamoureux and Joseph, "Toward Transformative Practice"; McIntyre et al., "Systems-Level Barriers"; Pilling, "Queer and Trans Madness"; Pilling et al., "Fragmented Inclusion"; Robertson et al., "The Experiences of Lesbian and Gay Adults."

5 Poole, *Behind the Rhetoric.*

6 Tew et al., "Social Factors and Recovery."

7 Davidson and Roe. "Recovery from versus Recovery in Serious Mental Illness"; Tew et al., "Social Factors."

8 Harper and Speed, "Uncovering Recovery"; Howell and Voronka, "Introduction"; Morrow, "Recovery: Progressive Paradigm or Neo-liberal Smokescreen?"; White and Pike, "The Making and Marketing."

9 Weisser, Jamer, and Morrow, *A Critical Exploration.*

10 Howell and Voronka, "Introduction," 4.

11 Mental Health Commission, *Changing Directions*, 12

12 The MHCC leaves the distinction between "problems" and "illnesses" intentionally vague, stating that it does not "attempt to draw a firm line between 'problems' and 'illnesses,' or to resolve all of the controversies surrounding the choice of terminology" (Mental Health Commission, *Changing Directions*, 11). The use of "problems" in addition to "illnesses" cannot therefore be characterized as a clear departure from the medical term "illnesses."

13 Morrow and Weisser, "Towards a Social Justice Framework," 31.

14 These implications will no doubt be made more explicit in the MHCC's 2016 *Mental Health Action Plan*, which is based on *Changing Directions.*

15 Mental Health Commission, *Changing Directions*, 57.

16 Ibid.

17 For example, the refusal to name racist state regulations, such as the ones governing foreign accreditation, as a factor in newcomer difficulties in obtaining employment matching their skill level and education (Mental Health Commission, *Changing Directions*, 60).

18 Mental Health Commission, *Changing Directions*, 68.

19 Fernando, *Mental Health, Race and Culture*, 110.

20 Mental Health Commission, *Changing Directions*, 68.

21 Jiwani, *Discourses of Denial.*

22 Mental Health Commission, *Changing Directions*, 68.

23 Connell, *Gender.*

24 There is a difference between arguing that hegemonic masculinity affects how men are perceived by self and others in relation to "mental illness" and arguing that men present signs of mental illness differently than

women. One acknowledges the socially real effects of constructs such as gender, while the other presents men as a universal group with essential characteristics.

25 Fernando, *Mental Health*; Metzl, *The Protest Psychosis*.
26 Mental Health Commission, *Changing Directions*, 68.
27 GLADD, "Media Reference Guide."
28 Bauer et al., "'I Don't Think This Is Theoretical,'" 353.
29 Jagose, *Queer Theory*.
30 Mental Health Commission, *Changing Directions*, 68.
31 Ibid.
32 Ibid.
33 Ibid.
34 Discrimination against LGBT people within the mental health system and society is also referred to as a historical phenomenon in *Toward Recovery and Well-Being* (Mental Health Commission of Canada), the document that outlines the framework for *Changing Directions* (Mental Health Commission of Canada), 44.
35 Mental Health Commission, *Changing Directions*, 68.
36 Ibid.
37 Bauer et al., "'I Don't Think This Is Theoretical.'"
38 Mental Health Commission, *Changing Directions*, 68.
39 Rossiter and Morrow, "Intersectional Frameworks in Mental Health," 314.
40 King et al., "A Systematic Review of Mental Disorder," 70; Meyer, "Prejudice, Social Stress, and Mental Health," 674; Morrison, "Psychological Health Correlates."
41 Carr, "'The Sickness Label"; Chunn and Menzies, "Out of Mind, Out of Law," 306; Jackson, "In Our Own Voice," 11; Kanani, "Race and Madness"; Menzies and Chunn, "Race, Reason, and Regulation"; Menzies and Palys, "Turbulent Spirits"; Pilling, "Queer and Trans Madness"; Scholinski, *The Last Time I Wore a Dress*; Winters, "Gender Dissonance"; Yellow Bird, "Wild Indians."
42 Durazo, Bierria, and Kim, "Community Accountability."
43 See for example Cohen, "Death and Rebirth."
44 Burstow, *Psychiatry and the Business of Madness*; Fabris, *Tranquil Prisons*.

BIBLIOGRAPHY

Bauer, Greta R., Rebecca Hammond, Robb Travers, Matthias Kaay, Karin M. Hohenadel, and Michelle Boyce. "'I Don't Think This Is Theoretical; This

Is Our Lives': How Erasure Impacts Health Care for Transgender People."
    Journal of the Association of Nurses in AIDS Care 5 (2009): 348–61.
Burstow, Bonnie. *Psychiatry and the Business of Madness*. New York: Palgrave
    Macmillan, 2015.
Carr, Sarah. "'The Sickness Label Infected Everything We Said': Lesbian
    and Gay Perspectives on Mental Distress." In *Social Perspectives in Mental
    Health: Developing Social Models to Understand and Work with Mental
    Distress*, edited by Jerry Tew, 168–84. Philadelphia, PA: Jessica Kingsley
    Publishers, 2005.
Chunn, Dorothy E., and Robert Menzies. "Out of Mind, Out of Law: The
    Regulation of Criminally Insane Women inside British Columbia's Public
    Mental Hospitals, 1888–1973." *Canadian Journal of Women and the Law* 10,
    no. 2 (1998): 306–7.
Cohen, Cathy. "Death and Rebirth of a Movement: Queering Critical Ethnic
    Studies." *Social Justice* 37, no. 4 (2011/2012): 126–32.
Connell, Raewyn. *Gender*. 2nd ed. Cambridge, UK: Polity Press, 2002.
Daley, Andrea. "Being Recognized, Accepted, and Affirmed: Self-Disclosure
    of Lesbian/Queer Sexuality within Psychiatric and Mental Health Service
    Settings." *Social Work in Mental Health* 8, no. 4 (2010): 336–55.
Daley, Andrea, and Nick Mulé. "LGBQTs and the DSM-5: A Critical Queer
    Response." *Journal of Homosexuality* 61, no. 9 (2014): 1288–312.
Davidson, Larry, and David Roe. "Recovery from versus Recovery in Serious
    Mental Illness: One Strategy for Lessening Confusion Plaguing Recovery."
    Journal of Mental Health 16, no. 4 (2007): 459–70.
Durazo, Ana Clarissa Rojas, Alisa Bierria, and Mimi Kim. "Community
    Accountability: Emerging Movements to Transform Violence." *Social Justice*
    37, no. 4 (2011/2012): 1–12.
Fabris, Erick. *Tranquil Prisons*. Toronto, ON: University of Toronto Press, 2011.
Fernando, Suman. *Mental Health, Race and Culture*. New York: Palgrave
    Macmillan, 2010.
GLADD. "Media Reference Guide, Transgender Glossary of Terms." Accessed
    February 16, 2017. https://www.glaad.org/reference/transgender.
Harper, David, and Ewen Speed. "Uncovering Recovery: The Resistible Rise
    of Recovery and Resilience." *Studies in Social Justice* 6, no. 1 (2012): 9–26.
Howell, Alison, and Jijian Voronka. "Introduction: The Politics of Resilience
    and Recovery in Mental Health Care." *Studies in Social Justice* 6, no. 1
    (2012): 1–7.
Jackson, Vanessa. "In Our Own Voice: African-American Stories of
    Oppression, Survival and Recovery in Mental Health Systems."
    International Journal of Narrative Therapy and Community Work 2 (2002): 11–31.

Jagose, Annamarie. *Queer Theory: An Introduction*. New York: New York University Press, 1996.

Jiwani, Yasmin. *Discourses of Denial: Mediations of Race, Gender, and Violence*. Cambridge, UK: Cambridge University Press, 2006.

Kanani, Nadia. "Race and Madness: Locating the Experiences of Racialized People with Psychiatric Histories in Canada and the United States." *Critical Disability Discourse* 3, (2011): 1–14.

King, Michael, Joanna Semlyen, Sharon S. Tai, Helen Killaspy, David Osborn, Dmitri Popelyuk, and Irwin Nazareth. "A Systematic Review of Mental Disorder, Suicide, and Deliberate Self Harm in Lesbian, Gay and Bisexual People." *BMC Psychiatry* 8, no. 1 (2008): 70–87.

Lamoureux, Alexandra, and Ameil J. Joseph. "Toward Transformative Practice: Facilitating Access and Barrier-Free Services with LGBTTIQQ2SA Populations." *Social Work in Mental Health* 12, no. 3 (2014): 212–30.

McIntyre, John, Andrea Daley, Kimberly Rutherford, and Lori E. Ross. "Systems-Level Barriers in Accessing Supportive Mental Health Services for Sexual and Gender Minorities: Insights from the Provider's Perspective." *Canadian Journal of Community Mental Health* 30, no. 2 (2012): 173–86.

Mental Health Commission of Canada. *Changing Directions, Changing Lives: The Mental Health Strategy for Canada*. Calgary, AB: Mental Health Commission of Canada, 2012.

Mental Health Commission of Canada. *Toward Recovery and Well-Being: A Framework for a Mental Health Strategy for Canada*. Calgary, AB: Mental Health Commission of Canada, 2009.

Menzies, Robert, and Dorothy Chunn. "Race, Reason, and Regulation: British Columbia's Mass Exile of Chinese 'Lunatics' Aboard the Empress of Russia, 9 February 1935." In *Regulating Lives: Historical Essays on the State, Society, the Individual, and the Law*, edited by Robert Menzies, Dorothy Chunn, and John McLaren, 196–230. Vancouver, BC: UBC Press, 2002.

Menzies, Robert, and Ted Palys. "Turbulent Spirits: Aboriginal Patients in the British Columbia Psychiatric System, 1879–1950." In *Mental Health and Canadian Society: Historical Perspectives*, 149–75. Montreal, QC: McGill-Queen's University Press, 2006.

Metzl, Jonathan. *The Protest Psychosis: How Schizophrenia Became a Black Disease*. Boston, MA: Beacon Press, 2009.

Meyer, Ilan. "Prejudice, Social Stress, and Mental Health in Lesbian, Gay, and Bisexual Populations: Conceptual Issues and Research Evidence." *Psychological Bulletin* 129, no. 5 (2003): 674–97.

Morrison, Melanie A. "Psychological Health Correlates of Perceived Discrimination among Canadian Gay Men and Lesbian Women." *Canadian Journal of Community Mental Health* 30, no. 2 (2012): 81–98.

Morrow, Marina. "Recovery: Progressive Paradigm or Neo-liberal Smokescreen?" In *Mad Matters: A Critical Reader in Canadian Mad Studies,* edited by Brenda Lefrançois, Robert Menzies, and Geoffrey Reaume, 323–34. Toronto, ON: Canadian Scholars' Press, 2013.

Morrow, Marina, and Julia Weisser. "Towards a Social Justice Framework of Mental Health Recovery." *Studies in Social Justice* 6, no. 1 (2012): 27–43.

Pilling, Merrick Daniel. "Queer and Trans Madness: Biomedical and Social Perspectives on Mental Distress." PhD diss., York University, 2014.

Pilling, Merrick, Meg Howison, Tyler Frederick, Lori Ross, Chyrell d. Bellamy, Larry Davidson, Kwame McKenzie, and Sean a. Kidd. "Fragmented Inclusion: Community Participation and Lesbian, Gay, Bisexual, Trans, and Queer People with Diagnoses of Schizophrenia and Bipolar Disorder." *American Journal of Orthopsychiatry* 85, no. 5 (2017): 606–13.

Poole, Jennifer. *Behind the Rhetoric: Mental Health Recovery in Ontario.* Winnipeg, MB: Fernwood Publishing, 2011.

Robertson, Jennie, Helen Pote, Angela Byrne, and Francisco Frasquilho. "The Experiences of Lesbian and Gay Adults on Acute Mental Health Wards: Intimate Relationship Needs and Recovery." *Journal of Gay & Lesbian Mental Health* 19, no. 3 (2015): 261–84.

Rossiter, Kate, and Marina Morrow. "Intersectional Frameworks in Mental Health: Moving from Theory to Practice." In *Health Inequities in Canada: Intersectional Frameworks and Practices,* edited by Olena Hankivsky, 312–30. Vancouver, BC: UBC Press, 2011.

Scholinski, Dylan. *The Last Time I Wore a Dress: A Memoir.* New York: Riverhead Books, 1997.

Tew, Jerry, Shula Ramon, Mike Slade, Victoria Bird, Jane Melton, and Clair Le Boutillier. "Social Factors and Recovery from Mental Health Difficulties: A Review of the Evidence." *British Journal of Social Work* 42, no. 3 (2012): 443–60.

Weisser, Julia, Brenda Jamer, and Marina Morrow. *A Critical Exploration of Social Inequities in the Mental Health Recovery Literature.* Burnaby, BC: Centre for the Study of Gender, Social Inequities and Mental Health, Simon Fraser University, 2011. https://www.researchgate.net/profile/ Marina_Morrow/publication/264877917_The_Recovery_Dialogues_A_ Critical_Exploration_of_Social_Inequities_in_Mental_Health_Recovery/ links/5a2d66e6aca2728e05e2e06e/The-Recovery-Dialogues-A-Critical -Exploration-of-Social-Inequities-in-Mental-Health-Recovery.pdf.

White, Kimberley, and Ryan Pike. "The Making and Marketing of Mental Health Literacy in Canada." In *Mad Matters: A Critical Reader in Canadian Mad Studies*, edited by Brenda Lefrançois, Robert Menzies, and Geoffrey Reaume, 239–52. Toronto, ON: Canadian Scholars' Press, 2013.

Winters, Kelley. "Gender Dissonance: Diagnostic Reform of Gender Identity Disorder for Adults." *Journal of Psychology and Human Sexuality* 17, nos. 3–4 (2006): 71–89.

Yellow Bird, Pemina. "Wild Indians: Native Perspectives on the Hiawatha Asylum for Insane Indians." 2017. http://www.power2u.org/wild -indians-native-perspectives-on-the-hiawatha-asylum-for-insane-indians -by-pemima-yellow-bird/.

8 Homage to Spencer: The Politics of "Treatment" and "Choice" in Neo-liberal Times

MEGHANN O'LEARY AND LIAT BEN-MOSHE

At the heart of this essay is the personal account of the first author recounting the psychiatrized life and eventual death of her friend Spencer. We offer his story and that of Meghann's and weave our analysis of his predicament in regular typeface. We do not aim to make Spencer into a modern day martyr for the movement but instead offer his story as one out of thousands of similar narratives floating in the world. We are offering an analysis of Spencer's lived reality as psychiatrized, Meghann's account of him (from her positionality) as well as her account of her own psychiatrization and how it intersected and differed from Spencer's. But we would also like to propose an analysis of what is *not* in the narrative but lies beneath the surface, the structures of oppressions shaping lives and notions of "choice"[1] in the contemporary United States.

We also offer this narrative with a personal aim – we want to remember him, and many people like him, as flesh and blood, as precarious, fallible but also unique and multi-dimensional. We want not so much to narrate Spencer as aim to analyse the discourse surrounding his public perception and that of people similarly situated. What we aim to show is the violent nature of psychiatrization and notions of "choice" under global racial capitalism in its current formation, which we will sometimes refer to as *neo-liberalism* for shorthand. *Neo-liberalism* refers to a certain regime of social economic governance that includes privatization, free market economy and a variety of austerity measures. Here, we also want to add the specific ways that neo-liberal models of choice create a regime of violence that is not necessarily coercive but instead appears as if we can be all we want to be and in fact should aspire to do so, without taking into account the restrictions put forth by oppression caused by racism, class inequality, gender/sexuality, and disability/mental difference, differences whose consequences are made worse by the same neo-liberal forces. Neo-liberalism as a discourse reduces our beings into calculations of cost-effectiveness, measurable outcomes of productivity and growth, which become the only benchmark of value in a racial capitalist system. We are arguing that neo-liberalism seemingly offers individuals limitless choices and possibilities, while constructing and constraining the paths one must choose to create a life of supposed value. Under the guise of freedom, neo-liberalism actively creates and sustains systematic oppression, blaming individuals for not making the right choices. This becomes particularly harmful for individuals wrapped up in the psychiatric system who face the mandate of recovery often with minimal resources and support and with no alternative recourse for the imperative to *get well*.

People like Spencer's subjectivity is often subsumed under not only his psychiatric diagnosis but also coercive neo-liberal notions of "personal responsibility" and popular psy-discourses of betterment and "recovery," which are made simultaneously unavailable and compulsory under racial capitalist settler regimes of power and governance. In many ways, the responsibility of recovering his life was placed squarely on Spencer's shoulders, so society was able to absolve itself of any responsibility it had in his passing. Given Spencer's precarious position of poverty and limited access to resources, we would like to illustrate not only the impossibility of such a task but the violence such frameworks inflict on psychiatrized individuals who are also marginalized and privileged in other ways. We offer this analysis after Meghann's narrative. We should also point out that it is impossible to narrate another person's life, even if they are known intimately.

> To many, Spencer was nothing special. Another "troubled youth" wrapped up in the mental health system. His story is actually not that rare and could be easily summed up in a paragraph. Committed to a psychiatric ward at the age of 21 with the diagnosis of bipolar psychosis, he spent years trying to rebuild his life. After his release he stayed at a half-way house and then moved into a studio apartment of his own, with the support of his mother. He attended classes at the local community college, took his prescribed dosage of lithium diligently, and did his best to avoid alcohol, although he was not always successful. He continued to smoke pot regularly and worked hard to form a band, playing often at local music venues. He worked at various low-wage jobs, including unloading deliveries at Goodwill and working at a local arthouse movie theatre, which he seemed to enjoy the most. He tried intermittently to attend therapy but

never really followed through; the process was arduous and the available staff fluctuated. At the age of 23 he committed suicide. There were rumours that he had stopped taking his medication. A common story, seemingly easy to read and understand. A tragic narrative of an individual who could not take responsibility for his life. If only we had known sooner and the signs were clear, his death would have been preventable, the story goes. We could have treated him better, more directly, made him go to therapy, seek help, seek treatment. To me, and many others who knew him, Spencer and his story are much more complicated.

It is so hard to take the essence of someone, explain their brilliance, their humour, and explain them in words. I can tell you things Spencer said and did, like when he showed up at a Halloween party with his face painted red, white, and blue, with some vampire fangs in his mouth. His explanation: "I just figured there's nothing scarier than unbridled patriotism." I can tell you that he was well loved and well known in his local community and that his presence at music shows, his head bobbing relentlessly, his 6'4" frame jumping in the air, his thick bangs bouncing against his sweaty forehead, his eyes alight, his pure bliss, is still missed. There is a music venue in my hometown that I still can't go to without wishing he were there.

I can tell you he was my first serious boyfriend, that I loved him, and that we spent nearly every day together for nine months, until I went back to school in New York. Afterwards we talked, until the long distance just didn't work anymore. Then we stayed friends. I can tell you that he was one of the most creative people I have ever known. When I speak of him this way, his suicide becomes a true loss, a gap in the community that can never be filled. Not to romanticize his passing though; his death was violent: hit by a train. His long battle with various psychiatrizations, his struggles with being labelled bipolar, schizoaffective by doctors, "crazy" by acquaintances, "troubled" by concerned adults, was now over.

The news of Spencer's death overwhelmed me. I was 21 and had no real response, no coping strategies in place, except a steady stream of alcohol, cigarettes, and tears, long talks with friends over beers, but nothing that really abated the feeling of absence and loss. Death means different things to different people. For me, it was often just the simple fact that I would never see Spencer again. The stress of the situation, the excessive amounts of alcohol, the travel (I was in London at the time, and afterwards in Boston for a week), the impending warm weather after a long, dreary New York winter all collided and propelled me into what some term mania, others distress, some just plain "going nuts." In any case, the euphoria I experienced three years prior returned, interspersed by outbursts of grief. Hygiene fell by the wayside. I couldn't focus long enough to heat up a piece of toast, much less take a shower. But I was happy, ecstatic, brilliant, witty, and articulate. The universe and my relationship to it finally made perfect sense. Yet, some things were amiss. I began to have trouble dialling phone numbers; I was busy racking up long distance minutes, calling all my friends and extended family. It was all strangely familiar; similar behaviours had landed me in the hospital three years before, and it was escalating.

I have trouble explaining to people, even to my closest friends, how truly "crazy" I am. Anything they see in the media or read about bipolar disorder makes them assume that I have a "mild version," because, in fact, I do function quite well. I could tell them that if I did not take my daily cocktail of medications that at some point I would experience delusions, auditory and visual hallucinations, and extreme paranoia, and likely be sent straight to a psychiatric hospital, that I do in fact have a "severe" form of bipolar disorder. But I also believe there is a danger in relating this information, because I either come across as incredibly fragile, dangerous even, or some superhuman survivor, someone who "overcame" their illness.

Spencer and I were both white and lived in the university area. I fully acknowledge the privilege we both experienced as a white heterosexual couple pursuing our educations. We did not have to deal with the trauma of racism or homophobia and neither of us were jailed during our experiences of psychosis and distress, as so often happens to people of colour. I will never be able to fully understand the experience of the transgender woman of colour I spoke to who was told that her desire to be a woman was a manifestation of her bipolar disorder. Still, it was our shared experience of both madness and psychiatrization as white heterosexual individuals that brought Spencer and I together. And, yet, because of my higher class status and Spencer's position of poverty, our process of psychiatrization differed markedly. I was able to access resources that were not available to Spencer and in fact to the majority of psychiatrized people.

He was currently on medication, while I, with the support of my doctor, was slowly weaning myself off. But that is where our stories diverge, our stark class differences affecting everything from peer attitudes and societal acceptance to support and treatment. I grew up in an upper-middle-class household with two parents who worked in lucrative careers. Spencer was raised by his mother who often struggled to make ends meet. After my hospitalization, my dad flew out to New York as quickly as he could, and after 24 hours, took me out of the hospital "against medical advice" (an official term often referred to as AMA) because he observed that I was actually getting worse instead of better. While Spencer was checking himself back into a psychiatric hospital because he knew he needed help and logically thought that was the best place to get it, my parents took me to a private appointment with my psychiatrist in my hometown, who informed them that if they could manage it, they should take some time off work. My parents' jobs were flexible and lucrative enough where they could do this. Spencer did not have this option. This also served to keep my experience quiet, so that only my closest friends and family knew what had really happened. Spencer's experience was widely known. His ex-girlfriend even worked at the mental health hospital where he was stabilized with medication before moving to a halfway house. More than a few times I heard the whispers, saw the prolonged stares: "You see that dude, he's fucking crazy."

Terrified of another trip to the hospital, I willingly took the antipsychotics prescribed for bipolar disorder, with my psychiatrist's guidance, in very small doses, as needed, a crumb here, a crumb there. My doctor listened to my concerns regarding the side effects, was attentive, made suggestions instead of giving orders. We were in fact a team. But such attention comes at a steep price that few can afford. Literally. My psychiatrist does not accept insurance and her current rate is $210 an hour. (Even if Spencer wanted to, which is a big unknown, he would not have access to such forms of costly treatment.)

Although she refused to overmedicate, the crumbs that I would nibble took their toll. It was a gradual shift, and barely perceptible, but I became sluggish, dulled, the colour slowly left my cheeks, the light behind my eyes faded, my joints swelled, and I couldn't understand why I was so tired. Walking my dog became a chore rather than enjoyable exercise, as my legs moved slowly, feeling like they were slogging through water. I slept, a lot, whenever I could, and there were days when I simply could not get the energy to get out of bed. I would call in sick to work, feigning a stomach illness or a migraine, feeling horribly guilty and lazy afterwards. "Everyone feels like this at some point," I thought. "I must just be lazy, have poor coping skills." I highly doubt though that I could call into work and say I couldn't come in because my bipolar disorder was acting up without serious repercussions and questioning of my competency to perform my job.

While I would characterize my expensive psychiatrist as good, and the treatment that I received as better than what many people experience, I also have to admit that what she could and did do for me was very limited. I was an individual, receiving therapy and medication in the vacuum of her office, my own little Foucauldian space existing out of time and context. Never did she encourage me to seek accommodations in school or in the workplace, and the isolated nature of the treatment prevented me from forging a community of resistance with other Mad-identified and disabled people. It was only after I moved to Chicago and discovered a disability community that in fact encourages disclosure as both a means to accommodation and access and a form of resistance to oppressive norms that I was able to process my own experience and the experience of Spencer as a violent abjection, our choices for recovery dictated by forces beyond our control, our experiences marginalized and medicalized.

One day my dad commented, "He [Spencer] just seemed to struggle so much with ... life." Yes, it is true, but I also wonder if it is a certain type of life that he struggled with, the normative expectations of a society where efficiency, productivity, organization, and executive function are championed over creativity, sensitivity, kindness, and social justice. I saw it with my students, diagnosed with autism and in a special education program that worked to include them in the general education classes. They were very creative, brilliant, and passionate in their own way, but too often stigmatized, chided, and ridiculed by peers and teachers, because they couldn't organize their agendas and folders, or write neatly, because their bags overflowed with library books, instead of iPods and cell phones. I wonder, if we lived in a society that valued difference and responded to struggles with understanding, patience, and support, how well Spencer and millions of others would fare. I would like to look beyond framing Spencer's story as a common tragedy that resulted in his failure to take his medication and attend therapy. Such a limited discourse not only ignores his brilliance, creativity, and subjectivity, but also the continued injustice he faced as others looked to him to recover his life. Yes, his story is a tragedy, but it is the tragedy of a dysfunctional, neo-liberal, racial settler capitalist society that both creates and exploits people's vulnerability. At the end, all I know is that I miss Spencer terribly and that I think the world was a far better place with him in it.

Psychiatric Power

Without discounting the benefits of therapy or medication per se or the existence of "useful" psychiatrists, as Meghann's narrative shows, we contend that psychiatry as a practice and an institution is so deeply embedded in discourses of settler racial capitalism and neo-liberalism ("free choice"), discourses that directly inflict violence on marginalized people labelled as deviant, that it is beyond remediation and reform. Much like special education and the prison industrial complex, of which we would add psy-knowledge plays a large part, the institution of psychiatry must be resisted from without, rather than reformed from within.

As a medical practice that has historically struggled to legitimate itself, psychiatry wields immense power over minds considered deviant. When you are a patient in extreme crisis and distress, your only options for so called treatment is through biopsychiatry, even if this route is not actually financially, geographically or culturally attainable or desirable to you, the imperative when one is mentally struggling is to "see a doctor." And if you are actually sitting in a psychiatrist's office explaining your symptoms, it is not hard to recognize where the power and agency lie.

Despite the common-sense belief in biopsychiatry as a science and field of medicine, as Michel Foucault argues, the power that psychiatry wields is not based on a linear history of scientific discovery and progress concerning the workings of the mind in regards to madness.[2] As Foucault illustrates, public fear of the Other, and its resulting confinement was the impetus for a medical and juridical understanding and treatment of madness. In his description of the "Ship of Fools" the Mad are physically set adrift without boundaries, but they are also in the liminal places of society's imagination, unseen and excluded, they rest at the borders, but there is always the constant threat of their encroachment. When the Hôpital Général was established in Paris in 1656, madness came under the purview of the medical establishment and was codified as "mental illness." Once a disturbance of the soul and the spirit, mental illness was now understood as an affliction of the mind.[3] But the new authority that medicine claimed over madness should not be considered a historical progression any more than Pinel and Tuke's celebrated releasing of the Mad from the physical chains that bound them. Moral treatment became the prerogative in which Mad patients would ostensibly be treated "humanely." However, the patients were still confined in a separate space, an asylum that existed anachronistically, outside of time, outside of history.[4] The physical chains had been replaced by invisible moral chains absorbed into their very consciousness through a process of self-monitoring.

Becoming psychiatrized does not just mean that you are labelled as "crazy." It also means that you are no longer seen as legible and as capable; your own insight and abilities are constantly questioned, and there is a definitive medical explanation for all your behaviours and feelings. Yet at the same time you are expected to take full responsibility for your life, to function in society as others deem fit. It is a tenuous balance to maintain. Expectations are low, and while you are prescribed medication and encouraged to find stable employment to pay rent and buy food, you are often not given the dignity to fail and make mistakes. The maintenance of your security and safety becomes the priority, often at the expense of your agency and that of others who are made even more precarious. The "choices" you must make always involve some sort of surveillance imposed by others. For us, psychiatrization is tied with both docility making (anatamo-politics) and biopolitics – state management on the level of populations, which we explain below.

These moral chains, the imperative to be happy and productive, or seek treatment when not functioning under these normative expectations, infiltrate one's sense of being, and not just for those psychiatrized. British social theorist Nikolas Rose argues that we all, and we would add "we" in racist capitalist regimes, are constrained by societal institutions that dictate such practices as how to properly raise children, what products to consume, how to consume them, and how to form a lifestyle that will satisfy the ever-elusive promise of well-being and happiness.[5] Psy-discourses construct us as particular subjects – seeking professional expertise for inner transformation, emphasizing what we could become versus what we are. As Rose argues:

> The government of the soul depends upon our recognition of ourselves as ideally and potentially certain sorts of person, the unease generated by a normative judgment of what we are and could become, and the incitement offered to overcome this discrepancy by following the advice of experts in the management of the self.[6]

But the violence of psychiatrization is even more insidious, possibly because it is more explicit. Yes, all of our souls are governed, but some embody this governance and oppression more than others. When you are given a label of *severe mental illness*, you are immediately positioned as dangerous and incompetent. The "incitement" Rose mentions to reconcile the apparent "discrepancy" between what one is and what one could become, although impossible for anyone to achieve, is especially elusive yet mandatory for psychiatrized people. We are still held responsible for initiating and following the path to recovery, a path that is actually defined and dictated by others. Expectations for psychiatrized people's betterment and fulfilment may be low, but any deviance from the prescribed path, especially suicide, is framed as a personal failure.

Biomedicalization of the Psyche

Constructing mental difference as purely biological sickness does very little to alleviate suffering, especially since much of it comes from social and political structures that are then blamed on individuals as personal faults or deficiencies. A key tactic used by many mental health advocacy organizations in the United States, such as the National Alliance on Mental Illness, is to frame mental illness as a brain disorder,[7] similar to other chronic medical conditions like diabetes. The organization's definition of mental health conditions is "medical conditions that cause changes in how we think and feel and in our mood. They are not the result of personal weakness, lack of character or poor upbringing."[8] Framing mental illness as a treatable medical condition ostensibly helps to combat stigma, which is one of the organization's stated goals. A series of online comics on BBC *Newsbeat* entitled "Mental Health Week: How Drawings on Social Media Are Changing the Conversation" depicted a series of people experiencing various medical conditions such as the flu, food poisoning, an amputated limb, and diabetes, with others standing by telling them to "make an effort," accusing them of "not even trying." One person tells another who is injecting insulin into his side that it is not healthy that he has to take medication everyday just to feel normal. The author of many of the cartoons, Robot Hugs, says, "People still need to tell people that their mental illnesses are legitimate conditions."[9] This is an understandable tactic, but it uses faulty logic: no brain scan or blood test will indicate a person has schizophrenia or bipolar disorder, so the comparison does not hold much weight. Despite attempts to forge strict medical classifications of symptoms indicative of specific "mental illnesses," mostly through the *Diagnostic and Statistical Manual of Mental Disorders*, which is currently in its fifth edition, *diagnosis* and *treatment* are biopolitical constructs and not neutral terms.

Foucault discusses biopolitics as a specific power technique exerted by the state to govern the physical and political body on a population level (as opposed to disciplinary power, which is exerted on an individual, anatomic level).[10] This is where race and disability converge. Foucault claims that with the advent of biopolitical control (i.e., management of whole populations, not just regarding individual bodies and abnormalities but the creation of a *healthy* populace), the state uses racism as a mechanism to differentiate between those worthy of living and those who are dispensable to the healthy activity of the state. This can be conceived of as a mechanism of biological warfare of sorts, which is used not against an enemy but against a perceived threat to the whole population. Note that Foucault's conceptualization of race is in the delineation of categories, a way to sort out or partition populations, and not only in relation to colour, creed, ethnicity, and so on. "Abnormalities" (criminals, Mad people, etc.) were conceptualized as and in racist terms and were made dispensable.[11]

In addition to Foucault's use of the term *biopolitics*, we also want to note that any meaning assigned to mental difference as illness (especially biology) is inherently political, hence our understanding of mental difference coded as a medical condition is biopolitical in nature. Many scholars and activists have demonstrated how psychiatric diagnoses are more indicative of attempts to control social and cultural upheaval and, therefore, change drastically throughout history. For example, the work of American studies scholar Jonathan Metzl reveals how schizophrenia transitioned from a diagnosis given to white housewives to "angry Black men" during the civil rights era in the United States.[12] This makes any understanding of psychiatric diagnosis as objective medical classification especially problematic.

Treatment "Adherence" and Notions of Choice

In popular discourse on mental health, it is assumed that the key to successful treatment is medication adherence and therapy (see Kay Redfield Jamison for example).[13] We want to be careful here not to redraw the binary between "I choose to take psychopharmaceuticals" and "I choose not to." This illusion of binary decision making in a vacuum and the complexity of choice is what we want to foreground here, not individual actions. Even if some perceive or take medication as a way to alleviate distress, it still does nothing to treat *oppression* and often becomes another form of oppression.

We suggest that this so-called solution simplifies a systemic problem embedded in neo-liberal discourses of independence, choice, and responsibility, implying that we are all individual actors in a free market economy, rational actors in a democratic society with equal opportunities. American studies scholar Lisa Duggan argues that neo-liberalism has managed to dictate and infiltrate culture by focusing on the economic agenda of privatization and the social agenda of personal responsibility. Both agendas uphold neo-liberalism in society, which Duggan claims is a ruse of neo-imperialism, "founded on force and coercion."[14] Duggan argues that despite the election of Democratic president Bill Clinton in 1993, the neo-liberal themes of privatization and personal responsibility were further cemented and became cultural common sense disguised as economic discourse leading to freedom and democracy. Characteristics like self-esteem, independence, and competition were touted as essential to "personal responsibility," while entitlement, dependence, and irresponsibility were seen as social ills embodied in (specific) individuals.[15] While espousing a supposedly colour- and gender-neutral agenda, these neo-liberal demands for "personal responsibility" actually expanded the racist classist patriarchal core of the US settler state. As Duggan puts it, "The sexual practices and household structures of poor women, especially black women, are the central causes of poverty and of associated social disorder and criminality."[16] Meanwhile, the male dominated arenas of law and order were espoused – for example, through zero tolerance policies and the war on drugs.

The insidious coercive practices of US society are also held in place by psychiatric discourses. The so-called democratic society that is founded on principles of freedom and equality is actually a settler racial capitalist state embedded in psy-discourses. Rose argues that we are all embedded in the power dynamics of "psy sciences and their associated bodies of expertise."[17] While the power of psy-knowledge dictates the "choices" of society as a whole, including those with the most social and economic capital, we argue that the violence implicit in the power of psy-knowledge and practices is most evident when applied to marginalized populations, people of colour, trans and queer people, and people living in poverty. This can be gleaned from common stereotypes surrounding welfare recipients, particularly single Black women,[18] as well as the high incidence of alcoholism, drug abuse, domestic violence, and suicide on Indigenous reserves, in essence scapegoating individuals without deep acknowledgement of the political and economic factors leading to such social abandonment. Racism, sexism, colonization, and genocide are rarely acknowledged in such neo-liberal discourses. Take, for example, an incident in Albuquerque, New Mexico, where both Meghann and Spencer grew up. A homeless man, diagnosed as mentally ill, was shot and killed by two police officers in 2014.[19] He was apparently camping out in the foothills, known to be a space of economic wealth with little diversity. What is overlooked is the pernicious nexus of gentrification and criminalization that continues to create precarious populations and then marginalizes them in violent ways, which is a continuation of land theft and dispossession that came with settler colonialism (especially evident in New Mexico as it is now called). Such oppressions often intersect and the increased surveillance of, as well as the physical and psychic violence inflicted on, for example, trans people of colour or people in poverty who are labelled as mentally ill make notions of "recovery" and "choice" problematic at best and deadly at worst. In sum, although the consequences of neo-liberal psyche governance under settler racial capitalism will differ significantly based on a person's rank in the pecking order, it is a violent discourse that underlies the lives of people like Spencer, as well as those who don't share some of his privileges (he was white) or marginalization (because of his class and disability status).

Another area where this phenomenon is particularly apparent is in the prison industrial complex. As Dylan Rodriguez and other prison abolitionists suggest, it is impossible to espouse, discuss, or practise abolition without an understanding of racial captivity as a core function of carceral logics.[20] The availability of (especially) Black bodies (in what we call the United States) and Indigenous bodies (especially in what we call Canada) for capture in carceral settings is not about over-representation but is a key feature of the carceral racial state. As suggested elsewhere, the disabling nature of, and which bodies are available for, capture should be understood as a core feature of incarceration.[21] People with disabilities are over-represented in every aspect of criminalization and imprisonment. Incarceration does not target or affect people equally. The majority of prisoners are poor and are people of colour. Poverty is known to cause a variety of impairments and disabling conditions so that disability in prison or jail is more the rule than the exception. In addition, the prison environment itself is disabling; even if someone entered prison without a disability or mental health diagnosis, they are likely to get one.[22]

In a variety of carceral settings (psych hospitals, prisons, and out-patient regiments) psy-experts regularly prescribe sedating medications, such as Seroquel, and other antipsychotics under the guise of "treatment."[23] Understandable responses to imprisonment, such as increased anxiety and anger, are medicalized and pathologized as indications of a disorder.[24] Kilty explores the medicalization and psychiatrization of imprisoned women as a form of moral regulation, very similar to the self-monitoring that was induced among patients by Pinel and Tuke.[25] But it is a regulation that exposes the tension between neo-liberal discourses of choice and personal responsibility, while at the same time arguing that mental illness is a disease beyond a person's control:

> The process of psychiatrization exists in tension – on one hand it seeks to label criminalized women by identifying their individual barriers to reformation (i.e., whatever mental illness or diagnosis they are viewed as suffering from), and on the other, it operates within the neo-liberal carceral constraints that lay all responsibility for change on the hands of prisoners themselves.[26]

But as Kilty points out, such a response to distress and crisis on the part of psy-experts is common outside prison walls as well. This is what Fabris terms "chemical incarceration."[27]

The term *medication adherence* implies that people have a choice about how they will respond to crisis and distress in their lives and to the diagnosis of a mental illness. In a consumerist society that prizes the sanist notion of rationalism, *choice* and *adherence* are in fact an illusion. The question is not whether people will adhere to medication regimes but which medication they will take and for how long. If they choose not to take medication, how will they regulate their body/mind and be efficient and productive citizens so they can avoid the surveillance and violence imposed by psy-expertise? But avoidance is also an illusion. If psy-knowledge and expertise cannot explicitly dictate what a person chooses to do, the implicit messages of consumer improvement in a neo-liberal society will induce moral self-monitoring.

Recovery: It Gets Better – For Whom?

Prominent disability and mental health advocate Patricia Deegan discusses the experience of being labelled as schizophrenic at the age of 17 and told that if she took medication her whole life and avoided stress, she might be able to "cope":

> My teenage world in which I aspired to dreams of being a valued person in valued roles – of playing lacrosse for the U.S. women's team or maybe joining the Peace Corps – I felt those parts of my identity being stripped from me. I felt I was given not a diagnosis, but a prognosis of doom.[28]

Deegan's expectation that she will merely cope with medication and avoidance of stress, is a common experience for psychiatrized people that we want to underscore here. As we discussed earlier, it becomes a both unrealizable and imperative mandate, made worse for those psychiatrized. Yet it should be noted that the aspects of Deegan's identity that make her a "valued person" in "valued roles" are already imbued in circuits of racial capital. Lacrosse is a Native American sport, appropriated by settlers and often played by whites of upper-middle class. Deegan's other example of value, joining the Peace Corps, reproduces a colonial and imperial project (what some refer to as a *white saviour complex*). Deegan's experience comes from a specific lens of possible privilege not often afforded those who struggle daily to survive the oppression of poverty, racism, colonization, and genocide. The point is not to vilify Deegan but to point to the ways we place value, which have little to do with her inherent humanity and instead with jobs and pursuits approved, encouraged, and even dictated by both settler colonial racial expectations and neo-liberal discourses of success and functioning. Deegan is expressing very acutely the insidious violence of neo-liberalism, which dictates "choices" that will make a person valuable and then denies those so-called choices to psychiatrized individuals. Personal responsibility remains paramount, but access to valued social and economic positions is ever elusive. It is this systemic discourse of power that must be resisted so that value is accorded differently, including for those who are inherently deemed as invaluable under racial settler capitalism.

Deegan's "prognosis of doom" is, again, familiar to many who have been psychiatrized, but it is also an experience shared by those who are (or get marked as) non-normative in other ways because of race, sexuality, gender, religion, nationality, disability, and more (or any intersection of those). While we don't want to assume that as a woman Deegan did not encounter the violence of doom and devaluation previously, her experience of being psychiatrized made these feelings particularly salient. We do want to hold the fact that this itself is a form of privilege (to not feel the full effects of this devaluation before psychiatrization and the ability to access mechanisms that provide such diagnosis and prognosis, as we discuss below). As critical disability studies scholar Rachel Gorman points out, adopting a Mad identity can be construed as a privilege that racialized people who live in poverty cannot afford. It is easier for people who do not live under other juridical surveillance, such as racism and classism, to claim a Mad identity as a form of resistance. For many racialized people madness is perceived as the result of poverty or trauma and is accorded a different perspective.[29]

This critique is related to recent debates on futurity in queer theory (and disability studies). Specifically, it is related to the barrage of queer of colour critique of the It Gets Better campaign initiated in 2011 by advice columnist Dan Savage. The campaign was a response to the high number of suicides of LGBTQ and gender variant teens in the United States. Don't give up now, the campaign says, "it" will get better. "It" here is a person's life chances, progress, proximity to assimilation (i.e., success), as opposed to "it" – the material conditions of oppression that will be eliminated. But for those with literally no future this affirmation is nonsensical at best and offensive at worst. It only gets better from a certain privileged locale.[30] If Crip theory is "haunted by the disability to come," Puar's important intervention suggests that such discussions of futurity "also disavow the debility already here."[31] In other words, disability and Mad Studies and communities need to be anchored more in the understanding "that in working-poor and working-class communities of colour, disabilities and debilities are actually 'the norm.'"[32]

In this chapter, while we try to convey the importance of a supportive disability and Mad community that resists neo-liberal notions of choice and freedom as forms of recovery, we want to acknowledge the complexity of this issue and the ways in which claiming membership in an oppressed identity category as a form of resistance may not work for everyone. In bringing these issues to the forefront we want to avoid framing Spencer and Meghann's story as the essential and universal story of psychiatrization and violent oppression, as both identify, or identified, as white, straight, and cisgender. In framing this narrative, we want to be clear that our intention is not to reify the production of an "identity-based Mad movement that reproduces a white, Western Mad Subject" a dangerous pitfall that Gorman highlights.[33] Rather we want to stress the ways in which psychiatrization is embedded in neo-liberal racial settler capitalist frameworks that dictate and enforce one's value and opportunities in society. In her book *The Right to Maim* Jasbir Puar discusses the difference between disablement and debilitation as "the slow wearing down of populations instead of the event of becoming disabled."[34] While disability or madness and their accompanying pride discourses become ways of identification that are useful to enact new ways of understanding people's worth and value beyond neo-liberal or normative demands, it is not a legible recourse for all. This is intentional because what some call madness, others call stress or life, in other words the slow wearing down of body/minds on a population level. Some paths to so-called liberation are foreclosed by the same mechanisms that seemingly open them for others. Puar terms this as "the tension between targeting the disabled and targeting to debilitate."[35]

Psy-Power and Intersectionality

We argue that psy-knowledge itself not only targets societal institutions but has become an institution itself that perpetuates capitalist and racist ideology in its practices. Contrasting the experiences of Spencer and Meghann with those absent from the narrative but who experience the violence of psychiatrization, governance of the soul, and the imperative to be productive and valued under racial settler capitalist ideals yields a fruitful analysis of such regimes while understanding the unequal consequences of living and dying under such regimes. Taking a broader approach, we argue that psy-discourse and practices are a key component of maintaining a racial settler capitalist regime, a term that addresses the ways in which capitalism promotes and sustains both anti-Black racism and Indigenous colonization and genocide. Gender and women's studies scholar and psychiatric survivor Louise Tam argues that we must recognize psy-knowledge's complicity in and perpetuation of racist and colonialist practices:

> By attending to (post)colonial and transnational governing structures like those described above, I argue that racial oppression is sustained through "madness" – through people's encounters with psy knowledge.[36]

Psy-knowledge and practice must be recognized not as sites of healing and recovery, but as structures of power that work to shape human subjectivity to embrace the needs of capitalist regimes of truth. As Puar notes: "Given the relationship of bankruptcy to medical care expenses in the United States, debt becomes another register to measure the capacity for recovery, not only physical but also financial. Debility is profitable to capitalism, but so is the demand to 'recover' from or overcome it."[37]

Value and Choice

What many people don't realize is that encounters with the psychiatric system, whether through enforced hospitalization or medication where one is rendered helpless and at the mercy and control of others, so often causes more violence and trauma than the experience of psychosis or distress itself. In his encounters with the psychiatric system, psychiatric survivor and activist Erick Fabris explores the violence inherent in psychiatrization, the direct and legitimated control enforced by others. He states:

> A body/mind that does not perform, that cannot represent itself in the language, lacks the order or value to be present and will be exempted from communication and decision-making. Moreover, while its slippage could easily be seen as freedom from order, order is imposed anyway, by "sound" right thinking people with more value.[38]

The issue we want to emphasize here is that it is not just "treatment" that becomes problematic under psychiatric regimes of racial settler capitalism, but also the very idea of a coherent rational actor embedded in all notions of neo-liberal governance. For people who are not perceived (or do not perceive themselves) as rational, and those psychiatrized are by definition precisely that, there can be no rational choice in a so-called free market. Stripped of rationality and value, the psychiatrized person becomes someone to contain and control by people with more value who know better. In some ways, our attempt here to create a coherent narrative of Spencer betrays the incoherence of the "psychotic" or *manic* experience described above. We don't want to rescue this experience and narrate it with the lens of reason but to offer a narrative example of why incoherence should be valued on its own terms as well.[39]

Through this narrative and analysis, we have attempted to demonstrate the ways in which neo-liberal regimes of truth have created and perpetuated ideals of "choice," "recovery," and "personal responsibility" as a way to treat individuals embedded in the mental health system. In this framework if such a treatment fails, as it did with Spencer, the fault rests with the individual. This absolution of responsibility is not only an easy out but also a perpetuation of violence on a people thought to have little value. Lisa Cacho, whose scholarship focuses on how intersectional identities work to assign human value, explores how certain racialized bodies that resist normativity are rendered illegible and exist in a space of social death.[40] In the final chapter of her book *Social Death*, she grapples with assigning value to her cousin Brandon, who died in a car accident and in his life did not meet the heteronormative expectations of racial settler capitalist neo-liberal success: "Rather than repudiating non-normative behaviour and ways of being, we would read non-normative activities and attitudes as forms of 'definitional power' that have the potential to help us rethink how value is defined, parcelled out, and withheld."[41] As an unmarried drug user without a college degree, who worked at low-wage jobs, Spencer was accorded little value in a neo-liberal capitalist regime that creates and sustains vulnerability and then individualizes the tragedy that results. As we noted earlier, Spencer's racial and gendered privilege as a white heterocis man made him inherently more valuable than many other marginalized individuals, and we do not aim for his story to be a meta-narrative that represents the experience of all psychiatrized people. However, we do want to highlight the ways in which Spencer's class status and disability still made him particularly vulnerable to the violence of racial settler capitalism. Our aim is to interrogate and reconstruct a common narrative of personal choice and individual tragedy based on neo-liberal discourses. Hopefully, this narrative is a step in not only reframing Spencer's story but reimagining his life, and that of others like him, their pursuits, and their humanity as valuable.

NOTES

1 We use many scare quotes throughout this chapter because we want to be clear that we are arguing that recovery, treatment, and mental illness (the terms we use them on most in the chapter) are social constructs and that we are using them in the ways they appear with psy- and some lay discourses, not to affirm their validity. We also question the notion of choice under neo-liberal discourses.
2 Foucault, *History of Madness*, 273.
3 Ibid., 220.
4 Ibid., 491.
5 Ibid., 4.
6 Ibid., 11.
7 The National Alliance on Mental Illness (NAMI) has been recently reframing its message to incorporate environmental factors as possibly contributing to diagnoses of "mental illness." See NAMI, "Learn More."
8 Ibid.
9 Morse, "Mental Health Week."
10 Foucault, *The Foucault Reader*, 263.
11 Foucault and Ewald, *"Society Must Be Defended."*
12 Metzl, *The Protest Psychosis*.
13 Jamison, *An Unquiet Mind*.
14 Duggan, *The Twilight of Equality?*, 70.
15 Ibid., 14.
16 Ibid., 16.
17 Rose, *Governing the Soul*.
18 Rousseau, "Social Rhetoric and the Construction of Black Motherhood."
19 Ohlheiser and Izadi, "Judge: New Mexico," 1.
20 Rodríguez, "(Non)Scenes of Captivity."
21 Ben-Moshe, Chapman, and Carey, *Disability Incarcerated*.
22 Ben-Moshe and Stewart, "Disablement, Prison and Historical Segregation," 87.

23 Chapman, Carey, and Ben-Moshe, "Reconsidering Confinement."
24 Kilty, "Governance through Psychiatrization."
25 Ibid.
26 Ibid.
27 Fabris, *Tranquil Prisons.*
28 Deegan, "Recovery and Empowerment," 16.
29 Gorman, "Mad Nation?", 269.
30 There had been immense critique of the privileged position assumed in the idea of "it gets better" and the campaign itself from queer of color and other critical frameworks such as Puar, "In the Wake," and Goltz, "It Gets Better." See also Kafer, *Feminist, Queer, Crip* for a critique of the original assertion by Edelman, *No Future* regarding "no future" for queers and especially for crips (people with disabilities).
31 McRuer, *Crip Theory*, 207; Puar, "Coda," 152.
32 Puar, "Coda," 153.
33 Ibid., 270.
34 Puar, *The Right to Maim,* xiv.
35 Ibid., xxi.
36 Tam, "Whither Indigenizing the Mad Movement?", 286.
37 Puar, "Coda," 154.
38 Fabris, *Tranquil Prisons,* 26.
39 See also Ben G., "On Radical Empathy and Schizophrenia."
40 Cacho, *Social Death,* 38.
41 Ibid., 167.

BIBLIOGRAPHY

Ben-Moshe, Liat, Chris Chapman, and Alison C. Carey, eds.. *Disability Incarcerated: Imprisonment and Disability in the United States and Canada.* New York: Palgrave Macmillan, 2014.
Ben-Moshe, Liat, and Jean Stewart. "Disablement, Prison and Historical Segregation: 15 Years Later." *Disability Politics in a Global Economy: Essays in Honour of Marta Russell.* New York: Routledge, 2016.
Cacho, Lisa Marie. *Social Death: Racialized Rightlessness and the Criminalization of the Unprotected.* 1st ed. New York: New York University Press, 2012.
Chapman, Chris, Alison C. Carey, and Liat Ben-Moshe. "Reconsidering Confinement: Interlocking Locations and Logics of Incarceration." *Disability Incarcerated: Imprisonment and Disability in the United States and*

Canada, edited by Liat Ben-Moshe, Chris Chapman, and Alison C. Carey, 3–24. New York: Palgrave Macmillian, 2014.

Deegan, Patricia E. "Recovery and Empowerment for People with Psychiatric Disabilities." *Social Work in Health Care* 25, no. 3 (1997): 11–24.

Duggan, Lisa. *The Twilight of Equality? Neo-liberalism, Cultural Politics, and the Attack on Democracy.* Boston, MA: Beacon Press, 2012.

Edelman, Lee. *No Future: Queer Theory and the Death Drive.* Durham, NC: Duke University Press, 2004.

Everett, Barbara. *A Fragile Revolution: Consumers and Psychiatric Survivors Confront the Power of the Mental Health System.* Waterloo, ON: Wilfrid Laurier University Press, 2000.

Fabris, Erick. *Tranquil Prisons: Chemical Incarceration under Community Treatment Orders.* Toronto, ON: University of Toronto Press, 2011.

Flemming, Walter C. "Getting Past our Myths and Stereotypes About Native Americans." *Education Digest* 72, no. 7 (2007): 51–7.

Foucault, Michel. *The Foucault Reader,* edited by Paul Rainbow. New York: Pantheon Books, 1984.

Foucault, Michel. *History of Madness,* edited by Jean Khalfa, translated by Jonathan Murphy and Jean Khalfa. London, UK: Routledge, 2006.

G., Ben. "On Radical Empathy and Schizophrenia." In *Criptiques,* edited by Caitlin Wood, 219–28. New York: May Day, 2014.

Goltz, Dustin Bradley. "It Gets Better: Queer Futures, Critical Frustrations, and Radical Potentials." *Critical Studies in Media Communication* 30, no. 2 (2013): 135–51.

Gorman, Rachel. "Mad Nation? Thinking through Race, Class, and Mad Identity Politics." In *Mad Matters: A Critical Reader in Canadian Mad Studies,* edited by Brenda Lefrançois, Robert Menzies, and Geoffrey Reaume, 269–80. Toronto, ON: Canadian Scholars' Press, 2013.

Jamison, Kay Redfield. *An Unquiet Mind: A Memoir of Moods and Madness.* New York: Vintage Books, 1996.

Kafer, Alison. *Feminist, Queer, Crip.* Bloomington: Indiana University Press, 2013.

Kilty, Jennifer M. "Governance through Psychiatrization: Seroquel and the New Prison Order." *Radical Psychology* 9, no. 1 (2011). http://radicalpsychology.org/vol9-1/kiltys.html.

McRuer, Robert. *Crip Theory: Cultural Signs of Queerness and Disability.* New York: New York University Press, 2006.

Metzl, Jonathan. *The Protest Psychosis: How Schizophrenia became a Black Disease.* Boston, MA: Beacon Press, 2009.

Morse, Felicity. "Mental Health Week: How Drawings on Social Media are Changing the Conversation." *BBC Newsbeat*, February 18, 2016. http://www.bbc.co.uk/newsbeat/article/35564616/mental-health-week-how-drawings-on-social-media-are-changing-the-conversation.

National Alliance of Mental Illness. "Learn More." Accessed, April 29, 2016. https://www.nami.org/Learn-More.

Ohlheiser, Abby, and Elahe Izadi. "Judge: New Mexico Police Officers Will stand Trial for 2014 Fatal Shooting of a Homeless Man." *Washington Post*, August 18, 2015, 1.

Puar, Jasbir K. *The Right to Maim: Debility, Capacity, Disability*. Durham, NC: Duke University Press, 2017.

Puar, Jasbir K. "Coda: The Cost of Getting Better Suicide, Sensation, Switchpoints." *GLQ: A Journal of Lesbian and Gay Studies* 18, no. 1 (2012): 149–58.

Puar, Jasbir. "In the Wake of It Gets Better." *Guardian*, November 16, 2010. https://www.theguardian.com/commentisfree/cifamerica/2010/nov/16/wake-it-gets-better-campaign.

Rodríguez, Dylan. "(Non)Scenes of Captivity: The Common Sense of Punishment and Death." *Radical History Review* 2006, no. 96 (2006): 9–32.

Rose, Nikolas. *Governing the Soul: The Shaping of the Private Self*. London, UK: Routledge, 1990.

Rousseau, Nicole. "Social Rhetoric and the Construction of Black Motherhood." *Journal of Black Studies* 44, no. 5 (2013): 451–71.

Tam, Louise. "Whither Indigenizing the Mad Movement? Theorizing the Social Relations of Race and Madness through Conviviality." In *Mad Matters: A Critical Reader in Canadian Mad Studies*, edited by Brenda Lefrançois, Robert Menzies, and Geoffrey Reaume, 281–97. Toronto, ON: Canadian Scholars' Press, 2013.

9 Indigenizing the Narrative: A Conversation on Disability Assessments

PRIYA RAJU AND NICOLE PENAK

Priya: It is such a beautiful fall day, Nicole.

Nicole: It really is, Priya. The sun is shining and offers a kind of relief to the cold wind blowing past us. And look, the leaves have already started to turn colour, vibrant reds, browns, and yellows.

Priya: It's a perfect day for one of our walks. One of our walks ... with a tape recorder *(laughter).* Today we've decided to record and transcribe an ongoing discussion we've been having, as two colleagues at an Indigenous health centre. Despite our personal perspectives on colonialism and systemic violence, we're finding that our work forces us to replicate that violence in surprising ways, even though we're supposed to be in "helping" roles. It's a conflict that we're each working through on our own and together.

Nicole: It's interesting because this is not the beginning of this story and it is definitely not the end either.

Priya: Yeah, it's like we're parachuting our audience – anyone reading this – into our story, into a chapter somewhere in the middle. They're plopping right into this ongoing conversation taking place in the traditional territory of the Huron-Wendat, the Anishinaabe Nation, and Haudenosaunee Confederacy, which is now called Toronto, Canada. It's a long conversation, so hopefully our reader decides to continue along this path with us for a while.

Nicole: Well you know, stories do need an audience. The written word has transformed the process of storytelling, text being a sort of self-contained thing. However, storytelling, from an Indigenous approach, is an innately relational activity. Indigenous storytelling, which is predominantly based on oral delivery and aural reception, requires relationship, an active audience, listener, or reader. With this understanding, our new joiners, the readers of this transcript – yes, you guys! – your contribution to this story is of great importance too. The strength of stories is in their ability to touch us where we are, today, here, in our bodies and hearts, to challenge us to think, to examine our emotional reactions, and to reflect on a story's connectedness to our own lives and spirit, and extend that connectedness to the rest of creation. This connection is made not only through a storyteller's relationship to the topic of their tale, but also through a storyteller's ability to develop a relationship with their audience.

Priya: Well, I guess it makes sense then to begin building a relationship with the readers by introducing ourselves and our connection to this story we're unpacking. Nicole, want to get us started?

Nicole: Sounds great. This importance of relationship really stems from my identity as a Maliseet and Mi'kmaw First Nations woman. In my culture we have a clan system, not unlike other Indigenous cultures around the world. Ours too is hereditary and describes a person's family relations along with roles and responsibilities that people are raised with. The Anishinaabe word for clan, *dodem* – some may have heard another pronunciation, *totem* – derives from the word *dodosh,* "our breast," and literally translates to "that which you draw nourishment from." Your clan is a place you belong to, a community, teachings, skills, that you have even before you are brought to this earth. Each clan carries particular roles and knowledge for their community or nation. Bird clans, like the Eagle, are our leadership and governance clan. We can see this in the highly sophisticated communication and council systems which we have learned from crows, leadership and organization from migratory birds, and in birds of prey how they form long-standing relationships with their partners, and coordinate caregiving duties of their young. So for my family, as Eagles, we carry knowledge and responsibilities about councils, governance, and leadership in a good way. But what this boils down to is carrying relationship teachings – healthy relationship being the foundation to things like good leadership and governance. As a social worker in the mental health system, and with my understanding of systemic violence in the mental health system, I focus on relationships.

As an Indigenous woman from this place we now call Canada, I am no stranger to the impacts of systemic violence, namely the ongoing process of colonization. Colonization that began over four hundred years ago with land theft, disease, forced relocation, efforts to exterminate our cultures and populations, environmental destruction, and a continued assault on individuals and families through systems like child welfare, criminal justice, and mental health. There may be many different definitions of colonialism that we find in various books or disciplines, but in my view, an Indigenous understanding of colonialism is the destruction or dismantling of relationships – a divisive process that not only continues to isolate people from their families, culture, and community but has also dismantled people's sense of self. This process has had a profound impact on Indigenous communities and it continues to affect all of us, Indigenous and non-Indigenous – as individuals, our families, and our communities. We have all been a part of a process that has destroyed our relationships to each other, to the land, to nature, and also dismantled our relationships within ourselves, our peace of mind, our health, our spirits. So maybe, just maybe, the answer lies in strengthening and restoring the healthy relationships between us. And so, it's no surprise that when considering a methodology for our contribution to this book *Madness, Violence, and Power*, we would support an approach that is grounded in and builds relationship, like dialogue and storytelling.

Priya: This is a fascinating approach for me, because as a child of recent immigration, and also as a psychiatrist, stories are at the core of my being too. The roots of my family tree go several generations deep into the soil of a small Telugu-speaking village region in south India. Because I'm the first of my line to be born so far away, on this territory that we call Canada, I've grown up hungry for those stories that get told and retold within the family, tying us to each other, creating and re-creating the past and the present. I was raised with Hindu legends that have no real end, that have many versions, that spin off into side stories and circle back again. In my family we basically live and breathe stories. Increasingly, I can see how these stories link to various types of colonialism as well. There's my family's privilege within the oppressive caste system, our connection with the fight against the British for Indian independence, then the process of migration and becoming a "minority" community overseas, the impacts of which are hugely buffered by our having money. This brings me to our present reality: to add to my family's complex experiences with oppression, we are also settler colonialists living on stolen Indigenous land. So, I'm still working through my own story, really. I think that's one of the things that brought me to my career as a psychiatrist, where I pretty much work with stories full-time. I get to do even more building of story, justice, spirit, and relationship when I work in Indigenous health and healing environments, like where I work with you, Nicole – although sometimes that's a really difficult and problematic process.

Nicole: And that's what we're here talking about. Given both of our connections to relationship and story, and the meaning that we each get from working at an Indigenous health centre, it makes sense that we both have a hard time when the job seems to require disrupting other peoples' stories. In particular it's jarring when clients need our help to apply for disability benefits. There are many layers of violence to this process.

Priya: Actually, our relationship with each other has really grown from our conversations about this issue. It was during these walks on our lunch breaks – in this very park – that we learned that we each had similar challenges with disability assessments and applications. So, this dialogue is a foundational one for our friendship! ... But it's not as familiar to everyone, so first I'll describe the disability system for our readers. For each province's low-income social assistance program, there's an application process to get additional assistance for people with disabilities. In Ontario the service is called ODSP, or the Ontario Disability Support Program. It provides income supplementation, as well as access to job training programs. It's a lot more than regular welfare, although it's still not enough to rent an average one-bedroom apartment in downtown Toronto. To access ODSP, a person has to "prove" that they have a disability that prevents them from working. And this is where the violence of the process comes in.

Nicole: In the Indigenous health centre where we work, we have both been called upon in our roles to support people with their ODSP applications. You, as a psychiatrist here, are called to complete psychiatric assessments, which may result in a mental illness diagnosis that this person would use in their disability application. And I, as a social worker, working with people often over a longer period, to come to know more about them, their families, and communities, which often informs these assessments, and has been used in ODSP applications to describe how the psychiatric diagnosis may be impacting a person's day-to-day life. So even though our professional approaches are different, we end up working together in these applications.

Priya: It seems simple, but it's actually very complicated. Working on these applications has definitely been part of a relationship-building process, because there are so many apparent divides between the two of us. There's our professional disciplines, our world views, our personal roots and backgrounds and all the dynamics related to that ...

Nicole: Yes, two different people from two different worlds, professionally and culturally – working with the same people.

Priya: Completely different worlds sometimes! My contribution is obviously highly medical. In my assessment, I have to go through the person's story and decide if they have a mental illness diagnosis. And from the perspective of my training, the answer may be *yes*. Many of the people I see – while they are creative, resourceful people – may have major mental and emotional difficulties that fit a diagnosis, which in my opinion will make it hard to participate in the job market, at least anytime soon.

Nicole: But then layer that with this specific community, the Indigenous community, and we are dealing with structural barriers that will complicate this even further.

Priya: Are you talking about barriers to finding work and moving forward, or the other inequities upstream from that?

Nicole: The ability to participate fully in society! Indigenous people in Canada, and of course Ontario, are over-represented in every social determinant of poor health or unwellness. From housing, education, health services, exposure to crime and violence, social support, societal attitudes such as racism, access to mass media, residential segregation, access to nutritious food and clean water, never mind the ongoing project of colonization and struggles for self-determination.

Priya: Well, that's it, that's exactly what I'm struggling with. All the things you just mentioned have a lot to do with why this person – let's say an Indigenous woman for example – is now sitting in my office. The link between her oppressive colonial situation and her specific current issues may be obvious. Or it may be indirect, showing up in her early life story or her parents' situations. But it's almost always there. She is living in a disabling *experience*, and I am being asked to frame that as a particular mental illness that *she has*. I have to describe her quote-unquote *symptoms*, meaning some aspect of her feelings or behaviour that show her to be *ill*. Sure, I can tell her backstory – her upbringing, her family's life, the context of residential schools, the reserve system, even colonialism in general. But at the end of my report I have to make my diagnosis, always. The way my story ends takes over the whole tale, irrespective of what kind of narrative I was trying to explain before it. I feel like that just violently rearranges her whole story, her whole lived experience, conveniently removing the colonial roots of her issues, and using medical language to describe her present. So, this is when I come to you and I end up ranting about it on my lunch break! I'm always like, "Oh man, there's this and that going on for her, and I'm supposed to write down "in conclusion ... this woman has depression?'"

Nicole: (sigh) Yeah – way to simplify.

Priya: And that simplification feels really, really wrong to me. I keep wondering, what is the impact of describing this woman's struggles this way?

Nicole: Yeah. At what cost? At what cost are people obtaining these assessments, these subsidies?

Priya: And so, I keep thinking ... am I the only one this doesn't seem right to? That's why I was so relieved to start discussing this with you, Nicole. How do *you* relate to this issue?

Nicole: Well, on the one side, I agree that it's disturbing to have to boil things down from colonization, ongoing racism and oppression, to individual symptomatology. It is a strange, violent, and depoliticizing process. On the other side, my profession as a social worker, like yours, can also perpetuate oppression. It is rooted in colonization. We are agents of social control, really, you know deployed –

Priya: The front-line of the colonial –

Nicole: The front-line of the colonial empire. Meaning that we both work for the state, and our fields serve as "hidden" ways that the state extends its power – the power to describe people, and tell them what they have to do. As you may or may not know, social work in North America is a dynamic tale of imperialism and resistance. Its story is one plagued with the reproduction of the colonial project, a divisive process that continues to isolate Indigenous people not only from their families, culture, and community, but one that has dismantled people's sense of self. It's not uncommon for Indigenous Peoples to see social workers as the enemy. That's important to know. It was social workers who came into our homes to take away our children and place them in the state's care, in an effort to assimilate and exterminate our communities. As a First Nations woman and registered social worker, engaging this story at times has ripped me into pieces.

Priya: I can't even imagine. I'm understanding that relationship more and more. At this agency I notice that many people are perfectly happy seeing me as a psychiatrist and yet are terrified of involving a social worker. Even though I personally see major violence in having your colonial experience being translated into mental illness and disability language, psychiatrists seem to be a less legendary threat compared to social workers for the Indigenous clients at this agency. So, I do find that some people here seek out the medical language and see it as helpful. It's kind of interesting to me.

Nicole: But a tradition of helping does exist in an Indigenous perspective too. Concepts around living a good life, coupled with the space that is made to use Indigenous knowledge here has a powerful potential. Yet these assessments push us to say things like *struggle*, or *issue*, or *mental illness*, or *disability*. Those are all of course terms based in *unwellness*.

Priya: Mmm-hmm. That's the medical orientation.

Nicole: Well, it may be important then to look at the question, What is wellness? What is it that we are trying to achieve? You know, all our units at this health centre have traditional Anishinaabe names. They can help us to see the Indigenous lens of the work that we are doing. We went to the traditional people in our community and asked, you know, we're going to open a mental health unit in our centre. What could be a name for it? A name that could help us understand this work that we're doing, to work towards mental health?

Priya: Right. By the time I joined, it was called the Babishkhan unit.

Nicole: Yes, and that word, *Babishkhan* comes from drum teachings. There are many different drum teachings, and they change from community to community, since we're not a homogenous people. But the Anishinaabe word *Babishkhan* for me, refers to the ties at the back of a drum, which hold it together. The drum came from a time when we were unwell, fallen out of relationship with one another, with creation, there was fighting, starvation, illness, environmental degradation. A young girl went out fasting and asked for something to bring back to her community to bring peace and wellness, and she was given the drum. When the people played the drum, the community began to heal. The drum is about relationships, it is a treaty that reminds us of our responsibilities to one another and with the rest of creation. Even in the small drum, there are 12 rawhide ties at the back. All coming together: that music, that beauty, that life, that wellness that comes from the drum, are possible only with those 12 ties forming relationship with one another. So that's an important message to keep at the forefront of our minds: wellness or unwellness is not an individual thing. Only by addressing all these relationships can we pull that rawhide over the drum frame. Only by having that relational view of wellness can we begin to heal again.

Priya: Absolutely. It's a powerful image. In fact, my own cultural and spiritual traditions are also quite different from the individualized medical model. In my community people are often viewed and defined in terms of their relationships. And in Hindu spirituality, one tries not to be too attached to any one desirable way of being or frantically pursue the notion of being "fixed." Obviously it's not this simple, but there are these trends inside of me. It's funny, Nicole – when it comes to these assessments, both of our backgrounds feel out of step with our professional roles.

Nicole: Yes. And what you're saying about your work with these assessments is a huge challenge. To have to boil down personal and historical trauma, family violence, oppression, racism, poverty – to boil those things down and label it as individual pathology, a disability belonging to one person, would be incongruent – to use strong words – it would be incongruent with an Indigenous world view. It's not how I understand myself and my own instincts either, and yet it's being asked of me as part of my job, to assist that process as a social worker.

Priya: Mmm-hmm. I'm sure it feels incongruent for you. I think it's a dilemma that goes right to the core of having a psychiatrist at this centre in the first place, for disability applications and beyond. I know the idea is to balance the world views, but in my head, I'm like, this is – there is an impasse here, with me as a medical specialist. Medicine and psychiatry are given a lot of power in society. It's colonialism all over again – privileging one way of seeing things, violently replacing people's ways of telling their own stories. I often think about my own history and world views and compare them to my identity and work as a psychiatrist. I can relate to that feeling you described of being ripped apart, as a colonized person doing this kind of work. The discordance is always there, but it becomes so painfully obvious when I'm applying a mental illness diagnosis and supporting the disability program for an Indigenous person. That is not the life work that I had planned for myself. It's a very painfully and densely packed process for me. I try to make it a more responsible and authentic interaction, but I'm still doing that work, which is a bare fact that I just avoid thinking about most days.

Nicole: Interesting how this story not only is violent towards the people we work with, the clients of this health centre, but is violent towards us as practitioners. And yet many of us are still engaging in this process, validating a story that is hurting us all.

Priya: It can feel quite awful. But then I listen to the perspectives of some activist friends and organizations, as far as I understand them. Most, like us, will acknowledge that the government disability system doesn't recognize discrimination. But overall, their argument seems to come back to the fact that people need to have their struggles recognized and accommodated as disability, and they do not have humane living conditions otherwise, and they need support. That it is not my place to decide whether someone is "able," to gatekeep who should apply for or get ODSP, or try and talk anyone out of applications, which – let me clarify – I don't do. I *do* the assessments, and I encourage people to apply, appeal, whatever – I'll help if I can.

Nicole: Mmm-hmm.

Priya: So, it feels problematic for me to even question the use of a tool that could make things slightly better for a marginalized person. Of course, I'm sure true accommodation is a whole other vision aside from disability payments, but at least fighting poverty feels like a compelling argument to me.

Nicole: For me, the past-present connections here are alarming, how much this modern discourse sounds like a past one that the Indigenous community, we've come across before. This neo-liberal, capitalist narrative. If you look back to the time of the postwar welfare state, it's probably an era that most Canadians look fondly on, the creation of our social safety net. My profession, social workers, had a lot to do with bringing universal social welfare programming to people across Canada, this anti-poverty push, because of how hard communities were hit postwar. The challenge is, specifically for Indigenous people, how we have been brought into this liberal discourse. Before this, although clearly not perfect, there was the idea of a nation-to-nation relationship, between Indigenous nations and the federal Government of Canada. And this was a time when that idea began to disappear from political discourse. The overt forms of colonization and oppression against Indigenous nations began to shift and change in the postwar era. This is when the term *the Indian Problem* was coined. Our "problem" was seen as our inability to access and fully participate in society – namely, the economy – like other citizens of Canada. And so that began shifting the focus of systematic interaction with Indigenous people, it shifted to be about welfare in a broad way – child welfare, family services, adult education, and economic welfare as well.

So, moving into the fifties, we saw the creation of Section 87, now Section 88 of the Indian Act, which for the first time ever opened up Indigenous communities, reserve territories to provincial welfare programming. This had never been heard of before, you know? The province has nothing to do with the nation-to-nation relationship that exists between Canada and the Indigenous people of this territory. And now, this move to open up our communities to social workers and the welfare system, to correct this *Indian Problem* ... the theory being that it would change all the damage that had been done in our communities, and why we were in such ill health and poverty. But by doing this, applying that liberal lens that's very much about the individual, about equality – although not equity-based equality – this very universalizing lens, locates the problem and solution of Indigenous wellness in our people's participation in the Canadian economy. So, what does this do? It obscures our treaty relationships. It obscures concepts around self-determination. It obscures the history of colonization. Government intervention is what caused this state of utter despair, unwellness, poverty. But somehow, with more interference and more intervention, it could be corrected? This is extremely problematic for Indigenous Peoples. It is a violent act that removes Indigenous people from our story, our context. It erases our history, places a universal Canadian citizenship upon us, and instead of asking, What's wrong with this system? it asks What's wrong with you Indigenous people?

Priya: Exactly. Like, who are you not to be able to participate?

Nicole: Like, here's your bag, or your suitcase, of rights as a Canadian (not an Indigenous person). And if you're not capable of operationalizing these, of being a successful individual in Canada, then this is your own problem. And we're setting up social welfare systems to assist you in participating in the economy. So, what's wrong with you?

Priya: It locates the problem in the individual. Something's wrong with you, or you must be ill not to be able to participate, and so on.

Nicole: Totally erasing our history. And how poverty for Indigenous people in Canada is unique. It is rooted in this very systematic denial of our sovereignty and treaty relationships in Canada.

Priya: Right. So, you're saying that this differential history of poverty, Indigenous versus mainstream, makes a universal anti-poverty strategy inappropriate. And specifically, an approach that promotes disability programs as a way to combat poverty.

Nicole: Most definitely. I think so. I think if we move forward with an anti-poverty lens, it has to have an Indigenous lens, an anti-colonial lens also, that has to be part of the discussion. Because to simply work for Indigenous people to gain access to the economy is, in a sense, the exact colonial project that Canada has worked towards: to continue to remove our sovereignty, erode our communities, and have us assimilate as just any other Canadian, on the one hand; and on the other hand, it removes blame and responsibility from the system, from the provincial and federal government, for having engaged and continuing to engage in this colonial process. It instead places blame and shame onto individuals.

Priya: That's right. You know, when I hear you shake up that idea of the neo-liberal poverty and state welfare lens, and how it violently universalizes people, it makes me think of the shared roots between that and the problems with the mental health or psychiatric lens. It's just as ahistorical and depoliticizing. So, for Indigenous people, this psychiatric-disability-assessment thing is a double whammy.

Nicole: Completely.

Priya: I think the anti-poverty language and the mental illness language can be really convincing because on the face of it, poverty, as well as "illness" – say, what I call depression or schizophrenia – may *look* similar between Indigenous and non-Indigenous people. It's easy for the neo-liberal project to promote universal solutions. It's scary how similar the narratives are in both economic and health domains.

Nicole: Versus a person's experience of whatever this phenomenon is. It violently severs Indigenous Peoples from our own story, it disappears any potential alternative narrative of what is happening in this person's universe.

Priya: This issue of narrative violence is all over our current system, although psychiatry is such an obvious culprit. But more specifically, I think we're putting our finger on why psychiatric assessments for disability applications are a particular problem from an Indigenous perspective. And why even the idea of this process being a way to address Indigenous poverty is itself a problem. It's not a perspective that I've heard a lot and it gives me a lot to think about. Although it's most obvious when it comes to Indigenous people, when I think about it, this is actually a mechanism of violence for everyone – cutting anyone off from their own stories and solutions.

Nicole: Exactly. You know, in my teachings we have fixed storied beings as well as ever-changing beings that live in our stories. This helps us to understand that stories are not always set in stone, such as stories of historical accounts, but that stories are alive and that we are a part of various living stories, ongoing relational creative processes that we are always engaging with. And I think it's important that these stories are alive and that we are able to be a part of this process of storying our own experience. Is it that we believe mental illness or disability truly exists, or is it that we have not yet heard other narratives? Is it that we believe the government's explanation for poverty? Or that we don't have access to other stories or understandings about what this could potentially be? And if it is unwellness, that we don't have alternative narratives about how potentially these things can be worked through or moved through? You know, that is a violence ... on our knowledge and world view –

Priya: A whole way of explaining or storytelling –

Nicole: You know, it's been delegitimized. And then we're stuck having to work in these rigid frameworks like when we write up these disability applications together. So Priya, given that you see this narrative violence also, how is it that you navigate this in your work?

Priya: Well, I can at least aim for transparency. I make it clear to people how I see what we are doing together, when we are doing an assessment that may lead to applying for ODSP. I'd say something to this woman, like, "We are telling the version of your story that may describe you as disabled." Then we also try and deliberately use the space to look at other versions of her story, which are just as valid. We look at her strengths and resourcefulness. We look at her upbringing, oppression, and so on. Often we go through the *family* story and make links if there is trauma that trickled down the generations, along with the gifts that have also been handed down. Even beyond this, I have had a handful of patients who are up for discussing the clear campaign against Indigenous Peoples in this country, and how it is not a coincidence that they have these struggles and are entering a system of now being reliant on social assistance. Not everyone sees it that way, but many people do, and they're able to relax in an assessment once they feel we are relatively more on the same page.

Nicole: Likewise, I find myself working in alternative stories with the people I work with. We often work together to Indigenize their narratives of unwellness, of poverty, or of disability. Working to remove an individual sense of deficiency, shame or guilt and instead tie their experience to the larger story of colonization in Canada. Including the experiences and worldview of the person's family, community or their nation has really presented a variety of alternative accounts, alternative stories that people use to heal their relationship with themselves and build an understanding of the other relationships in their lives that can be included in their healing journey.

Priya: Honestly, I think that is the real healing that is needed here – and I don't think that psychiatric assessments *or* disability applications will have a place in that process. The way I do it can help, I think, but I don't feel like it resolves these issues … and that's not within my ability. It's a way for me to negotiate my relationship to my patient, and build story authentically about our positions in the room. It's also my negotiation with the mandate of this agency, and my collaboration with my colleagues here – exploring different ways of telling these stories.

Nicole: If we are all part of a living story, that story is a place we can meet, to share and explore. A story is not a solid thing in and of itself, a self-enclosed or discernible point or object in the universe. It is like a constellation that presents itself in the sky, made up of the connections of light emanating from the relationship between stars, and between these stars and the sky, space, the moon, the distance from the earth, and the human eye. Stories embody this relational core of an Indigenous world view, a story is a collection of relationships – between people, community, context, place or setting, storyteller, audience and reader, past, present, and future – hundreds of factors forming a web of relations that we discern as "a story." What better way to work to understand the relationships involved in your patients unwellness, what better way to build stronger relationships with them, and what better way to build relationship between yourself and other practitioners working towards the healing of unwellness you are concerned with?

Priya: You're right. I think it's only through these stories and these relationships that this work can change. Obviously, on top of this, there's a lot that needs to change at the structural levels of these relationships. So that part of the story is yet to be told.

Nicole: Well, the story is the path, not the destination. It is a process of relationship building. This is the connection between knowing and being, theory and practice. To do differently, we need to be able to *conceive* of things differently. Including our response to these oppressive structures. By working together, and building relationship through story making, we work to create things into being. Storying new possibilities, opening our imagination to create alternative paths to wellness that did not exist before, not even in our minds. Like we are doing now, together.

Priya: So, this is how it starts – what we are doing now, this process of walking together, sharing, talking, forming relationship. This is the process of beginning to address the multiple forms of violence embedded in these psychiatric disability assessments and beyond.

Nicole: And maybe we have already begun to build more relationships through this story, with these people reading this transcript. Maybe you will continue in this story pathway with Priya and me, creating and bringing life to alternative possibilities.

Priya: Well, I'm pleased to be walking this path with you all, and with you, Nicole. When I look around the park we're in, I see all these other folks and community members around us, including some of the oldest trees in Toronto, towering over our heads. I realize that this is a conversation that has lots of witnesses and participants.

Nicole: Absolutely. Many more stories to be told. And the path, I see, is leading us right back to the office building – it looks like our lunch break is almost over.

Priya: Time to get to work?

Nicole: Time to get to work.

10 Madness, Violence, and Media

BRIGIT MCWADE

How are madness and violence represented in media culture? How is a "natural" or "causal" relationship between madness and violence imagined, produced, circulated, and resisted in media? This chapter reviews the existing literature on madness and violence in the media.[1] In disentangling madness, violence, and media, new perspectives and routes for action emerge.

Perspective I: The Media Is Stigmatizing

In 1996, Greg Philo and the Glasgow Media Group published *Media and Mental Distress*, reporting the findings of the first major study in the United Kingdom on media coverage of mental health/illness.[2] This research examined both the content of press, television, and films and how these related to public beliefs about mental illness. It involved an extensive content analysis and a series of focus group interviews with members of the general public, mental health service users, and their carers or family members. The research was developed in collaboration with Health Scotland, the Royal College of Psychiatrists, and Survivors Speak Out. In particular, it aimed to explore the media's role in perpetuating the myth that mentally ill people (especially those diagnosed with schizophrenia) were more prone to violence than others. The findings of the report were the following:

> The stigmatisation of those who are mentally distressed has a long history in our culture and obviously predates our contemporary media. It must also be said that the portrayal of mental illness in films, on television and in the press is not the only source of public information

and understanding in this area. Nonetheless, media coverage does have an important influence. Our study of the content of press and television showed that two-thirds of media references to mental health related to violence and that these negative images tended to receive "headline" treatment while more positive items were largely "back page" in their profile, such as problem pages, letter or health columns.[3]

In light of these findings, Philo et al. propose that "persistently inaccurate media presentations of mental illness" need to be changed via the development of guidelines for journalists and other media makers.[4] In particular, they argue that their findings have strong implications for mental health policy at the time of publication. The authors contended that myths about violent mental patients were undermining the success of "care in the community"[5] by fostering community hostility towards service users, impacting negatively in their social and support networks, and therefore increasing hardship and distress. Such stigmatizing media representations were also preventing people from seeking help from health services for mental distress.

Research carried out over several years by Otto Wahl and colleagues in Canada came to similar conclusions.[6] The realization of these guidelines for media producers can be found in most global north countries.[7] These guidelines promote "facts" about mental illness to correct what they construe as inaccuracies in media representations. For example, in addressing the association of violence with mental illness (specifically schizophrenia), the following "fact" about violence and mental health is widely circulated: "Over a third of the public think people with a mental health problem are likely to be violent – in fact people with severe mental illnesses are more likely to be victims, rather than perpetrators, of violent crime."[8] Underpinning this approach is a firm belief that once media representations adhere to the "facts" any stigma about mental health will magically disappear.

There are several problems with this research that need highlighting given their predominance in debates concerning media, violence, and madness. First, these work within a "media effects" paradigm in which "the media" are understood to cause effects in the general public. David Gauntlett has helpfully outlined a long list of problems with this idea.[9] Primarily, studies such as these approach social problems in a back-to-front way–they identify a problem (the stigma of mental illness) and then attempt to prove that the media are to blame (through misrepresentation of the "facts"). The objects of inquiry (stigma, violence, mental illness) remain discrete, pre-defined, and decontextualized.

For example, studies such as those by Philo and the Glasgow University Media Group and Wahl and colleagues work within the paradigm of mental *health and illness* to conduct content analyses – to identify all the instances of representations of mental illness in different media in a given timeframe.[10] These definitions are fixed and direct the analysis in particular ways, yet experiences of madness and distress are incredibly diverse and vary over time and in different places. Similarly content analyses of media violence work with set definitions of violence, such as "the overt expression of physical force (with or without a weapon) against self or other, compelling action against one's will on pain of being hurt or killed, or actually hurting or killing."[11] However, defining violence in this fixed way is problematic because "violence is not a singular thing which might grow cumulatively like poison inside people."[12] Like individualizing biopsychiatric definitions of mental illness, these definitions of violence tend to focus on individual physical violence and threat of violence.

What we count as violence and madness is important. We might want to ask why some kinds of violence (and their depiction) are understood to be problematic while others are not,[13] and equally why some kinds of madness and distress (and their depictions) trouble us. How can we broaden our definition of violence in ways that are "sensitive to who is violent, towards whom and in what context"?[14] What might different understandings of madness and distress, outside of the individualizing deficit model of biomedical psychiatry, bring to the discussion? As Harper has highlighted, the "equation of violence with immorality ignores both the violence of social oppression and the possibilities of violence as legitimate response to it."[15] Neither violence nor madness are individual; they are relational phenomena that cannot be reduced to the physical or biological but must also be understood as social, political, cultural, and institutionalized. In rethinking madness and violence this way, we can reveal everyday processes of normalization, legitimization, and the ideological and economic interests implicit in the madness/violence nexus.

The media effects model works with a concept of individuals taken from psychology that treats people as inadequate and incapable of doing anything but accepting the intended meaning of any media message. This is evident in Wahl's studies. These kinds of media analyses are easily put to service in conservative campaigns for more control of media, in this case, positioning psy-professions as the experts who should control and inform media messages about mental health and illness.[16] The example of the Glasgow Media Group's study is particularly interesting because they do a lot of work that attempts to move from a simplistic explanation of cause and effect to analysis that attends to the complexity of belief formation. They do this with a distinct methodology that combines content analysis with focus groups and interviews with media audiences. However, they arrive at the same conclusion – that the media must change and be more tightly controlled through codes of conduct.

In their literature review and the findings of their empirical study, Philo et al. highlight a particular ambivalence in public beliefs about mental illness – first, that it is a widely held belief that people in distress are unwell because of social and environmental factors and would benefit most from social support from friends, family, and community; second, that people who are mentally ill are also believed to be dangerous and unpredictable and have the potential for enacting violence, and that they are unsuited to work or other social roles. These beliefs were coupled with reluctance for closeness or intimacy with someone who is mentally ill. This is an important finding; however, the analysis presented does little to make sense of this suggested ambivalence. In part, this is because the researchers classify the former beliefs about mental illness as positive and sympathetic, and the latter as negative.

As I argue below, the distinction between positive and negative representations or beliefs about madness is problematic because it obscures the ways in which both can secure or reflect psy-discourse and power. In addition, although Philo et al. are careful to argue that "media exist within social cultures: they do not create the whole social world or how we think about it," they fail to acknowledge the political context within which representations and beliefs are co-constructed.[17] For example, they point to changing mental health policies with no acknowledgment of how these changes further secured powers of coercion and increasing reliance on biomedical explanations of madness and distress in tandem with the individualizing rhetoric of recovery discourse.[18] Furthermore, they point to the way in which the conflation of madness and violence are rooted in more generalized fears about living in a scary and unpredictable world, but do not account for the ways in which emotions are not natural individual feelings but deeply political phenomena.[19] Finally, they espouse a "fundamental truth about mental distress"[20] that draws heavily on a normative recovery discourse.

Perspective II: Psychiatric Media Cultures

Studies like Philo et al.'s and Wahl's obscure how psy-knowledge and practices, and national mental health policy and law, are strongly implicated in the stigmatization of madness and distress by diverting our attention to media representations. Their analyses begin and end with media. To better understand how the conflation of mental illness and violence is achieved, legitimated, and widely circulated, we need to develop our understanding of the *"relations of reciprocity* between [these] primary definers and the media."[21]

In her article "Making Bipolar Britney: Proliferating Psychiatric Diagnoses through Tabloid Media," Jijian Voronka provides us with a more comprehensive account of the relationship between the mental health system and media producers. Using the story of popstar Britney Spears's accrual of a diagnosis of bipolar disorder, Voronka shows how the tabloid press draws upon psy-expertise to narrate Spears's "descent into madness" in a way that reasserts the validity of psy-discourse. In doing so, possible alternatives to this dominant treatment paradigm are erased. Voronka argues that because psychiatry has been strongly contested both in terms of its scientific rigour and for its long history of patient abuse and torture, it needs to constantly promote itself to maintain and increase its market share of the mental health industry. She contends that it is because psychiatry "sits on a precarious credibility" that it depends on "constant re-legitimation in order to hold stable its assertions that madness is a problem of science and disease."[22] Britney Spears's public breakdown, her receipt of a diagnosis, and her ensuing treatment all serve as stories through which psy-expertise can be circulated. Both stories of going mad and stories of recovery can be manipulated to serve this purpose. The logic proceeds thus: if she is ill, she must be treated; if she recovers, it is proof that the treatment works; if she does not recover, it is because she did not adhere to her treatment. The "facts" of bipolar disorder frame Spears's life experiences, making them legible only in psychiatric terms.

Tasha Dubriwny adds to this perspective with an analysis of TV news reporting on postpartum depression and psychosis.[23] Dubriwny proposes that postpartum distress has the potential to challenge widely held beliefs about what constitutes "essential/good motherhood." Dubriwny argues that the dominant concept of motherhood is shaped by patriarchal capitalism, in which it is understood that it is in all women's nature to want to have children, that they are biologically able to do so, and that they have a selfless predisposition to nurture those children once they are born. Furthermore, it is white, middle-class women who are married to the father of their children that are idealized as "good" mothers. In this context, postpartum depression and psychosis must be "domesticated" to neutralize its threat to these dominant and oppressive ideals.[24] Dubriwny demonstrates this is done "through the reliance on psychiatric experts who speak from within a biomedical paradigm and the use of white, upper-class women to provide anecdotal information about postpartum disorders."[25] Postpartum depression and psychosis must be construed as diseases or illnesses that are temporary and can be treated biomedically. The psychiatric experts describe and define the illness, while the women's stories of recovery through treatment give an authenticity to the science. Lucy Costa and colleagues have documented and analysed this current trend within the mental health system in Canada in which intimate and personal stories of madness and recovery are commodified.[26] They argue that while telling stories is a central part of user and survivor organizing and activism, this has been co-opted by powerful organizations who seek to secure their access to resources by asserting their effectiveness through patient testimonies.

Costa and colleagues, Dubriwny, and Voronka all demonstrate that not only do psy-discourse and media work together to reproduce psy-power but that these medicalized representations also depoliticize marginalized people's dissent. Crucially, it is often through positive media reporting that this work is done, such as the stories of recovery told by women in treatment for postpartum depression analysed by Dubriwny. In contrast to Wahl's focus on negative representations of mental illness, or Philo et al.'s exploration of contradictory positive and negative representations and public beliefs, this work reveals that we must pay attention to the way in which both negative and positive representations play a part in securing psy-dominance in common knowledge about madness and distress. Indeed, the distinction between negative and positive representations is misleading. Furthermore, these representations strengthen and maintain gendered, racialized, and classed norms through the conflation of the white, middle-class, liberal individual with the ideal subject of those recovery stories that shore up psy-power.

In *Policing the Crisis: Mugging, the State, and Law and Order*, cultural theorist Stuart Hall and his co-authors detail this relationship between dominant ideologies and the everyday practices of making the news.

They argue that it would be inaccurate to argue that the media are in some way controlled by those with vested interests (e.g., psychiatry). Nonetheless, rules governing journalists and the structure of news reporting mean that the media "tend, faithfully and impartially, to reproduce symbolically the existing structure of power in society's institutional order."[27] In upholding ideals of balance and impartiality, and distinguishing between fact and opinion, the media strongly rely upon "experts" to provide their stories with credibility. Thus, those endowed with institutional expertise, in our case psychiatrists and psychologists, are the go-to people for stories on madness and distress; they are the "primary definers."[28] When counter-perspectives are sought in the name of balance, the "primary definers" have already set the limits of what is possible to say about that particular news item: "Arguments *against* a primary interpretation are forced to insert themselves into *its* definition of 'what is at issue' – they must begin from this framework of interpretation as their starting-point."[29] So the values of journalism entail the reproduction of dominant discourses *without necessarily being explicitly controlled by those in power*.

Hall and colleagues develop these ideas to think about how journalists do crucial work in translating expert knowledge into "public idiom," making it accessible and investing it "with popular force."[30] At times, editorials will even claim to "speak for the public," to express what the collective consensus is assumed to be on a particular issue.[31] In what Hall and colleagues describe as "spirals of amplification" this media expression of "public opinion" then feeds back into legitimizing official expertise and dominant discourses on the matter.[32] The authors closely detail the relationship between control culture (law and order) and representation (media) through the example of increased reporting of muggings in the 1970s in Britain. They argue that

> violence is perhaps the supreme example of the news value "negative consequences." ... The use of violence marks the distinction between those who are fundamentally of society and those who are outside it. It is coterminous with the boundary of "society" itself. ... The state, and the state only, has the monopoly of legitimate violence, and this "violence" is used to safeguard society against "illegitimate" uses. Violence thus constitutes a critical threshold in society.[33]

If we use this provocation to think about the association of violence with mental illness in media, we get a different perspective to that proposed by studies such as Philo et al.'s and Wahl's. We can see that the association of violence and mental illness works to mark those living with mental illness diagnoses as outsiders. The point is that "the media" are not solely responsible for stigmatizing madness and distress, but rather reproduce stigma by working in tandem with existing psy-knowledges, which are themselves stigmatizing.

British mental health nurses Bates and Stickley argue that the mental health system – comprising law, policy, and professional practices – is a form of "institutionalised stigma."[34] In their consideration of the dilemma of anti-stigma campaigns, they conclude that mental health "legislation which removes a person's rights, coerces them into treatment and focuses extensively on diagnosis and risk factors may perpetuate stigma and social exclusion."[35] Similarly, some evidence shows that medical models of madness and distress produce more negative and stigmatizing perceptions of people with mental health conditions than do social explanations.[36] But this "institutionalised stigma" also sets the terms through which violence perpetrated by those living with a diagnosis of mental illness will be read.

Stigma – in this case, the association of mental illness and violence – is integral to the ethos of mental health systems in most global north countries. For example, in the United Kingdom, mental health policy and law can be understood as practices of state-making, in which the risk to violence is one of the key "critical thresholds" that determines the nation-state's insiders and outsiders.[37] Stigma is a specific boundary marker that legitimates state-enacted violence (being sectioned under the Mental Health Act, receiving forced treatment, and experiencing the resulting impoverishment and marginalization). Dominant debates about media representation and anti-stigma campaigns are part of these practices of state-making. Stigma and anti-stigma are not concerned with individuals but rather have political currency in producing inequalities on a national and global scale.[38]

How do we refuse the primary definers' terms when we think about the relationship between madness and distress, violence, and media representations? We could begin with those "facts" that are widely circulated. Let us take, for example, the one in four statistic intended to make people understand that mental health and illness are facts of life, universal experiences, and to some extent "normal." What is effaced here is that, in our current system, *who* you are matters in terms what happens to you when you experience madness and distress. For example, if you are Black or Black British in the United Kingdom you are more likely to be detained and forcibly treated under the Mental Health Act 1983/2007.[39] Representing mental health as everyone's business belies the significant inequalities inherent in our current system. Similarly, if we begin to unpick the claim that "people with severe mental illnesses are more likely to be victims, rather than perpetrators, of violent crime,"[40] we also encounter problems. The anti-stigma statistic about violence is offered as reassurance *for members of the public*; it tells them that *they* are safe. The statistic is not a call to action around the inequalities of the violent victimization of Mad people. This *fact* does important work in silencing such questions with the promise that once we understand the facts of mental illness, stigma will be eradicated. It also conflates violence with violent crime, again drawing our attention away from structural and state-enacted violence, enforcing a divisive logic through the cultural economy of fear.

Conclusion

There are different perspectives on the relationship between madness, violence, and media. The dominant narrative currently circulating is one proposed by anti-stigma campaigners and especially those who have professional investment in mental health services, alongside some user-led organizations. Their argument is that the media stigmatize mental illness by portraying "the Mentally Ill" as violent and dangerous. Their solution to this problem is that media should address stigma by learning the facts of mental illness (drawn from psychology and psychiatry) and the "reality" of lived experience through the first-person testimonies of those who have a mental illness.

A counter narrative to this, gaining momentum through mental health service-user/psychiatric survivor activism and (latterly) Mad Studies, is that it is psy-knowledges and practices that are stigmatizing; the values underpinning media making work to reproduce psy-discourse and power. The solution to this is that media should circulate critiques of and present alternatives to psy-discourse. There is a long history of such alternative media representations from *Madness Network News* in the USA and *Phoenix Rising* in Canada, to contemporary examples, such as *Asylum Magazine* in the UK and Robert Whitaker's *Mad in America* blog.[41] Here we find counter-discourse covering such issues as the lack of evidence for the "chemical imbalance in the brain" argument and reporting on the violence of a system that entails forced treatment.

While I agree with the latter perspective, I want to push our thinking further here. It is not just that media reproduce or circulate psychiatric discourse as facts, nor are media biased per se. It is that *psychiatry is culture* and media representations of mental illness/madness are part of this. How we come to know ourselves is mediated through psychiatrized media cultures. In many ways, Philo and the Glasgow Media Group propose a useful methodology for making sense of the complex ways in which media shape beliefs about, and even override direct experience of, madness and distress. However, because they continued to work within the dominant paradigm of mental health and illness and did not provide an analysis of the political context, the radical promise of the project has yet to be realized. It is my hope that this work can be pursued in the future with a view to enriching our understandings of the political and cultural economies of madness and distress.

NOTES

1 This chapter focuses on media from the global north. I select a few studies to highlight in particular, rather than offering an extensive and in-depth review of all the literature. It should be noted that this is an under-researched area of inquiry. There is plenty of research on media effects and violence, and clinical studies concerning mental illness and violence, but there is little that focuses specifically on madness, violence, and media together.

2 A note on terminology. I use the terms that are specific to what I am discussing. In this case, anti-stigma campaigners talk about "mental health" and "mental illness." If I am writing from a mad activism perspective, I would use "madness and distress." I do this for consistency and clarity but also because language matters; it reveals particular sets of values and beliefs.

3 Philo and Glasgow University Media Group, *Media and Mental Distress*, 112.

4 Ibid., 13.

5 The deinstitutionalization conceived as "care in the community" took a very long time to implement in the United Kingdom and arguably has never been achieved. For more details see McWade, "Recovery-as-Policy."

6 Wahl, "Mass Media Images"; Wahl, "Mental Health Consumers' Experience of Stigma"; Wahl and Roth, "Television Images "; Wahl and Lefkowits, "Impact of a Television Film"; Wahl, "News Media Portrayal."

7 Time to Change, "Media Advisory Service."

8 Time to Change, "Violence and Mental Health."

9 Gauntlett, "Ten Things Wrong."

10 Philo and Glasgow University Media Group, *Media and Mental Distress*; Wahl, "Mass Media Images"; Wahl, "News Media Portrayal"; Wahl and Lefkowits, "Impact of a Television Film"; Wahl and Roth, "Television Images."

11 Gerbner et al. cited in Weaver and Carter, *Critical Readings*, 4.

12 Barker and Petley, *Ill Effects*, 3.

13 Weaver and Carter, *Critical Readings*.

14 Harper, *Madness, Power and the Media*.

15 Ibid., 48.

16 I will refer to psychiatry, psychology, and psychoanalysis as "psy" disciplines or professions. This is because the mental health system is a multidisciplinary field and it would be inaccurate to focus solely on psychiatry. Furthermore, all three disciplines are heterogeneous, and I do not want to represent them reductively as this would undermine the argument I present here.

17 Philo and Glasgow University Media Group, *Media and Mental Distress*, 103.

18 See for example McWade, "Recovery-as-Policy"; Spandler and Calton, "Psychosis and Human Rights."

19 See for example Davies, *The Happiness Industry*; Tyler, *Revolting Subjects*.

20 Greg Philo and Glasgow University Media Group, *Media and Mental Distress*, 113.

21 Hall et al., *Policing the Crisis*, 74.

22 Voronka, "Making Bipolar Britney."

23 Dubriwny, "Television News Coverage."

24 Ibid., 289.

25 Ibid.

26 Costa et al., "'Recovering Our Stories.'"

27 Hall et al., *Policing the Crisis*, 58.

28 Ibid.

29 Ibid., 57.

30 Ibid., 61.

31 Ibid., 61.

32 Ibid., 63.

33 Ibid., 67–8.

34 Bates and Stickley, "Confronting Goffman," 574.

35 Ibid., 572.

36 Read, "Why Promoting Biological Ideology"; Read and Harré, "The Role of Biological."
37 McWade, "Recovery-as-Policy."
38 This argument is partly drawn from Imogen Tyler's current work-in-progress concerning stigma. For more details see Tyler, "The Stigma Doctrine."
39 Health and Social Care Information Centre, "Inpatients Formally Detained."
40 Time to Change, "Violence and Mental Health."
41 *Madness Network News*; Psychiatric Survivor Archives of Toronto, "Phoenix Rising Annotated"; *Asylum*; *Mad in America*.

BIBLIOGRAPHY

Asylum: An International Magazine for Democratic Psychiatry. Accessed February 13, 2017. http://www.asylumonline.org/.
Barker, M., and J. Petley. *Ill Effects: The Media/Violence Debate.* 2nd ed. London, UK: Routledge, 2001.
Bates, L., and T. Stickley. "Confronting Goffman: How Can Mental Health Nurses Effectively Challenge Stigma? A Critical Review of the Literature." *Journal of Psychiatric and Mental Health Nursing* 20, no. 7 (2013): 569–75.
Costa, L., J. Voronka, D. Landry, J. Reid, B. Mcfarlane, D. Reville, and K. Church. "'Recovering Our Stories': A Small Act of Resistance." *Studies in Social Justice* 6, no. 1 (2012): 85–101.
Davies, W. *The Happiness Industry: How the Government and Big Business Sold Us Well-Being.* London, UK: Verso Books, 2015.
Dubriwny, T. N. "Television News Coverage of Postpartum Disorders and the Politics of Medicalization." *Feminist Media Studies* 10, no. 3 (2010): 285–303.
Gauntlett, David. "Ten Things Wrong with the 'Effects Model.'" In *Approaches to Audiences: A Reader,* edited by Roger Dickinson, Ramaswani Harindranath, and Olga Linné, 120–30. London, UK: Arnold, 1998.
Hall, S., C. Critche, T. Jefferson, J. Clarke, and B. Roberts. *Policing the Crisis: Mugging, the State, and Law and Order.* London, UK: Macmillan, 1978.
Harper, S. *Madness, Power and the Media: Class, Gender and Race in Popular Representations of Mental Distress.* Basingstoke, UK: Palgrave Macmillan, 2009.
Health and Social Care Information Centre. "Inpatients Formally Detained in Hospitals under the Mental Health Act 1983 and Patients Subject to

Supervised Community Treatment, England, 2014 to 2015." October 23, 2015. https://www.gov.uk/government/statistics/inpatients-formally-detained -in-hospitals-under-the-mental-health-act-1983-and-patients-subject-to -supervised-community-treatment-2014-to-2015.

Mad in America: Science, Psychiatry and Community. Accessed February 13, 2017. https://www.madinamerica.com.

Madness Network News. 2014. Accessed February 13, 2017. https://books. google.ca/books/about/Madness_Network_News_Volume_1 .html?id=pQLIBAAAQBAJ&redir_esc=y

McWade, Brigit. "Recovery-as-Policy as a Form of Neo-liberal State-Making." *Intersectionalities: A Global Journal of Social Work Analysis, Research, Polity, and Practice* 5, no. 3 (2016). https://journals.library.mun.ca/ojs/index.php/IJ/ article/view/1602/1331.

Philo, Greg, and Glasgow University Media Group. *Media and Mental Distress.* London, UK: Longman, 1996.

Psychiatric Survivor Archives of Toronto. "Phoenix Rising Annotated." Accessed February 13, 2017. http://www.psychiatricsurvivorarchives.com/ phoenix.html.

Read, John. "Why Promoting Biological Ideology Increases Prejudice against People Labelled 'Schizophrenic.'" *Australian Psychologist* 42, no. 2 (2007): 118–28.

Read, John, and N. Harré. "The Role of Biological and Genetic Causal Beliefs in the Stigmatisation of 'Mental Patients.'" *Journal of Mental Health* 10, no. 2 (2001): 223–35.

Spandler, H., and T. Calton. "Psychosis and Human Rights: Conflicts in Mental Health Policy and Practice." *Social Policy and Society* 8, no. 2 (2009): 245–56.

Time to Change. "Media Advisory Service." Accessed May 3, 2016. https:// www.time-to-change.org.uk/media-advice.

Time to Change. "Violence and Mental Health." Accessed May 3, 2016. https://www.time-to-change.org.uk/news-media/media-advisory -service/help-journalists/violence-mental-health-problems.

Tyler, Imogen. *Revolting Subjects: Social Abjection and Resistance in Neo-liberal Britain.* London, UK: Zed Books, 2013.

Tyler, Imogen. "The Stigma Doctrine." Accessed February 13, 2017. https:// thestigmadoctrine.wordpress.com.

Voronka, J. "Making Bipolar Britney: Proliferating Psychiatric Diagnoses through Tabloid Media." *Radical Psychology* 7, no. 2 (2008): 1–23.

Wahl, Otto F. "Mass Media Images of Mental Illness: A Review of the Literature." *Journal of Community Psychology* 20, no. 4 (1992): 343–52.

Wahl, Otto F. "Mental Health Consumers' Experience of Stigma." *Schizophrenia Bulletin* 25, no. 3 (1999): 467–78.

Wahl, Otto F. "News Media Portrayal of Mental Illness Implications for Public Policy." *American Behavioral Scientist* 46, no. 12 (2003): 1594–600.

Wahl, Otto F., and J. Y. Lefkowits. "Impact of a Television Film on Attitudes toward Mental Illness." *American Journal of Community Psychology* 17, no. 4 (1989): 521–8.

Wahl, Otto F., and R. Roth. "Television Images of Mental Illness: Results of a Metropolitan Washington Media Watch." *Journal of Broadcasting* 26 (1982): 599–605.

Weaver, C., and C. Carter. *Critical Readings: Violence and the Media.* Maidenhead, UK: Open University Press, 2006.

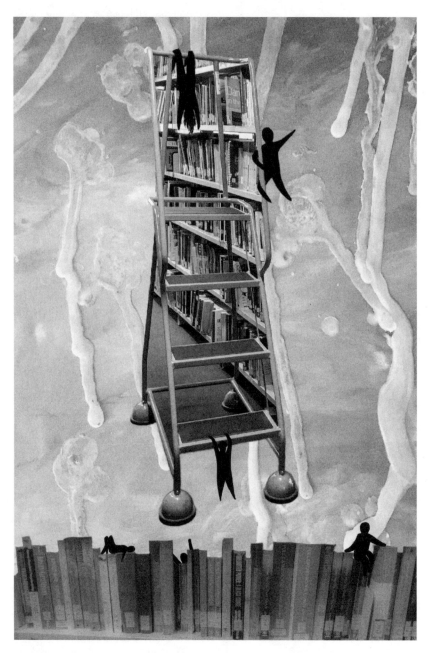

Figures playing among university library books, by Rachel Rowan Olive. Digital collage: acrylic paint, candlewax, photographs, and digital image work.

PART III

Law as Violence

Part III examines the relationship between law, policy, violence, and power as structurally authorized by the state and in relation to race, gender, and disability. Law itself can be implicitly violent with modes of enforcement and exercises of power that reinforce hierarchies and orders of patriarchal power. The chapters in Part III take us through local and international examples of how and to whom this happens. Given that law is continually bound up with its own need for legitimation, it falls into the dilemma of self-preservation despite calls for reform and thus perpetuates inequality and subordination of mental health service users and survivors via symbolic gestures of justice, as opposed to materialist change. By discussing the limitations of legal intervention and discourses of justice, these authors bring to the fore legal structural violence as an issue deeply tied and embedded in history and forms of identity representation.

We begin with Ameil Joseph's work on the ways in which familiar eugenic themes creep into and contribute to reproducing familiar prejudice, racism, and colonialist ideas in three recent pieces of Canadian legislation: the Canadian Faster Removal of Foreign Criminals Act, the Not Criminally Responsible Reform Act (NCR Act), and the Anti-terrorism Act. Joseph argues that the incarceration, treatment, and deportation of precarious and racialized bodies as authorized through these legislative initiatives, re-perpetuate bio-governance via "regimes of whiteness." Recognizable race, ability, illness, and criminality tropes once again permeate, infuse, and promote public moral panics through this legislation. Drawing on Slovoj Žižek's work, Joseph articulates the complex role of structural violence in maintaining subjective and invisible violence(s) experienced by those simultaneously targeted and harmed by relations of power and domination through the state. More importantly, chapter 11 forces readers to consider the confluence of law in nationalist agenda building through "threats" of the damaged and biologically inferior "Other." The underlying assumption that "citizenship" should exclude "risky foreigners" and that public space is saved for a sanitized few raises important questions and potential calls to action.

Chapter 12 brings together the personal and political in a discussion that looks at the need to re-examine reproduction narratives that constitute the pregnant Mad body as a "risky and dangerous" body needing surveillance. Tobin LeBlanc Haley argues that social policies and practices that seek to define and cultivate a world whereby reproduction is impermissible for Mad women, is in her summation, a form of epistemic violence. She draws from feminist political economy as a theoretical framework that challenges norms maintained through assumptions about sex, gender, and social roles in the neo-liberal economy. Haley also argues that violence is propagated further by medical and psychiatric powers being allowed to create social policies that both mark women's bodies as unsafe and simultaneously limit solutions to the prevalent problem of scarce social services and supports for pregnancy and child-rearing. This chapter offers and pushes us beyond the well-established history of women's violent psychiatric past (e.g., through sterilization narratives) towards a more nuanced understanding of how the surveillance and regulation of women's sexual autonomy persists today, despite understandings of its inhumane past.

Chapter 13, Uncovering Law's Multiple Violences, considers the 2007 death of teenager Ashley Smith in the Grand Valley Institution for Women in Ontario, Canada. Tess Sheldon, Karen Spector, and Mary Birdsell review Ashley's case and consider how violence was authorized and maintained in correctional and psychiatric institutions for youth (and young inmates) with mental health issues. Acting as counsel on behalf of a service-user advocacy organization for the inquest, the authors pose important questions about how law constitutes and controls "expert testimony" in court proceedings, given that the coroner in Ashley's inquest did not permit testimony from individuals with lived experience. Questions about the overuse of segregation, chemical and physical restraint, and body cavity searches are also raised in the chapter and remind us that much rethinking is still needed given the cavalier developments that have taken place so far. As an example, Sheldon, Spector, and Birdsell pose salient questions about the value of such inquests given that 104 of its recommendations have yet to be implemented. Correctional Service Canada rejected the jury's recommendations, and action is still required regarding the auditor general's ability to supervise, implement, and enforce inquest recommendations.

In chapter 14 Jen Rinaldi and Kate Rossiter take up similar issues of legal and state responsibility questioning what gains were achieved for abuse survivors of the Huronia Regional Centre. This institution, operated by the Government of Ontario, opened in 1876 to warehouse people with intellectual and developmental disabilities and was shut down permanently in March 2009. Rinaldi and Rossiter make the important point that legal frameworks are inadequate and harmful to institutional survivors of abuse – specifically as related to individuals with developmental disabilities. These processes, as the authors argue, are limited, exclusionary, and inevitably only further discursive violence. They offered insubstantial remedy for justice given the breadth and depth of horrific abuse that led to the class action suit representing 5000 former residents. Recognized as a landmark case, the legal settlement gave voice to the abuse endured by residents. However, the process of engaging, participating in, and voicing violence to suitably fit legal frameworks, and the subsequent processes for determining financial remedy, calls into question both the ethics and justice achieved through the arena of legal engagement.

Finally, chapter 15, the concluding chapter in this part, by Azeezah Kanji raises issues that are especially relevant in today's sociopolitical context regarding violence enacted by state actors advancing discourses on the war on terror. By reviewing the historical trajectory following the 2001 military campaign primarily led by the United States against individuals, organizations, and countries, Kanji discusses the ways in which racist policies and laws have led to unjust targeting of Muslims. She raises concerns about and offers analyses of the construction of Muslims as pathological and in need of psychiatric intervention via the administration of specially developed psychological assessment tools.

11 Contemporary Forms of Legislative Imprisonment and Colonial Violence in Forensic Mental Health

AMEIL J. JOSEPH

Introduction

This chapter is devoted to an understanding of how the confluence of violence within the different punishing regimes of Western biomedical psychiatrically dominated structures are sustained through policy and law to imprison difference, while simultaneously (re)creating ideas of whiteness, the pristine, the innocent, and the deserving. Specifically, through an examination of the Faster Removal of Foreign Criminals Act, the Not Criminally Responsible Reform Act, and the Anti-terrorism Act in Canada and their corresponding amendments to existing legislation, this chapter interrogates the deployment of racial and eugenic ideas for their replication of dehumanizing colonial discursive and rhetorical violence in everyday use, the institutionalization of violence within contemporary law, and the currently violent direct human consequences of these historically violent practices that ensure imprisonment of particular minds and bodies.

Punishing Difference: Regimes of Whiteness

The project of eugenics, specifically the idea that societies, people, and institutions could manipulate genetic variation to achieve desired characteristics, benefited greatly from the rise of enlightenment ideas and the scientific revolution pertaining to race, ability, mental illness, and human sexuality, which were simultaneously stratified by gender and class.[1] The context and use of eugenic and racial ideas within mental health systems and collaborative systems, such as the criminal justice system and the immigration system, have been documented and analysed for their contemporary descendants within practice policy and law.[2] Angus McLaren reminds us that the entire health care system in Canada is bound to a eugenic project, enshrined in policy and law.[3] Dr Helen MacMurchy was Ontario's leading public health expert in 1914 and "inspector of the feeble minded" from 1906 to 1916. MacMurchy sought to affect public health needs in the areas of infant mortality, maternal mortality, and feeblemindedness by advocating for segregation, sterilization, and restriction of immigration by arguing that feebleminded and defective children were costly and likely to commit crimes.[4] Similarly, in 1933, Canadian figure Tommy Douglas reasoned that "the mentally and physically subnormal" were the cause of a good deal of the distress of the great depression.[5] In his MA thesis, he traced the family trees of 12 "immoral and nonmoral women" to suggest that their 25 children and 105 grandchildren were "spreading disease, clogging up the school system, promoting crime and prostitution, burdening hospitals and overwhelming charitable institutions."[6] His recommendations were based on the idea of biological determinism, including restriction of marriage, segregation of the unfit, and sterilization. Finally, Dowbiggin documents how prominent medical and psychiatric figures advocated under eugenic rationale for the exclusion of foreigners as they were seen as the carriers of genetic defectiveness and a threat to the purity of the Canadian race. Prominent Canadian psychiatrist Charles Kirk Clarke, for example, advocated to government for changes to immigration and social care policy to inhibit the entry of immigrants, increase medical screening, and limit access to social support based on racial and eugenic ideas.[7] As such, by 1906, the Immigration Act was well developed with its eugenic and racial influence to include new reportable and inadmissibility criteria. Specifically, three classes of immigrants were delineated: (1) the physically or mentally disabled, (2) those with infectious or dangerous diseases, and (3) paupers or the destitute.[8]

The legacy of biomedical identification as a requisite for service acquisition continues to evoke a rationale of the deserving and undeserving while supplanting social problems with biological ones. The idea that mental and physical difference is bound to an Other or an immigrant and is burdensome to "Canadians" is both a product of colonial eugenic and racist ideas and a contemporary outcome of a social service system that sees differences in race, mental fitness, and physical ability as something external to the "normal," biologically determined, and wasteful of public expenditure. This is evident in current immigration law in Canada and required medical guidelines that state,

> **38.** (1) A foreign national is inadmissible on health grounds if their health condition
>
> (*a*) is likely to be a danger to public health; (*b*) is likely to be a danger to public safety; or (*c*) might reasonably be expected to cause excessive demand on health or social services.[9]

A Framework for Talking about Violence as a Confluence in Western Biomedically Dominated Mental Health, Criminal Justice, and Immigration Systems

Violence must be appreciated in all its forms. This includes the appreciation of the historical and contemporary violence within professions, professional technologies, practices, the knowledge disciplines that develop to support the work of professions, and how they collaborate and become enshrined within policy and law. Western psychiatric biomedicine, immigration regulation, and criminal justice systems must be considered within their historical confluence for their interdependent use and advancement of racial and eugenic ideas for projects of colonization and nation building. The processes and technologies of dehumanization have always been necessary for colonial and imperial projects. For exploitation, slavery, indenture, the colonization of lands, the upheaval of governments, and the imposition of religion to occur, a group had to be differentiated, subordinated into a general type, and seen through a lens of difference as an inferior group in need of Western civility, democracy, psychiatry, capitalism, and Christianity, and deemed worthy of violence and reasoned out of humanity.[10]

Specific professions and disciplines have taken a dominant role in implementing these racial and eugenic ideas in practice. For example, the Mental Health Act has etched within it the power and authority of psychiatry to diagnose, confine, and medicate without consent. The Criminal Code of Canada has engraved in it the delegation of power to psychiatry to assess criminal responsibility. The Immigration and Refugee Protection Act has also provided a notion of "serious criminality" and "threat to the public" to allow for legal, immigration, psychiatric, and professional authorities to use exceptional and non-transparent discretionary powers. This includes the authorization of violence to people identified as different, and the formulation of a dangerous Other that is biologically inferior with tendencies towards criminality, who is "not Canadian," and thereby undeserving of care.

Describing the historical and contemporary confluence of biomedicine and psychiatry, immigration regulation, and criminal justice systems of violence to engage with this complexity must of course, at the very least, use the complexity of analysis required for an understanding of the development of aspects of the confluence of identity and difference, to rationalize projects of human order, human hierarchy, to achieve dehumanization to rationalize subjugation and exclusion. As notions of undesirability were forged historically for colonial projects so were ideas of race, and ability, of mental health and mental illness, of acceptable and unacceptable, of deviant sexualities and the establishment of taxonomies of people and genders.

Slavoj Žižek offers a framework from which we can consider the confluence of violence enacted when analysing historical and contemporary projects of dehumanization that is individual, social, structural, and systemic.[11] Žižek describes various forms of violence:

1. Subjective violence takes in the most visible forms of violence, including physical, verbal, and organized violence perpetrated by individuals, states, and groups.
2. Objective violence contains two kinds: *symbolic* violence embodied in language and its forms, and *systemic* violence "the often catastrophic consequences of the smooth functioning of our political and economic systems."[12]

Symbolic violence "is not only at work in the obvious – and extensively studied – cases of incitement and of the relations of social domination reproduced in our habitual speech forms: there is a more fundamental form of violence still that pertains to language as such, to its imposition of a certain universe of meaning."[13] Systemic violence is "violence inherent in a system: not only direct physical violence, but also the more subtle forms of coercion that sustain relations of domination and exploitation, including the threat of violence."[14]

As Žižek states, "one should resist the fascination of subjective violence, of violence enacted by social agents, evil individuals, disciplined repressive apparatuses, fanatical crowds: subjective violence is just the most visible of the three."[15] As Žižek describes,

> the catch is that subjective and objective violence cannot be perceived from the same standpoint: subjective violence is experienced as such against the background of a non-violent zero level. It is seen as a perturbation of the "normal," peaceful state of things. However, objective violence is precisely the violence inherent to this "normal" state of things. Objective violence is invisible since it sustains the very zero-level standard against which we perceive something as subjectively violent.[16]

Žižek's framework allows for an analysis of physical violence, the structural violence of economic relations, and epistemic, cognitive, and rhetorical forms of violence as products and processes, as human creations, relations of power, and modes of domination, cultural and social factors of violence, and the dangers of violent means to achieve unpredictable ends. With respect to colonization, Žižek's framework accommodates a consideration of the violence in the writing of history or historiography, the violence reproduced from the master/slave relationship. It is a framework that facilitates appreciation of the oppression of people who have experienced the mental health system, psychiatric survivors, ex-patients, consumer survivors, people with lived experience of mental health issues, service users, system users, psychiatric prisoners, and the psychiatrically incarcerated and perspectives of Mad people or madness, while also attending to the violence of technologies, products and practices of race and colonization, eugenics and nation building. In this way, naming the act of imprisonment of a person, a people, through physical means, discursive means, and legislative means can all be achieved without separating the violence achieved: that is, the imprisonment of mind and body.

Contemporary Forms of Legislative Imprisonment and Colonial Violence in Forensic Mental Health

New legislation has been approved that requires an analysis of interdependence to appreciate the confluence of violence achieved through the working of criminal justice, psychiatric, and immigration laws, policies, and practices. The Faster Removal of Foreign Criminals Act received royal assent on June 19, 2013. It was originally tabled as Bill

C-43. The Act amends the Immigration and Refugee Protection Act and references the Canadian Security Intelligence Service Act, Protecting Canada's Immigration System Act Bill C-31, Bill C-38, and the Jobs, Growth and Long-term Prosperity Act. The stated summary provided by the Government of Canada professes that the Faster Removal of Foreign Criminals Act serves to "limit the review mechanism for certain foreign nationals and permanent residents who are inadmissible on such grounds as serious criminality."[17] It also "provides for the mandatory imposition of minimum conditions on permanent residents or foreign nationals who are the subject of a report on inadmissibility on grounds of security that is referred to the Immigration Division or a removal order for inadmissibility on grounds of security or who, on grounds of security, are named in a certificate that is referred to the Federal Court."[18] Bill C-31 limits the right to appeal a removal order or deportation order based on a finding of serious criminality even though permanent residents or foreign nationals may have humanitarian and compassionate grounds for appeal (i.e., how settled the person is in Canada, general family ties to Canada, the best interests of any children involved, and what could happen to the applicant if the request is not granted, including persecution, lack of social support, medical treatment, etc.).[19]

The Not Criminally Responsible Reform Act, which received assent April 11, 2014, is a piece of legislation separate from the Faster Removal of Foreign Criminals Act. It was originally tabled as Bill C-14. It amends the Criminal Code of Canada and the National Defence Act. In its summary, it states,

> This enactment amends the mental disorder regime in the *Criminal Code* and the *National Defence Act* to specify that the paramount consideration in the decision-making process is the safety of the public and to create a scheme for finding that certain persons who have been found not criminally responsible on account of mental disorder are high-risk accused. It also enhances the involvement of victims in the regime and makes procedural and technical amendments.[20]

A key differentiating amendment from the prior legislation is that Bill C-14 adds a new category of "high-risk offender" that ,when applied to a person, can limit any disposition that grants them freedom from incarceration in either a prison or a mental institution regardless of a finding of not criminally responsible by reason of mental disorder (NCRMD).[21]

Under the revision, a person found NCRMD who is deemed a "high risk" or a threat to the public can also be deemed too dangerous to ever leave inpatient treatment, incarceration, or confinement. The National Defence Act is amended to include a provision for those deemed "a significant threat to the safety of the public" rendering the high-risk offender" a national defence concern. A person found NCRMD is mandated via disposition to psychiatric treatment. If the person should recover and no longer be at risk to anyone's safety, a new provision in this act allows for any victims to be notified so they can challenge the release.

While victim impact statements were provided for previously in the Criminal Code, the power of victims to influence the decisions or dispositions of the Review Board has been increased exponentially. Specifically, when a person is now deemed high risk the victim is invited to provide an impact statement.[22] If the accused is given an absolute discharge the victim is notified and can request information on where the accused plans to live.[23] The victim can now inform the hearing as to where the accused can be prevented from going in terms of location, make restrictions to ensure no contact, and so on, even though no risk may be present to the victim.[24] Also, the Criminal Code was amended to redefine what a high-risk accused person or what "a significant threat to the safety of the public" means. Sections 672.5401 states that a significant threat to the safety of the public means "a risk of serious physical or psychological harm to members of the public – including any victim of or witness to the offence, or any person under the age of 18 years – resulting from conduct that is criminal in nature but not necessarily violent."[25]

Presently, written into law is the power of the victim of a crime (to which the accused has been found NCRMD) to state that since the public presence of the accused represents a potential psychological risk to them because of the crime that occurred (which may or may not have been violent) the accused can be deemed a "significant threat to the public" and not be granted a disposition that relieves them from imprisonment, involuntary hospitalization, or confinement. Any societal prejudice, bias, or discriminatory beliefs that perpetuate fear of harm from the accused (i.e., people with mental health issues are always dangerous) are permitted to affect the freedom of the accused.

This puts the impact of criminality in the forefront and considerations of risk to the public based on one's current status of mental wellness as secondary. The impact of the crime, even though a person is found not criminally responsible, again is reverted to a primary focus which the NCRMD finding was meant to remove to counter the effects of the discriminatory criminalization of people with mental health issues whether they have committed an offence or not. The initial reason for the NCRMD finding was so that people who committed crimes because of illness, who did not understand both the nature of the crime or the repercussions of what they had done, could seek help. The NCR Reform Act re-criminalizes even acts found to be NCRMD.

The Anti-terrorism Act received Royal Assent June 18, 2015. Originally tabled as Bill C-51, the act amends the Security of Canada Information Sharing Act, Secure Air Travel Act, Aeronautics Act, and the Canada Evidence Act; the Criminal Code of Canada; Canadian Security Intelligence Service Act; and the Immigration and Refugee Protection Act. The summary, while lengthy, contains a plethora of ambiguities offering extreme discretionary authority to security and government professionals. A first point of effect it that this Act authorizes the Government of Canada's "institutions" to share, disclose, or appropriate any information "*in* respect of activities that undermine the security of Canada."[26] This can affect one's ability to travel and what can be submitted as evidence, and allows for expanded "recognizance conditions" (reporting and surveillance requirements) to be applied to people: "Part 4 amends the *Canadian Security Intelligence Service Act* to permit the Canadian Security Intelligence Service to take, within and outside Canada, measures to reduce threats to the security of Canada, including measures that are authorized by the Federal Court."[27] It also gives exceptional powers to the Minister of Immigration to request and act upon information deemed of interest to national security and limits the ability for people to appeal or request a judicial review by the Federal Court of Canada.[28]

While seemingly new and separate pieces of legislation, passed at different times, these Acts carry out a very familiar project. Dowbiggin and McLaren have made clear that racial, eugenic immigration fears exemplified above within the delineation of the notions of undesirability and prohibited classes, enshrined within the 1906 Immigration Act and advanced by prominent figures such as MacMurchy and Clarke, consolidated the idea that "foreigners" were somehow burdensome to the public and carriers of hereditary forms of defectiveness, including mental illness, feeblemindedness, and inherent criminality.[29] The Faster Removal of Foreign Criminals Act, (re)invokes the idea that "foreigners" are a burdensome cost and threat to Canadian society. At the same time, it reproduces the idea that there is an inherent criminality (the unrehabilitatable) that exists in foreign bodies that must be handled swiftly (as of course no complexities of consideration would be congruent with this point of view) thus eliminating the need for considerations of appeals, even for humanitarian and compassionate grounds. Regardless of length of time in Canada, existence of family in Canada, or threat of persecution elsewhere, these people are deemed inadmissible based on the application of a finalized classification of "serious criminality" that is fixed and unchanging. The idea of a foreign threat who is "not our problem," inherently criminal, dangerous, and undeserving is relied upon in the Faster Removal of Foreign Criminals Act. It evokes historically established ideas of undesirability that assumed immigrants were carriers of hereditary defectiveness, and prone to poverty and criminality. These ideas were enshrined in law in the historical examples provided above: the Immigration Act of 1906 and the prohibited classes listed in the Act to Amend the Immigration Act of 1910. This notion of serious criminality depends upon these ideas of inherent criminality and foreign threat. Simultaneously the NCR Reform Act (re) invokes the idea of a dangerous mentally ill person who is a threat to society. It does so through the creating of a "high-risk" offender category that must be contained, confined, or forcibly medicated under supervision and prevented from release, even though they have been found not criminally responsible for their actions (the untreatable). The NCR Reform Act also relies on notions of hereditary defectiveness, and threat associated with people who are identified as having mental health issues by psychiatry. Together, notions of serious criminality and high risk rely on historically established ideas of undesirability based on eugenic and racial positions that were entrenched beginning with the 1906 Immigration Act; established as prohibited classes in the 1910 Act Respecting Immigration; and advanced by leading psychiatrists, political figures, and public health experts (Helen MacMurchy and C.K. Clarke) that promoted ideas that mental illness, disease, and crime were bound to inferior immigrants, genetics, and races.[30] These ideas continue to operate to ensure a depiction of a person is sufficiently dehumanized to justify any violence done to them. They are considered outside of humanitarian considerations, discursively described in fixed, unchanging terms of threat, deficit, and lack and are often positioned as undeserving because of foreignness or defectiveness.

The NCR Act also, through its revisions of "a significant threat to the safety of the public" makes a person with mental health system involvement a national defence concern. This national concern by virtue of the new Anti-terrorism Act makes personal mental health information a piece of "evidence" to be shared among government and security personnel to limit permission to travel, to issue more recognizance conditions, or to act on a detention or removal order through a third party agent, such as the Canadian Security Intelligence Service or Citizenship and Immigration Canada. As a result, a foreigner with a mental health concern can be continuously monitored as a threat, found to be burdensome (the undeserving alien), and forcibly confined or deported from Canada or ordered to comply with forced psychiatric treatment without appeal or annual review and subject to the discretion of immigration and security officials.

The three laws operating together as a confluence represent the continuation of a racial and eugenic project of nation building that establishes the Other as threat and danger, inherently and biologically inferior, while simultaneously constituting in law the idea of "Canadian" citizens as those who strive to keep the public safe and secure. This "public," no matter how long a person has been in Canada, cannot be permeated, reconsidered, or reformed with the inclusion of foreign bodies. The three laws operating together also create situations that permit the criminalization of immigrants, racialized people, those deemed sexually deviant, and people identified with mental health issues within all policies and their corresponding institutions. This situation continues the consolidated eugenics and racial colonial project that established the prohibited classes of "Persons mentally defective," "Diseased persons," "Persons physically defective," "Criminals," "Prostitutes or pimps," "Procurers," "Beggars and vagrants," "Charity immigrants," and "Persons not complying with regulations."[31] However, it now does so under the guise of protection for "the Canadian public," an idea that (re)produces fabricated ideas that associate people of colour, immigrants, and people with mental health issues with criminality and biological defectiveness and targets these *undesirables* as undeserving of public support or care and deserving of the confluence of violence imposed upon them. This violence makes possible the practice reported in April 2015 that "forty per cent of Ontario inmates who were locked away in solitary confinement for 30 or more straight days – twice the limit permitted under the United Nations' Nelson Mandela Rules – suffered from mental health issues or other special needs."[32] It makes possible the use of the Central East Detention Centre for the imprisonment of immigrants and to isolate them from receiving help and support.[33] In general, it makes it possible that a person who has lived in Canada on average 20 years, has been receiving mental health support for on average for seven or eight years, but who is not a Canadian citizen can be found to be too high risk or be too prone to "serious criminality" to stay in Canada and can be deported to their country of origin regardless of any humanitarian considerations.[34]

These forms of violence have not gone without resistance or dispute. In 2013 a coalition of organizations and agencies formed to dispute or amend the NCR Reform Act, pointing out that "this legislation is trying to correct a problem that does not exist and the changes are not evidence-based."[35] The coalition stated that the Act perpetuated stigma surrounding mental illness. Also, in September 2013, 200 immigration detainees at the Central East Detention Centre staged a protest and hunger strike. The detainees had been refused access to family and legal counsel, subjected to frequent lockdowns, and refused recreation and endured a number of other violations of dignities and rights.[36]

In terms of Slavoj Žižek's framework of violence, we must understand the *subjective* violence of imprisonment of mind (through the application of mandatory conditions of forced psychiatry treatment, reporting requirements, and perpetual surveillance). This includes the use of dehumanizing language. We must also consider the *objective* violence in both of its forms and the *symbolic* violence that orchestrates meanings though language that (re)establish notions of someone who is inherently criminal, divorced of historical, social, or political context, and who is biologically inferior and thereby dangerous and untreatable. We must also consider the (re)establishment of the association among foreign bodies, threat, burden, and disease. *Systemically*, we must consider the day-to-day violence that occurs through the regular practice of our policy and laws as though they were designed separately and are acting in a fair manner. The outcome is the rationalization of the identification of people (mostly of colour) as violent because of mental health issues and a threat to Canadian society, and therefore undeserving of Canadian care or inclusion because of consideration for the Canadian public. The outcome is also the increased surveillance, confinement, and forced treatment of those deemed foreigners (86% of whom are from the global south) through the application of racial and eugenic ideas that are embedded within policy and law and thereby in the regular lived experience of immigrants in Canada.[37]

These examples of violence within policy and law are indications of violence within institutions, practised by professions, and congruent with the historical colonial technologies and practices of human hierarchy and division used to rationalize violence. By attending to and focusing together upon the technologies and practices of violence as a confluence (interdependent and working together historically and currently to achieve historical, imperial, and colonial project outcomes), it is less likely that individual components of violence will be considered without also perceiving the violence that sustains the perception that there is a normal peaceful state of affairs in Canada. Notions and ideas of the "peaceful, safe, Canadian" were forged through violent means and achieve violent ends through the establishment and *reinvocation* of practices of dehumanization that recreate the idea of the untreatable, the un-rehabilitatable criminal, and the undeserving alien. As a result, violence is legitimized through the imprisonment of minds and bodies of difference. If we refuse to rationalize the use of violence of any kind on any person, we perhaps will disarm the historical and contemporary systems and structures of violence that sustain the idea that violence can be done to one person while another remains at peace.

NOTES

1 Littlewood and Lipsedge, *Aliens and Alienists*, 33; Dowbiggin, *Keeping America Sane*.
2 Chadha, "'Mentally Defectives' Not Welcome"; Chan, "Crime, Deportation"; Joseph, *Deportation*.
3 McLaren, *Our Own Master Race*.
4 Ibid., 30.
5 Founder of the Co-operative Commonwealth Federation, former premier of Saskatchewan and first leader of the Canadian federal New Democratic Party. Widely lauded for his support for universal public health care.
6 McLaren, *Our Own Master Race*, 8.
7 Dowbiggin, *Keeping America Sane*.
8 See Chadha, "'Mentally Defectives' Not Welcome"; Joseph, *Deportation*.
9 *Immigration and Refugee Protection Act* (S.C. 2001, c. 27).
10 See Fanon, *The Wretched of the Earth*; Said, *Orientalism*; Memmi, *The Colonizer*; Césaire and Pinkham, *Discourse on Colonialism*; Spivak, "Can the Subaltern Speak?"; Joseph, *Deportation*.
11 Some of this section on Žižek's violence framework is covered in chapter 2 of Joseph, *Deportation*.
12 See Žižek, *Violence*, 2.

13 Ibid.
14 Ibid., 9.
15 Ibid., 11.
16 Ibid., 2.
17 *Faster Removal of Foreign Criminals Act*, SC 2013, c 16.
18 Ibid.
19 Ibid.
20 *Not Criminally Responsible Reform Act*, SC 2014, c 6.
21 Ibid.
22 See below from Criminal Code of Canada Bill C14 (*Not Criminally Responsible Reform Act*, SC 2014, c 6):

> (3) Section 672.5 of the Act is amended by adding the following after subsection (13.2): Notice to victims – referral of finding to court (13.3). If the Review Board refers to the court for review under subsection 672.84(1) a finding that an accused is a high-risk accused, it shall notify every victim of the offence that they are entitled to file a statement with the court in accordance with subsection.

23 Notice of discharge and intended place of residence:

> (5.2) If the accused is discharged absolutely under paragraph 672.54(*a*) or conditionally under paragraph 672.54(*b*), a notice of the discharge and accused's intended place of residence shall, at the victim's request, be given to the victim within the time and in the manner fixed by the rules of the court or Review Board.

24 See 672.541 and 672.542 of the Criminal Code of Canada, Bill C-14.
25 See 672.541 and 672.542 of the Criminal Code of Canada Bill, C-14.

> Significant threat to safety of public: 672.5401. For the purposes of section 672.54, a significant threat to the safety of the public means a risk of serious physical or psychological harm to members of the public – including any victim of or witness to the offence, or any person under the age of 18 years – resulting from conduct that is criminal in nature but not necessarily violent.

26 *Anti-terrorism Act*, 2015, SC 2015, c 20.
27 Ibid.
28 Ibid.
29 Dowbiggin, *Keeping America Sane*; McLaren, *Our Own Master Race*.
30 See Chadha, "'Mentally Defectives' Not Welcome"; Dowbiggin, *Keeping America Sane*; McLaren, *Our Own Master Race*.
31 "An Act Respecting Immigration [1910]."
32 White, "Documents Reveal."
33 Keung, "Immigration Detainees."
34 Joseph, *Deportation*.

35 Registered Nurses' Association of Ontario, "Resolution 5."
36 Keung, "Immigration Detainees."
37 See Joseph, *Deportation*, 147.

BIBLIOGRAPHY

Legislation

Anti-terrorism Act, SC 2015, c 20.
Faster Removal of Foreign Criminals Act, SC 2013, c 16.
Immigration and Refugee Protection Act, SC 2001, c 27.
Not Criminally Responsible Reform Act, SC 2014, c 6.

Secondary Sources

"An Act Respecting Immigration [1910]." Early Canadiana Online. 2017.
  Accessed December 23, 2013. http://eco.canadiana.ca/view/oocihm
  .9_07184/2?r=0&s=1.
Ashcroft, Bill, Gareth Griffiths, and Helen Tiffin. *Post-Colonial Studies: The Key
  Concepts*. Abingdon, UK: Routledge, 2013.
Césaire, Aimé, and Joan Pinkham. *Discourse on Colonialism*. Marlborough, UK:
  Adam Matthew Digital, 2007.
Chadha, Ena. "'Mentally Defectives' Not Welcome: Mental Disability in
  Canadian Immigration Law, 1859–1927." *Disability Studies Quarterly* 28, no. 1
  (2008): 1–30.
Chan, W. "Crime, Deportation and the Regulation of Immigrants in Canada."
  Crime, Law and Social Change: An Interdisciplinary Journal 44, no. 2 (2005):
  153–80.
Dowbiggin, Ian Robert. *Keeping America Sane: Psychiatry and Eugenics in the
  United States and Canada, 1880–1940*. Ithaca, NY: Cornell University Press,
  1997.
Fanon, Franz. *The Wretched of the Earth*. New York: Grove Press, 1965.
Foucault, Michel. *Madness and Civilization: A History of Insanity in the Age of
  Reason*. New York: Pantheon Books, 1965.
Joseph, Ameil J. *Deportation and the Confluence of Violence within Forensic Mental
  Health and Immigration Systems*. Basingstoke, UK: Palgrave Macmillan, 2015.
Keung, Nicholas. "Immigration Detainees in Lindsay Jail Stage Protest and
  Hunger Strike." *Thestar.com*, September 20, 2013. https://www.thestar

.com/news/immigration/2013/09/20/immigration_detainees_stage_
protest_and_hunger_strike.html.

Littlewood Roland, and Maurice Lipsedge. *Aliens and Alienists: Ethnic
Minorities and Psychiatry*. London, UK: Routledge, 1997.

McLaren, Angus. *Our Own Master Race: Eugenics in Canada, 1885–1945*.
Toronto, ON: Oxford University Press, 1990.

Memmi, Albert. *The Colonizer and the Colonized*. Boston, MA: Beacon Press,
1965.

Registered Nurses' Association of Ontario. "Resolution 5: Amend Bill C-54,
the Not Criminally Responsible Reform Act to Avoid Harm." Canadian
Nurses Association, 2013. https://www.cna-aiic.ca/~/media/cna/
page-content/pdf-fr/2013_resolution_5_e.pdf?la=en.

Said, Edward W. *Orientalism*. New York: Pantheon Books, 1978.

Spivak, Gayatri Chakravorty. "Can the Subaltern Speak?" In *Marxism and the
Interpretation of Culture*, edited by Lawrence Grossberg and Cary Nelson.
Chicago: University of Illinois Press, 1988.

White, Patrick. "Documents Reveal Troubling Details about Long-term
Solitary Confinement." *Globe and Mail*, April 24, 2016. https://
www.theglobeandmail.com/news/national/documents-reveal
-troubling-details-about-long-term-solitary-confiment/
article29746902/?cmpid=rss1.

Žižek, Slavoj. *Violence: Six Sideways Reflections*. New York: Picador, 2008.

12 The (Un)Writing of Risk on My Mad Pregnant Body: A *Mad* Feminist Political Economy Analysis of Social Reproduction and Epistemic Violence under Neo-liberalism

Introduction

While I write this, I am in the third trimester of my first pregnancy. As a Mad woman,[1] negotiating pregnancy has been an experience filled with joy, despair, anxiety, anger, and pride, as well as an overarching feeling of riskiness. Indeed, the one feeling permeating these last 38 weeks is an awareness that I am perceived, and perceive myself, as risky. In this short chapter I offer a feminist political economy analysis of the *epistemic violence* I have experienced in the *risky body* of a pregnant Mad woman living in Ontario, Canada, in neo-liberal times, proposing the need to *madden* the feminist political economy framework. By epistemic violence I mean "the violence done to people via particular knowledge claims,"[2] which Foucault links to the redefinition of sanity in the eighteenth century, but which is part of a broader production of the Other and the erasure of alternative forms of knowing and being central to the project of colonialism and ongoing practices of imperialism.[3] Specifically, in this case I am referring to the sanist processes involved in writing the Mad pregnant body as risky, but I recognize these as one element in the deepening of our collective dispossession in this late phase of capitalism. I am not offering here one prescription for change but attempting to make sense of my experiences with being coded as risky and to also make visible the ways in which I enact/ed this violence upon myself. In making sense of my own experiences with epistemic violence, I draw attention to and challenge the pervasive assumption that pregnant people with psychiatric diagnoses are risky and that our bodies are in need of close monitoring. This piece intervenes in, and seeks to disrupt in some small way, the processes involved in directing or limiting biological reproduction for the purpose of creating bodies and political subjectivities compatible with the (sanist) neo-liberal age.

As epistemic violence, writing the pregnant Mad body as risky through medicine and social policy is not the violence of physical abuse, experimentation, and sterilization so prevalent in the lives and histories of Mad people. It is violence nonetheless because the imposition of risk on the Mad pregnant person threatens to limit, and in many cases does limit, what spaces and roles we can occupy, and when, where, why, if, and how we reproduce. Moreover, the medical practices and social policies that simultaneously mark us as risky while limiting services and supports for pregnancy and child-rearing sometimes turns the pregnant Mad person into a tool of personal regulation, enacting this (often unseen) violence against themselves.

My Story

When I found out I was pregnant, I was initially excited. Then the feelings of anxiety and sadness crowded out the happiness, aggressively reasserting their status as the nucleus of my personality, that constant companion I had momentarily neglected. My anxiety was not related to the fear of an early term miscarriage, but that I, as a depressed, bulimic, and compulsive woman, would somehow hurt my fetus by self-harming, taking my meds, not taking my meds, or passing on my Mad traits through my genes or my behaviours. Gone from my mind were my tremendous efforts to minimize acts of self-harm, the community of people who support me, and the work I have done as a feminist and political economist to understand the social, political, and economic roots of Mad oppression. All of this gave way to the part of me that had been taught to think of myself as biologically and irrevocably broken. This was a part of me that I had arrogantly thought was long ago dealt with.

I had instead, however, allowed these feelings of pathology to be buried under my privilege. I am a white, cisgender, normatively physically abled graduate student in a heterosexual partnership who has a set of diagnoses and labels that run the gamut from common place and popularized (depressed) to glamorized (eating disordered). I have not fully metabolized my (past and current) experiences of pathologization because of the ease with which my privilege allows me to pass (much of the time) as "normal," to (often) avoid the biopsychiatric gaze, and to evade (for the most part) the medical and legal reach of Canada's mental health care systems.[4] My privilege allows me to avoid a great deal of the physical, structural, and symbolic violence Mad people experience.

Once pregnant, society's psychiatric gaze focused in on me in a new way, triggering that long buried, self-loathing part of my psyche, which shouts, "I am sick," "I will have a sick pregnancy and a sick fetus," and "If I survive this I will be a sick mother with a child just like me: sick." I was, and remain, terrified; taught through the fetishization and psychiatric pathologization of violent parents in the news and entertainment, as well as my own past experiences with mental health professionals, that there is a hidden switch inside me that just might be flipped on without warning. I began to think of myself in terms so prevalent in both psychiatry and in social policy: in terms of risk factors and riskiness.

At the same time, my insurance coverage for my psychotherapist and my medication was coming to an end. I felt I needed (free) support,[5] someone to help me deal with the fact that I felt like I was a risk to my fetus just by virtue of being me. Because of my perception that there is limited research on how selective serotonin reuptake inhibitors affect a fetus, I went off my meds and got a referral to a perinatal psychiatric outpatient program.[6] I now see a psychiatrist monthly. In our sessions, which last anywhere from 20 minutes to an hour, I am asked rapid fire about my eating (fine), my purging (pretty minimal), my anxiety (through the roof), if I am suicidal (no past attempts, no plans at the moment), my career (working on it and a major source of stress and self-loathing), my plans for maternity leave (I do not qualify for maternity benefits under Canada's employment insurance program), my wariness of the medical system (a conclusion drawn solely from my choice of midwife in lieu of obstetrician), if I have regrets about getting pregnant (occasionally), whether I want to go back on meds (I had a very bad bout of depression at about 20 weeks), if I will consider going back on my meds immediately after giving birth to fend off postpartum depression (not sure), and if I feel connected to and happy about the pregnancy (usually, life is stressful right now as I try to finish my PhD and find stable work).

When I am feeling good, the sessions are short, mostly, I suspect, because I refuse to take medication, and the doctor does not feel she has anything else to offer me. When I am raging, despairing, and stressed, when I am in the thick of it, I am asked if I want to take meds and am told that the exposure of a fetus to the chemistry of the depressed, anxious body may also cause problems. What I am being taught through this process of rapid monthly assessment is not how to navigate the social pressures on pregnant people, and, especially, pregnant Mad people, not how to look after myself and/or how to enjoy (to whatever extent possible) my pregnancy, but that pregnant Mad people like me are risky to themselves and the fetus, and, as I argue later, to the well-being of society as a whole.

And yet, I continue to go to these appointments because it's not all bad. My psychiatrist sometimes normalizes my anxiety and celebrates my victories. I have someone looking out for me who can prescribe medication and monitor the effects should the need arise. But in exchange for these services, I must accept the constant messaging that I, just by virtue of being me, pose a risk (by my behaviour or my genetics) to my fetus and, someday, to my child. To be a good and responsible person, parent, and citizen, I must be proactive about managing the risks I pose to my child and, by extension, to the well-being of a society that barely tolerates mad existence.

Turning to a psychiatrist was both a recognition that I need and want supports and an act of violence against myself. I am not trying to demonize my (or any) psychiatrist or dissuade any person from accessing whatever resources, strategies, or comforts perinatal psychiatric services or any medical or non-medical social services may offer. We, after all, must find ways to live in/with society. What I want to provide through the telling and analysing of my own story is a critique of the contemporary social, political, and economic processes through which Mad pregnant people are being constituted and read as risky. While modern forms of eugenics and the associated elimination of physical and mental diversity have been discussed, there is little analysis about how and why pregnant Mad (and disabled) bodies are read as risky and directed to internalize and self-manage those risks.[7] This issue merits attention, and the first step is to ask, how can we understand this phenomenon?

The "Social" Story

Before embarking on this discussion, however, I must address the issues of abuse and infanticide that beset the topic of mad reproduction and parenting. While the question of child welfare is very important, I have neither the space nor the expertise to untangle the complex intersection of behaviours that may bring harm to a fetus, or result in violence against children, and the psychiatric pathologization of these acts. Instead, what I want to deal with in this chapter are my own feelings of pathology, the treatment of me as risky because of my psychiatric diagnoses, and how I am coming to understand these feelings. I argue that the feelings of risk and pathology that surfaced during my pregnancy are not unique to me, nor can they be limited to my psychiatrist's office. My experiences are part of the insidious, often invisible, and self-directed limitations and disciplinary mechanisms imposed on Mad peoples' autonomy over our reproductive lives under neo-liberalism. This message of madness (as well as disability generally) as risk is visible in the shaming and criminalization of perinatal addiction, our collective fascination with and endless debate over the mental health of parents, and especially women, who kill their children, and the popularity of precautionary genetic testing.[8] This messaging, as I discovered during my doctoral research in Ontario, often supports such policy practices as a lack of high-support housing appropriate for families and the removal of children by the state.

To understand how Mad pregnant bodies have been constructed as risky, how they have become a subject of epistemic violence in this particular historical moment, we need a framework that contextualizes the social reading of Mad pregnant bodies as risky, and the demands that we take sole responsibility for and manage these risks, within the prevailing gendered arrangement of production for surplus, subsistence, and social reproduction. We need a Mad feminist political economy of social reproduction. To date, despite significant feminist and political economy scholarship about mental health and madness,[9] feminist political economists (and in particular scholars writing about social reproduction) have been fairly silent on mad issues.[10] Yet I argue that the theory of social reproduction can shed significant light on the neoliberal logic underpinning the social embedding of risk and undesirability onto Mad pregnant bodies.

Feminist Political Economy and Neo-liberalism

Feminist political economy is a theoretical approach or framework that challenges the neglect of sex and gender categories, norms, and roles in the broader field of political economy.[11] Specifically, feminist political economists analyse the organization, mobilization, and processes of legitimization of gender hierarchies and the sex/gender division of labour in capitalist production.[12] Put more simply, feminist political economists analyse how (ever-changing) sex and gender categories and norms and the associated division of labour between people labelled as men and women are perpetuated and serve the production of value through the exploitation of women, and especially working-class, poor, and racialized women.[13] Key to understanding how gender categorization and gendered exploitation serves the production of value is the concept of social reproduction.

Social reproduction is the deeply feminized and racialized paid and unpaid work of fulfilling bodily, emotional, and social needs that is necessary to the reproduction workers, future workers, people who do not work, and the social order necessary to capitalism. Social reproduction, under capitalism, contributes to the production of value through the consumption of the resources required by this socially necessary work, acquired through wage labour, state services, and community networks, and by performing this socially necessary work for free or for (typically) low wages.[14] Feminist political economists, therefore, seek to bring a gender analysis to political economy precisely because they understand the capitalist economy as comprising the interrelated processes of production for surplus and subsistence, as well as social reproduction, which is structured by the sex/gender division of labour.[15] In identifying the value of social reproduction, feminist political economists offer an analytic framework through which to unpack those policies, practices, and social norms that structure this socially necessary labour in historically and geographically contingent ways.

Under neo-liberalism, "the contested political rationality that weaves foundational commitments to market logics, individualization, economic calculations of efficiency, and multiple sites of authority into new public policies and regulatory fields and onto existing ones,"[16] public supports for social reproduction (e.g., early child care programs, funding for long-term-care facilities) are increasingly reduced or reorganized in a way that pushes this work into the private sector and, especially, onto the bodies of women.[17] As part of this privatization of responsibility for social reproduction, greater scrutiny is being exercised over the lives of those accessing remaining state supports.[18]

It is in this context we must theorize the ascription of riskiness to the Mad pregnant body. I argue that the constitution of the Mad pregnant body as risky is about limiting, or at least mitigating, the economic cost of individuals and families who might need to access social supports or who might (re)produce children who require supports. The welfare state, which in Canada includes psychiatric services, is one mechanism

that teaches us how to behave in a manner compatible with the prevailing economic ideology. States, often in cooperation with psychiatry,
have long advanced particular forms of social reproduction, and specifically biological reproduction, in an effort to maintain certain kinds
of social orders and populations (e.g., the mental hygiene movement
and natalist-style policies),[19] often using overtly violent tactics (e.g., the
sterilization of Mad, disabled, and racialized people).[20] The ascription
of risk to the Mad pregnant body that I experienced in Ontario under
neo-liberalism is part of this larger history.

Under neo-liberalism, Mad people who procreate (or are even perceived as able or desiring to procreate) are marked by the prevailing
social, political, and economic configuration as risky gestators and
future parents, because we are presumed unable to look after ourselves
and our children, and because we might pass on our "defects" to future
generations. This riskiness is directly linked to the *perception* that Mad
people are unable to participate in the labour market and perform
the tasks associated with social reproduction independent from ever-
declining public supports. Ignored are the experiences of workplace
inaccessibility, discrimination, and high rates of precarious employment among people labelled as disabled underpinning historical and
ongoing exclusions from, and marginalization within, the processes of
production.[21]

In my experience in Ontario, the mental health care and welfare-
state system is not stepping in to help us navigate this imposition of
riskiness on our bodies, but is rather enacting this epistemic violence
by teaching us to avoid the risks of procreation or at least that we must
assume sole responsibility for the risks we pose to our children and to
the future of society. At the same time, supports for social reproduction are being eliminated whenever possible while, as stated, public
scrutiny of pregnant bodies is articulated through the organization
of social service provisioning (e.g., Ontario's Family Risk Assessment
Descriptors Neglect Index[22]) and in public attitudes towards people
with mental illness labels, particularly those who are poor, racialized,
or disabled.[23] In many ways the very social services, although meagre,
that provide some of the necessary resources for social reproduction
to many people are the same services that enact "riskiness" on our
bodies.

The embedding of riskiness and limitations imposed on the Mad
pregnant body is not separate from the removal of children from poor,
racialized, or Indigenous families or from the public shaming of lone

parents accessing state-funded services. Each of these groups experience epistemic violence via discursive and policy mechanisms that cast them as undesirable reproducers while at the same time contending with a form of social reproduction that involves little state support and much individual responsibility, thus dissuading certain kinds of biological reproduction. In this way, the epistemic violence visible in the inscription of risk on (and sometimes by) Mad pregnant bodies is part of a broader attack on the ability of all people to exercise reproductive autonomy and to survive and thrive.

NOTES

1 I use the term "Mad" to refer to anyone with mental diversity, psychiatric diagnoses, experiences or identities that are constructed as "mental illness." See discussion in Reville, "Is Mad Studies Emerging"; Shimart, "The Tragic Farce."

2 Lefrançois, Menzies, and Reaume, *Mad Matters*, 336.

3 Spivak, "Can the Subaltern Speak?"

4 Mental health care in Canada is developed and administered by the provinces and territories, meaning there are 13 distinct systems.

5 Psychiatric treatment in Canada is covered by provincial and territorial health insurance programs.

6 My experience was one where the available research was very limited because of the difficulty of conducting clinic trials with pregnant people. For more information on lack of research, see Canadian Women's Health Network, "Taking SSRI Antidepressants."

7 Tremain, "Reproductive Freedom"; Rock, "Eugenics and Euthanasia," 126.

8 See recent research on the regulation of pregnant bodies in relation to drug and alcohol use, for example, Stone, "Pregnant Women," and the focus on reproductive technologies and pressures on parents to prevent disability, for example, in Karpin and Savell, *Perfecting Pregnancy*.

9 See for example Diamond, "Feminist Resistance"; Morrow, "Mental Health Reform"; Moncrieff, "Neo-liberalism and Biopsychiatry"; Wilton, "More Responsibility, Less Control."

10 See major texts on feminist political economy and social reproduction such as Bakker and Gill, *Power, Production, and Social Reproduction*; Bezanson, *Gender*; Bezanson and Luxton, *Social Reproduction*; LeBaron and Roberts, "Toward a Feminist Political Economy"; Rioux, "Embodied Contradictions."

11 Vosko, "The Past."
12 Luxton, "Feminist Political Economy."
13 Ibid., 36; Arat-Koc, "Whose Social Reproduction?"
14 Bezanson, "The Neo-liberal State," 175; Cameron, "Social Reproduction,"
    45; Laslett and Brenner, "Gender and Social Reproduction"; Bakker and
    Gill, "Ontology," 17–18.
15 Vosko. *The Past*, 59–60, 75; Cameron, "Social Reproduction," 46.
16 Brodie, "Canadian Family Policy," 1588.
17 LeBaron, "The Political Economy," 903.
18 Chouinard and Crooks, "'Because They Have All the Power'"; Vosko,
    Temporary Work, 238; McKeen and Porter, "Politics and Transformations,"
    115–17.
19 Dickinson, "Scientific Parenthood"; Caldwell, Caldwell, and McDonald,
    "Policy Responses."
20 Roberts, *Killing the Black Body*, 66–7.
21 Tompa et al., "Precarious Employment."
22 Ontario Ministry of Children and Youth Services, "Ontario Family Risk
    Assessment."
23 Although I chose to focus on Mad pregnant bodies, the ascription of
    riskiness is not limited to Mad pregnant people. Indeed, non-Mad
    pregnant people and parents whose behaviour is considered to be
    "outside" of the deeply classed, raced, and gendered model of the "good
    pregnant person" are also seen as risky gestators and reproducers and
    experience pathologization and control but this issue merits interrogation
    and analysis beyond the scope of this chapter.

BIBLIOGRAPHY

Arat-Koc, Sedef. "Whose Social Reproduction? Transnational Motherhood and
    Challenges to Feminist Political Economy." In *Social Reproduction: Feminist
    Political Economy Challenges Neo-liberalism*, edited by Kate Bezanson and Meg
    Luxton, 75–92. Montreal, QC: McGill-Queen's University Press, 2006.
Bakker, Isabella, and Stephen Gill. "Ontology, Method and Hypotheses." In
    *Power, Production, and Social Reproduction: Human Insecurity in the Global
    Political Economy*, edited by Isabella Bakker and Stephen Gill, 17–41.
    Basingstoke, UK: Palgrave Macmillan, 2003.
Bakker, Isabella, and Stephen Gill, eds. *Power, Production, and Social
    Reproduction: Human Insecurity in the Global Political Economy*. Basingstoke,
    UK: Palgrave Macmillan, 2003.

Bezanson, Kate. *Gender, the State and Social Reproduction: Household Insecurity in Neo-liberal Times.* Toronto, ON: University of Toronto Press, 2006.

Bezanson, Kate. "The Neo-liberal State and Social Reproduction: Gender and Household Security in the Late 1990s." In *Social Reproduction: Feminist Political Economy Challenges Neo-liberalism,* edited by Kate Bezanson and Meg Luxton, 173–214. Montreal, QC: McGill-Queen's University Press, 2006.

Bezanson, Kate, and Meg Luxton, eds. *Social Reproduction: Feminist Political Economy Challenges Neo-liberalism.* Montreal, QC: McGill-Queen's University Press, 2006.

Brodie, Janine. "Canadian Family Policy and the Omissions of Neo-liberalism." *North Carolina Law Review* 88, no. 5 (2010): 1559–92.

Caldwell, John C., Pat Caldwell, and Peter Mcdonald. "Policy Responses to Low Fertility and Its Consequences: A Global Survey." *Journal of Population Research* 19, no. 1 (2002): 1–24.

Cameron, Barbara. "Social Reproduction and Canadian Federalism." In *Social Reproduction: Feminist Political Economy Challenges Neo-liberalism,* edited by Kate Bezanson and Meg Luxton, 45–74. Montreal, QC: McGill-Queen's University Press, 2006.

Canadian Women's Health Network. "Taking SSRI Antidepressants during Pregnancy: Considerations and Risks." Accessed April 29, 2016. http://www.cwhn.ca/en/node/42353.

Chouinard, Vera, and Valerie Crooks. "'Because They Have All the Power and I Have None': State Restructuring of Income and Employment Supports and Disabled Women's Lives in Ontario, Canada." *Disability and Society* 20, no. 1 (2005): 19–32.

Diamond, Shaindl. "Feminist Resistance against the Medicalization of Humanity." In *Psychiatry Disrupted: Theorizing Resistance and Crafting the (R)evolution,* edited by Bonnie Burstow, Brenda Lefrançois, and Shaindl Diamond, 194–207. Montreal, QC: McGill-Queen's University Press, 2014.

Dickinson, Harley. "Scientific Parenthood: The Mental Hygiene Movement and the Reform of Canadian Families, 1925–1950." *Scientific Journal of Comparative Family Studies* 24, no. 3 (1993): 387–402.

Karpin, I., and K. Savell. *Perfecting Pregnancy – Law, Disability and the Future of Reproduction.* New York, NY: Cambridge University Press, 2012.

Laslett, Barbara, and Johanna Brenner. "Gender and Social Reproduction: Historical Perspectives." *Annual Review of Sociology* 15 (1989): 381–404.

LeBaron, Genevieve. "The Political Economy of the Household: Neo-liberal Restructuring, Enclosures, and Daily Life." *Review of International Political Economy* 17, no. 5 (2010): 889–912.

LeBaron, Genevieve, and Adrienne Roberts. "Toward a Feminist Political Economy of Capitalism and Carcerality." *Signs* 36, no. 1 (2010): 19–44.

Lefrançois, Brenda, Robert Menzies, and Geoffrey Reaume, eds. *Mad Matters: A Critical Reader in Canadian Mad Studies*. Toronto, ON: Canadian Scholars' Press, 2013.

Luxton, Meg. "Feminist Political Economy in Canada and the Politics of Social Reproduction." In *Social Reproduction: Feminist Political Economy Challenges Neo-liberalism*, edited by Kate Bezanson and Meg Luxton, 11–44. Montreal, QC: McGill-Queen's University Press, 2006.

McKeen, Wendy, and Ann Porter. "Politics and Transformations: Welfare State Restructuring in Canada." In *Changing Canada: Political Economy as Transformation*, edited by Wallace Clement and Leah Vosko, 109–43. Montreal, QC: McGill-Queen's University Press, 2003.

Moncrieff, Joanna. "Neo-liberalism and Biopsychiatry: A Marriage of Convenience." In *Liberatory Psychiatry: Philosophy, Politics, and Mental Health*, edited by Carl I. Cohen and Sami Timimi, 235–55: Cambridge, UK: Cambridge University Press, 2008.

Morrow, Mariana. "Mental Health Reform, Economic Globalization and the Practice of Citizenship." *Canadian Journal of Community Mental Health* 23, no. 2 (2004): 39–50.

Ontario Ministry of Children and Youth Services. "Ontario Family Risk Assessment Descriptors Neglect Index." In *Ontario Child Protection Tools Manual*, 33–7. Toronto, ON: Ontario Ministry of Children and Youth Services, 2016.

Reville, David. "Is Mad Studies Emerging as a New Field of Inquiry?" In *Mad Matters: A Critical Reader in Canadian Mad Studies*, edited by Brenda Lefrançois, Robert Menzies, and Geoffrey Reaume, 170–80. Toronto, ON: Canadian Scholars' Press, 2013.

Rioux, Sebastian. "Embodied Contradictions: Capitalism, Social Reproduction and Body Formation." *Women's Studies International Forum* 48 (2015): 194–202.

Roberts, Dorothy. *Killing the Black Body: Race, Reproduction, and the Meaning of Liberty*. New York: Pantheon Books, 1997.

Rock, Patricia. "Eugenics and Euthanasia: A Cause for Concern for Disabled People, Particularly Disabled Women." *Disability and Society* 11, no. 1 (1996): 121–7.

Shimart, Irit. "The Tragic Farce of Community Mental Health Care." In *Mad Matters: A Critical Reader in Canadian Mad Studies*, edited by Brenda Lefrançois, Robert Menzies, and Geoffrey Reaume, 144–57. Toronto, ON: Canadian Scholars' Press, 2013.

Spivak, Gayatri. "Can the Subaltern Speak?" In *Marxism and the Interpretation of Culture*, edited by Cary Nelson and Lawrence Grossberg, 271–313. Urbana: University of Illinois Press, 1988.

Stone, R. "Pregnant Women and Substance Use: Fear, Stigma, and Barriers to Care." *Health and Justice*, 3. no 2 (2015): 1–15.

Tompa, Emile, Heather Scott, Scott Trevithick, and Sudipah Bhattacharyya. "Precarious Employment and People with Disabilities." In *Precarious Employment: Understanding Labour Market Insecurity in Canada*, edited by Leah Vosko, 90–114. Montreal, QC: McGill-Queen's University Press, 2006.

Tremain, Shelley. "Reproductive Freedom, Self-Regulation, and the Government of Impairment in Utero." *Hypatia* 21, no. 1 (2006): 35–53.

Vosko, Leah. "The Past, Present (and Futures) of Feminist Political Economy in Canada: Reviving the Debate." *Studies in Political Economy* 68 (Summer 2002): 55–83.

Vosko, Leah. *Temporary Work: The Gendered Rise of a Precarious Employment Relationship*. Toronto, ON: University of Toronto Press, 2000.

Wilton, Robert. "More Responsibility, Less Control: Psychiatric Survivors and Welfare State Restructuring." *Disability and Society* 19, no. 4 (2004): 371–85.

13 Uncovering Law's Multiple Violences at the Inquest into the Death of Ashley Smith

C. TESS SHELDON, KAREN R. SPECTOR, AND
MARY BIRDSELL

Introduction

We consider here the structural violence enacted by legal, correctional, and psychiatric institutions on psychiatrized incarcerated women.[1] Ashley Smith resisted against the multiple violences enacted against her. Ashley was 19 years old when she died in a segregation cell at Grand Valley Institution in Ontario, Canada. She had been in prison for five years, almost the entire time in solitary confinement. We draw, in particular, on our role as counsel for the Empowerment Council (EC) at the inquest into her death.

EC is an autonomous, member-run body that represents recipients and former recipients of mental health and/or addiction services, including those with experiences of the correctional systems. It engages in outreach, education, community development, and systemic advocacy through law reform and litigation. As a party at the inquest into Ashley Smith's death, EC brought the unique voice of consumer/survivors of the psychiatric system who have been physically restrained, involuntarily detained, medicated without their consent, subjected to invasive searches, and secluded. EC's purpose at the inquest was to advocate for recommendations that supported community integration, since the diversion of psychiatrized incarcerated women out of the correctional system and into the psychiatric system cannot serve as a panacea. In fact, the mental health system also failed Ashley Smith.

We are exceedingly grateful to Jennifer Chambers, Lisa Walter, and Robert Cardish for many things, significantly for their willingness to relate their powerful experiences in work and life.

We define law's violence structurally, rather than reducing it to an individual issue. Our purpose is to broaden contextual understandings of the violence manifest in the lives of people who have had contact with the correctional, legal, and psychiatric systems. We pay particular attention to three modes of violence relevant to Ashley's life and death, as well as our experience at the inquest into her death: (1) law is directly violent by reproducing power imbalances, (2) law's implementation failures perpetuate that violence, and (3) law can violently work to silence the voices of psychiatrized people by failing to recognize lived experience as expertise and by denying the expertise that people with lived experience may have.

Ashley's Life and Death

Ashley Smith was first arrested when she was 14. She spent about four years in the youth justice system in New Brunswick. When she turned 18, Ashley was transferred into the custody of the Correctional Service of Canada (CSC). Immediately upon entry to the federal system, Ashley was placed on segregation status and maintained that status for most of her time under federal jurisdiction.

Ashley was never provided with a comprehensive mental health assessment or an appropriate treatment plan that addressed her needs. There was no consideration of the compounding impact of her solitary confinement on her mental health. While in the custody of CSC, she was transferred 17 times between eight institutions (three federal penitentiaries, two treatment facilities, two external hospitals, and one provincial correctional facility). During one transfer, Ashley was duct-taped to the seat of an airplane with a "spit hood" over her head. In March 2007, Ashley was assaulted by a correctional officer at the Regional Psychiatric Centre, which prompted another transfer.

Ashley had a history of self-harm. She secreted objects, like ligatures and pieces of glass, in her body cavities. Federal correctional staff were directed by management to not engage with Ashley during her self-harming behaviour, since it was characterized as "attention seeking." On three occasions, Ashley was admitted involuntarily to Grand River Hospital in Kitchener, Ontario, pursuant to Ontario's Mental Health Act. Ashley died on October 19, 2007, at the Grand Valley Institution for Women, in Kitchener, Ontario, strangled by a ligature as correctional officers videotaped but did not intervene.

An inquest into Ashley's death was initially scheduled to begin in 2010 but was terminated in 2011. A new inquest into Ashley's death was called in September 2012 with Dr John Carlisle presiding as coroner. The scope of the inquest was expanded to include all of Ashley's detention in the federal system. On September 24, 2012, EC was granted standing as a party to the inquest.[2]

The inquest jury of five women heard from 83 witnesses over 11 months. As a party to the inquest, EC proposed to call three experts. EC was only permitted to call Dr Robert Cardish, a psychiatrist at the Centre for Addiction and Mental Health (CAMH) working with people who self-harm. He testified that controlling and punitive responses to self-harm by institutions, including mental health facilities and correctional institutions, inevitably reinforce the very behaviour they are trying to stop. He testified that the most important element of treatment is the creation of a relationship to support the identification of the underlying reasons for self-harming behaviour. He testified that such a relationship could be made while self-harm continued, contrary to the view taken by the CSC that Ashley's self-harm needed to stop before she could receive any support. Warmth and connection are integral components of treatment whereas isolation may perpetuate abuse.

EC sought to dissuade the jury from making recommendations that presumed that the psychiatric system is an alternative or adjunct to the criminal system. EC argued that the tools that are used to address self-harm in the criminal system, including restraints, seclusion, and coercion, are also used in psychiatric detention. Diverting Ashley to the psychiatric system would not have served as a panacea to resolving all of the failings of the correctional system. EC recommended that CSC move women who self-harm into the community as soon as possible on the basis that offenders with disability-related needs have better outcomes in the community.

On December 19, 2013, the jury concluded that Ashley's death was a homicide and delivered 104 recommendations aimed at preventing future deaths in similar circumstances. Some of those recommendations drew from EC's proposals:

- that persons with lived experience contribute to CSC's training about restraints (Recommendation 91);
- that an independent rights adviser/inmate advocate be responsible for advising all incarcerated persons about the use of restraints, consent to treatment, and seclusion (Recommendations 73–75);

- that CSC move to a restraint-free environment (Recommendations 38*ff*);
- that decision making about the clinical management and interventions of incarcerated persons with mental health issues be made by clinicians in consultation with the incarcerated person, rather than by security management and staff (Recommendation 19); and
- that a mental health professional visit all incarcerated persons in seclusion daily, including to "assess ... the inmate's tolerance to segregation" (Recommendation 32).[3]

Violence Directed at Ashley

Law is made by those with power. The law defaults to the interests of those with more power, exacerbating entrenched patterns of inequality.[4] Prisons are "inherently violent" and "their primary purpose is the infliction of pain and exclusion."[5] CSC's law-like rules permit the use of solitary confinement, restraint, and non-consensual searches. CSC's culture of "lawlessness and inhumanity" means that prisoners are repeatedly subject to punitive measures, amounting to "incarcerat[ion] *as* punishment, not *for* punishment."[6]

Law's violent reproduction of power imbalances is affected in part by its failure to consider what underlies the social context of incarceration. Prisons, for example, "are designed to "disappear" people, along with the social problems that put them there."[7] By using violent, physically punitive means to attempt to control Ashley's behaviour, the law through CSC created or compounded Ashley's mental-health-related needs. That is, the very act of imprisonment has "severe mental health repercussions."[8] Including because of its impact on mental health, long-term solitary confinement may be considered to be abusive or a form of torture.[9]

Seclusion and Restraint

The conditions of Ashley Smith's confinement were oppressive. She lived in secure isolation and sensory deprivation. She was often given no clothing other than a smock. She had no mattress and no blanket, and slept with the lights on.[10] She was the subject of over 150 security incidents,[11] which sometimes resulted in the application of restraints, at times contrary to existing CSC policy.[12] She was also subjected to chemical restraints to manage her behaviour. Medication was used where it was "not clinically warranted" and without appropriate medical oversight.[13]

CSC's reliance on solitary confinement is directly violent. Solitary confinement is a "risk factor for suicide"[14] and "can create mental illness where none previously existed, or exacerbate pre-existing illness."[15] In 2012, the United Nations Human Rights Committee Against Torture stated that Canada should "abolish the use of solitary confinement for persons with serious or acute mental illness."[16] The jury cited the United Nations Special Rapporteur's 2011 *Interim Report on Solitary Confinement* to recommend the prohibition of solitary confinement of more than 15 days.[17] Nevertheless, in its *Response to the Inquest Touching the Death of Ashley Smith*, CSC found that it was "unable to fully support" the jury's recommendations about solitary confinement.[18]

EC's recommendations were directed at ensuring that the jury understood that patients are segregated and restrained in psychiatric settings. EC pointed to the inquest into the death of Jeffrey James as an example.[19] EC also recommended that CSC consult with external partners, including persons with lived experience, towards the goal of a restraint-free environment. The jury agreed and recommended that "CSC move toward a restraint-free environment by implementing a least restraint policy."[20]

Searches

The authority of health care providers to perform body cavity searches was also relevant to the inquest. Ashley was certified pursuant to Ontario's Mental Health Act on a number of occasions, often effected for the purpose of forcing her to undergo body cavity searches in order to remove ligatures used for self-harm.[21] Ashley was searched on three occasions at Grand River Hospital. After the body cavity search was conducted, Ashley returned to the prison. She was voluntarily admitted to hospital.

At the inquest, EC raised questions about Ashley's consent to the searches. A hospital cannot search a person in the normal course unless there is an admission. A voluntary patient must consent to a search of the body.[22] An involuntarily admitted patient may be searched without consent only if there are "reasonable and probable" grounds to believe an illegal or a contraband item exists.[23] Reasonable grounds cannot include a "suspicion"[24] and are different from the criteria for involuntary admission.

The jury recommended that body cavity searches only occur with the woman's consent or in "exceptional circumstances in the absence of consent."[25] The jury further clarified that all examinations should be "performed by a licensed medical professional at an external medical facility in a manner most compatible with the inherent dignity of the inmate."[26] In its response, the CSC is silent on the jury's recommendation about body cavity searches.[27] As set out in the next section, CSC's failure to enforce the jury's recommendations perpetuates additional violence.

Violence of Neglect to Adopt Trauma-Informed Approaches

CSC's response to Ashley's struggles was to confine her longer, in ever more barren circumstances. Even though CSC management was aware of Ashley's conditions of confinement, no one ensured that she was treated in a humane and lawful manner.[28] Pollack points to CSC's "violence of neglect":

> Ethical and human rights violations may occur not only as a result of overt participation in violence, such as the interrogation of military prisoners, but as a result of "the violence of neglect" ... *Certain imprisoned groups may be more susceptible to the inaction or neglect of the authorities, such as Indigenous people, women, and those with mental health issues.*[29]

EC highlighted the trauma of Ashley's confinement, including management's refusal to permit correctional staff to build a relationship with Ashley. The "treatment" offered to Ashley was to "withhold warmth" and companionship, even to the point of watching her die alone in her cell. EC emphasized the effects of trauma, and the value of programs, spaces, and policies that place priority on trauma survivors' safety, dignity, choice, and control.[30] CSC's violent failure to adopt trauma-informed approaches is also enacted in psychiatric settings:

> The culture of psychiatric hospitals has been such that strong emotions are often treated as symptoms that must be contained. People showing strong feelings can even end up restrained, sometimes a trauma in itself.[31]

The jury adopted EC's proposed recommendation that CSC provide a broad range of trauma-informed supports.[32] Institutional treatment teams are to develop management plans that take into account past experiences of trauma, and the potentially traumatic effects of being incarcerated, segregated, or restrained.[33] The jury supported EC's recommendations that CSC staff should be trained in providing trauma-informed care to federally sentenced women who may have experienced trauma during their detention.[34] In its response, CSC baldly asserted that correctional programs already "delivered to women offenders are trauma-informed and women-centered."[35]

In general terms, the legal process and procedure did not respond to Ashley's resistance against the injustices perpetrated against her. Legislative safeguards requiring thorough, timely, independent reviews of her solitary confinement were not met. Her grievances about the conditions of her detention were inadequately addressed. Indeed, CSC did not open the last of her seven complaints until two months after her death.[36] Ashley's life and death illustrates the law's violent impact on psychiatrized incarcerated women. In contrast with the psychiatric evidence put forward at the inquest, EC sought to establish that any mental-health-related needs that Ashley may have had were inextricably linked to the way she had been treated in the prison system.

CSC's Violent Rejection of the Jury's Recommendations

CSC's violent rejection of the jury's recommendations further perpetuates in death the violence that Ashley experienced during her life. Without recognition and implementation of the recommendations made after hearing from 83 witnesses over almost a year of testimony, the violence enacted against Ashley, and defended as "necessary," is reproduced.

During the inquest, CSC "did everything they [could] to shield prisons from criticism."[37] About CSC's "bunker" mentality, Moore pointed to CSC's repeated attempts to block evidence about Ashley's maltreatment. For example, CSC objected to the bringing into evidence video footage of the airplane transfer where Ashley was duct-taped to the seat, and another depicting Ashley being repeatedly given forced injections of medication as she is physically restrained on a gurney by both straps and several guards.[38] Rather than resolving to address the "deep and longstanding problems with the structures of punishment," the CSC's "wagons were quickly circled."[39]

Law's Violence Is out of Sight

The law works through multiple channels, beyond legislation and court decisions. Law is enacted and implemented informally by organizations, like the CSC, which enact their own "law-like organizational rules." In that way, the law operates behind closed doors and beyond accountability. Law's violence is also obscured by its slow operation. Law's violence is, at times, elusive and invisible, and its obscurity and incremental nature perpetrate violence. We draw on the concept of "slow violence" from environmental law scholarship about the "elusive violence of delayed effects":

> Slow violence ... is a "violence that occurs gradually, and out of sight, a violence of delayed destruction that is dispersed across time and space, an attritional violence that is typically not viewed as violence at all." ... Instead, slow violence is incremental and accretive, and it jumbles expected connections between spatial and temporal scales.[40]

Similarly, the law's operation is obscured by the disjuncture between law on the books and law in practice. Critical accounts of the law abound with references to law's "everyday indeterminacy."[41] A law may be "positive on paper" while in practice fall short because of a "lack of monitoring and accountability mechanisms."[42] The dissonance between law on the books and law in action is also the subject of mental disability law scholarship.[43] Ontario routinely fails to enforce legal protections owed to persons involved in the psychiatric system.[44] The significant protections in Ontario's Mental Health Act are "often neglected or intentionally avoided in the day-to-day operation of hospitals."[45]

CSC's Refusal to Implement the Jury's Recommendations

The jury recommended that the auditor general review the CSC's response to the recommendations.[46] The auditor general had refused to comment on its plans.[47] There are open questions about the authority, ability, or willingness of the Coroner's Office and the auditor general to monitor, implement, and enforce inquest recommendations. The Coroner's Office lacks the resources to monitor compliance and has no authority to enforce them.

The CSC delayed its response to the jury's recommendations. When it did respond, the CSC rejected most of the recommendations made by the jurors.[48] In particular, CSC rejected recommendations to limit the use of solitary confinement and refused independent oversight.[49] Because the jury's recommendations are not binding, CSC has no requirement or incentive to implement the recommendations. These implementation failures perpetuate additional structural violence:

> A regime of government crime policy predicated on mass incarceration continues, so a rebellious teenage girl who persists in committing very minor offences and not complying with rules set by guards remains at least as likely as today to face the same escalating series of charges as Smith did in 2007."[50]

Political pressures influence the implementation of jury recommendations. There are emergent questions about the federal government's willingness to implement recommendations from the inquest regarding the restriction of the use of solitary confinement and the treatment of those with mental health issues.[51] A mechanism to oversee the responsiveness to or enforcement of jury recommendations would alleviate reliance on the political pressures of the day to ensure their implementation.

The Failure to Implement Recommendations from Other Inquests

Tragically, the CSC's failure to implement the jury's recommendations following the inquest into the death of Ashley Smith is not unique. In 1996, in a Commission of Inquiry into certain events at the Prison for Women in Kingston, Ontario, Madame Justice Louise Arbour provided a "scathing critique" regarding the exercise of discretionary power in Canadian prisons, where she condemned "the wanton disregard for prisoners' rights."[52] Kinew James died in a federal prison in 2013, under similar conditions as Ashley, and Bobby Lee Worm, a young Aboriginal woman, was held in solitary confinement for more than three and a half years.[53] Prisons are almost never held to account for their actions "except in the most egregious of circumstances."[54]

In Ontario, there have been a number of coroner's inquests into the deaths of psychiatrized persons.[55] Recommendations from those inquests are not always effectively implemented.[56] Following the 2008 inquest into the death of Jeffrey James, the jury recommended that the coroner automatically hold an inquest whenever a patient dies in a psychiatric facility where physical restraints are used. This recommendation has yet to be adopted.[57] The inquest recommenda-tions following the police killing of Edmond Yu, a racialized man in crisis, were "almost identical" to the recommendations made less than five years prior, in response to the police killing of Lester Donaldson in 1998.[58] The recommendations from the Donaldson inquest were "never effectively implemented due to budget constraints, which contributed to the killing of Yu."[59] Since and including the Yu Inquest, EC has been granted standing at most inquests in Toronto involving police killings of persons with mental health issues. Following EC's participation, direct education by consumer-survivor organizations has been delivered to every uniformed officer in Toronto. Reliance on jury recommendations may improve the experience of persons with mental health issues, but implementation is not guaranteed.

Violent Failure to Recognize Lived Expertise

Here, we explore questions of violence, power, and authority inher-ent in the coroner's decision not to recognize the legitimacy of expert-witnesses with lived experience of the psychiatric system. This violence circumscribed the inquest's transformative potential. The integrity of the coroner's process required that the voices of those most directly affected be heard.

Epistemological Violence

The law operates to eradicate the voices of people marginalized by the law. Correctional practices rely on the "orthodoxy" of evidence, and lived experience is one of the "disqualified forms of knowing since they do not conform to the scientific standards."[60] These "silencing pro-cesses" make invisible the social contexts of people who have experi-enced criminalization and "leaves little if any room for self-definitions and conversations about racialization, poverty, the role of violence against women, and the violence of the state."[61] Epistemic violence includes the "eradication of perspectives and subjectivities of criminal-ized women."[62] Legal processes also disqualify psychiatrized people as "legitimate knowers" because they do not fit into the "boundaries of what is considered evidence."[63] Liegghio defined epistemic violence as the "very denial of a person's legitimacy as a knower – their knowledge and their ways of knowing – that renders that person out of existence, unable to be heard and to have their interest count."[64]

EC's Proposed Experts

EC was granted standing at the inquest because it was determined to have "expertise" and a "unique perspective" with respect to "issues of mental health care and in particular mental health care of inmates in the justice system and corrections *from the point of view of the actual patients/ inmates*."[65] EC proposed to call three experts to give evidence: Dr Robert Cardish is a senior psychiatrist at CAMH; Jennifer Chambers, coordinator of the EC, who works with individuals involved in the criminal justice and mental health systems; and Lisa Walter, a person with lived experience in the psychiatric system and who was proposed to be similarly situated to Ashley with respect to her experience in the psychiatric system.

On September 10, 2013, the coroner ruled that Dr Cardish would be permitted to testify as part of an expert panel with other psychiatrists. The coroner found that Jennifer Chambers's proposed evidence was not relevant to the scope and focus of the inquest, since it was "non-expert opinion of an advocate that the mental health system has problems."[66] In so ruling, the coroner disregarded the findings of previous coroners and juries who had found Chambers' evidence foundational for many recommendations ultimately adopted. No other inquest had denied the relevance of her testimony when she sought to testify. The coroner found that Lisa Walter's proposed evidence, which "includes an account of her own experience of self-harming behaviour and its management," was not relevant to the scope and focus of the inquest. He could not "find a basis for accepting the proposed witness as an expert in any field" and stated that Walters had "[n]o reported academic qualifications or degrees."[67] EC requested an evidentiary hearing.[68] The coroner heard EC's submissions and those of other parties with respect to EC's two proposed witnesses on September 18, 2013.

EC's Arguments in Support of Its Experts

EC argued that the most effective way to approximate the voice of the person who died is to hear directly from those who are impacted by the inquest's outcome. To EC, relevant "lived experience" is an example of expertise. People with relevant lived experience can hold an equally significant type of expertise as people who have completed formal education or have extensive work experience. The admissibility of expert evidence does not depend upon whether the expert's skill was derived from specific studies or practical training experience. Expertise flowing from lived experience provides a unique and unequalled window into and perspective regarding the experience, impact, and outcomes of the operations, practices, and systems that are being assessed. While evidence of the experience from the person who died is unavailable, that of those with similar and relevant lived experience will provide the best available evidence.

EC argued that the coroner's ruling appeared to presume that a "lack of academic qualifications" excludes someone from being recognized as an expert. *R v Mohan* set out the four-part test for the admissibility of expert testimony: relevance, necessity in assisting the trier of fact, the absence of any exclusionary rule, and a properly qualified expert.[69] *Mohan* sets out that expert evidence will be considered necessary if it provides information likely to be outside the knowledge or experience of a judge or jury.[70] In discussing the fourth requirement ("a properly qualified expert"), the Supreme Court further stated that decisions about "expertise" should not be solely based on academic credentials but also based on experience.[71] The *Mohan* criterion were further elaborated upon in *Dulong v Merrill Lynch Canada Inc.*, where Ducharme J. observed that a proposed expert witness' "special" or "peculiar" knowledge can be acquired in a variety of ways. Practical training can be the source of an expert's "special" knowledge: "one can acquire the necessary knowledge through formal education, private study, work experience or *other personal involvement with the subject matter.*"[72] Justice Ducharme referred to the "old hunter" example offered by Falconbridge C.J. in *Rice v Sockett*:

> The derivation of the term "expert" implies that he is one who by experience has acquired special or peculiar knowledge of the subject of which he undertakes to testify, *and it does not matter whether such knowledge has been acquired by study of scientific works or by practical observation.* Hence, one who is an old hunter, and has thus had much experience in the use of firearms, may be as well qualified to testify as to the appearance which a gun recently fired would present as a highly-educated and skilled gunsmith.[73]

Persons with lived experience have also been recognized as experts to give expert evidence about that experience. In *Lane v Adga Group Consultants Inc*, the Ontario Human Rights Commission proposed to call Philip Upshall to testify at the hearing. The Human Rights Tribunal of Ontario found that although Upshall did not have any academic or professional credentials, he was qualified as an expert based on his lived experience.[74]

In addition, lived experience does not render a proposed expert biased. EC argued that the coroner's ruling about the admissibility of evidence with respect to Chambers appeared to presume that direct experience with the group most affected rendered the proposed evidence biased or partial. In *R v RDS*, the Supreme Court held that a Black female judge's comments about interactions between police officers and "non-white" groups was not biased or even reasonably apprehended as biased. An individual's personal experience or direct experience with persons directly affected does not render them biased.[75] Rather, such personal understanding and experience can have the opposite effect, enhancing their credibility, impartiality, and ultimately their expertise.

Inquest juries regularly recommend the inclusion of persons with lived experience in their recommendations to direct various organizations to consult with persons with lived experience in the development of policies. In particular, in the inquest into the death of Mathew David Reid, 2010, the jury recommended that "the Ministry of Children and Youth Services, in consultation with youth with lived experience in the child welfare system, work with Children's Aid Societies to develop best practice guidelines that will enhance the voice of the child in all aspects of service delivery."[76] The coroner stated that the reason for this recommendation was that "the jurors ... felt that young people should be included in this process in recognition of the importance of providing them with a voice in their own affairs."[77] EC submitted that to allow a jury to make recommendations supporting the important role that person's with lived experience play in the development of policies on the one hand, yet exclude such evidence at the inquest undermined the true impact of any such recommendations.

On October 4, 2013, the coroner dismissed EC's applications to qualify Walter and Chambers as experts.[78] The decision failed to recognize the relevance of Chambers' long-standing advocacy, and the value of Walter's personal and powerful experience of the psychiatric system and of the impact of various responses to self-harming behaviour. As a result, EC faced challenges ensuring the inclusion of the voice and perspective of those most directly affected. There was no witness, among 83, who could provide evidence to the jury about what it is like to experience self-harming behaviour, seclusion, restraint, invasive searches, or other of the complex experiences that Ashley Smith endured. This epistemological violence circumscribed the inquest's potential to result in a full public airing of the issues and limited its transformative potential.

Collective Voices

EC pointed to the value of the courts' attention to the lived experience of psychiatrized persons. A legal analysis that is faithful to a claimant's "whole story" is more likely to yield a just remedy. Critical accounts of the law, including feminist legal scholarship, emphasize the importance of lived experience as a basis for critical knowledge.[79] Critical accounts of the law are concerned with the "lived experience" of the legal system including "everyday legal consciousness."[80]

In particular, EC pointed to the value of attention to the collective experience of psychiatrized persons, rather than individuals here and there who can represent only themselves. That is, lived experience cannot be calculated outside of complex social conditions and identities of members of marginalized communities. We acknowledge that any strategy must resist essentializing the Mad/psychiatric disability identity. We draw on feminist disability scholarship, which "aims to denaturalize disability" and invites exploration of the "intricate relation between bodies and selves [and] the social processes of identity formation."[81] Disability is a state of being experienced but not experienced in exactly the same ways.[82]

We remain alert to pitfalls of the deployment of lived experience of psychiatrized persons. EC has long fought for the inclusion of the voice of lived experience in mental health practice and policy development. While recent attention has been paid to the value of "user perspective," this has not always played out in practice.[83] The emergence of "peer workers" is an example of the co-opting of the language of lived experience. Davidow finds that peers that are hired by, directed by, and accountable to existing systems "set out to do atrocious things that hardly do more than replicate what has been done over and over throughout the years."[84] Pollack is also troubled by "gender sensitive" correctional practices, characterizing them as "strategies for "'managing' women in prison." Understandings of the "lived experience" of criminalized women have been "absorbed by correctional logics to support the prison industrial complex."[85]

Conclusion

We explored questions of violence, power, autonomy, and dependency that underlie the governance of psychiatrized incarcerated women. We paid particular attention to three modes of violence: (1) law is directly violent reproducing power imbalances, (2) law's implementation failures perpetuate that violence, and (3) law violently works to render invisible the voices of psychiatrized people by failing to recognize "lived experience" as expertise. Rather than reducing it to an individual issue, we have adopted a structural lens to examine the multiple violences enacted by legal, correctional, youth justice, and psychiatric systems on psychiatrized incarcerated women. Our attention is focused broadly on "structural violence."[86] We recognize the concern that a broad definition of *violence* may obscure the responsibility of individual actors. Instead, our ultimate purpose is to broaden understandings of violence including the "contextual determinants of that violence."[87]

Attention to the "contextual determinants of violence" in the lives of psychiatrized incarcerated women is necessary to avoid characterizing Ashley Smith as an outlier. Efforts to characterize Ashley's death as extraordinary act to shield the individual, collective, and social pains of imprisonment from public view. According to Shoshana Pollack, a refusal to see the "social disorder signified by mass incarceration" violently "sidestep[s] the question of why the state responds to abused women with punishment." She continues:

> Reorienting our focus to institutions, structures, ideologies, and practices
> of punishment that normalize prison as a response to social inequalities
> exposes the violence of imprisonment.[88]

Ashley should not be portrayed as uncomplicated. The CSC defended their treatment of Ashley as "necessary" because her self-harm required the special measures of restraint, isolation, and solitary confinement. In her life, Ashley was described as a "large tyrannical child"[89] and "incorrigible while incarcerated."[90] One witness at the inquest described her: "She was a big girl. She was aggressive. She was strong. She was combative."[91] Some reports assert that "not diagnosing Ashley as mentally ill was the problem" and assumed that Ashley's "mistreatment was because she was mentally ill."[92] However, those arguments "diminish the argument that Ashley's behaviours might have been intentionally resistant and/or coping behaviours in an intolerable situation."[93]

Alternative characterizations of Ashley include her "intentional resistance" to the conditions of her detention.[94]

In closing, we identify opportunities for action to remedy the law's violence.

- First, legal and policy work will continue to challenge the direct violence enacted by the CSC on psychiatrized incarcerated women, including by the application of environment, chemical, and physical restraints. Tragically, Ashley's experience was "hardly isolated."[95] The experiences of federally sentenced women form part of the basis of two separate constitutional challenges to the use of solitary confinement.[96]
- Second, additional advocacy will improve the enforceability of jury recommendations. Law reform strategies may include the Coroner's Office direct report to the Legislature.[97]
- Finally, further work should identify creative and coordinated ways to push decision makers to recognize the legitimacy of expert witnesses with lived experience.

EC brought to the inquest the unique perspective of people who have been physically restrained, involuntarily detained, medicated without their consent, subjected to invasive searches, and secluded. For Ashley, these experiences took place in both correctional and psychiatric settings. EC's purpose at the inquest was to draw attention to the fact that psychiatric settings are not always the ideal solution. Ashley was not a person to be fixed. Instead, the focus needs to be on the provision of individualized community-based supports and services. Further work will support the realization of inquests' potential to illuminate the dark places behind the high walls of the institutional systems governing psychiatrized incarcerated women.

NOTES

1 During the inquest proceedings, Tess Sheldon and Karen Spector were employed by Justice for Children and Youth.

2 *Smith (Re)*, 2012 CanLII 101203 (ON OCCO), https://canlii.ca/t/ghfw7 (September 24 2012), wherein the coroner found that EC had standing on the issues of "Criminal and corrections issues including use of, effects of, and alternatives to the use of restraints and seclusion for people in

distress," "The effects on mental health of being in a system where rights to consent and refuse to consent to treatment are in issue," and "How correctional officers can relate to persons with mental health issues."

3   *Smith (Re)*, 2013 CanLII 92762 (ON OCCO), https://canlii.ca/t/g7cqv [Verdict].
4   See Miles and Sunstein, "The New Legal Realism"; Silbey, "After Legal Consciousness," 323, comments: "Why do people acquiesce to a legal system that, despite its promises of equal treatment, systematically reproduces inequality?"
5   Brown, *The Culture of Punishment*, 138.
6   Moore, "Ashley Smith Case."
7   National Film Board, "Interactive Portrait."
8   Pedlar, Yuen, and Fortune, "Incarcerated Women and Leisure," 24.
9   Grassian, "Psychiatric Effects," 325.
10 Sapers, *A Preventable Death*.
11 A stark contrast to the persistent state of sensory deprivation, a security incident would often involve multiple correctional staff barging into her cell, sometimes in riot gear, to control a situation.
12 Sapers, *A Preventable Death*.
13 "Ashley Smith's Sedations."
14 Sapers, *A Preventable Death*.
15 British Columbia Civil Liberties Association, "Solitary Confinement Backgrounder."
16 UN Committee against Torture, "Consideration of Reports."
17 Verdict, *supra* note 3 at 27: "That, in accordance with the Recommendations of the United Nations Special Rapporteur's 2011 Interim Report on Solitary Confinement, indefinite solitary confinement should be abolished."
18 Correctional Services Canada, *Response to the Inquest Touching the Death of Ashley Smith*, December 2014, 8, CSC http://www.csc-scc.gc.ca/ publications/005007-9011-eng.shtml.
19 *James (Re)*: 2008 CanLII 89705, https://canlii.ca/t/fzs0n.
20 *Smith (Re)*, 2013 CanLII 92762 (ON OCCO), https://canlii.ca/t/g7cqv [Verdict] at "Recommendation 38."
21 Perkel, "Mental Health Act; according to testimony at the inquest, involuntary admission to psychiatric settings "was their way of getting a cavity search done."
22 Dykeman, "Search and Seizure."
23 Mohri, "Guidelines for Searching."
24 Psychiatric Patient Advocacy Office, "Searches: Person and Property," Toronto, ON: PPAO, January 2009.

25 *Smith (Re)*, 2013 CanLII 92762 (ON OCCO), https://canlii.ca/t/g7cqv [Verdict]: "exceptional circumstances will only exist when, "in the opinion of a physician, there is a risk of death or serious bodily harm to the inmate or another person and the risk cannot be mitigated through any other reasonably available means."

26 *Smith (Re)*, 2013 CanLII 92762 (ON OCCO), https://canlii.ca/t/g7cqv [Verdict]: "Correctional Service of Canada staff escorting the inmate to the external facility is to request that the examination be conducted by a female."

27 Correctional Services Canada, "Response."

28 Sapers, *A Preventable Death.*

29 Pollack, "An Imprisoning Gaze," 109 [emphasis added].

30 Chambers, "What Do Client Rights."

31 Chambers, "Addressing Trauma."

32 *Smith (Re)*, 2013 CanLII 92762 (ON OCCO), https://canlii.ca/t/g7cqv [Verdict], at 4.

33 Ibid., at 23.

34 Ibid., at 89.

35 Correctional Services Canada, "Response," 20.

36 Sapers, *A Preventable Death.*

37 Moore, "Ashley Smith Case."

38 Ibid.

39 Ibid.

40 Nixon, *Slow Violence.*

41 McEvoy, "A New Realism," 433: "Authors in this mode [of New Legal Realism] characteristically analyze law as it works in reciprocal interaction with adjacent realms of social experience. The environment in which they situate their analysis is in an active, causally potent one. Legal consciousness suffuses that environment, organizing people's thought, their behavior, and their culture."

42 Law Commission of Ontario, *Framework for the Law*, 1.

43 Perlin, "Half-Wracked Prejudice," 23: "There is a wide gap between law-on-the-books and law-in-action. There is probably such a gap in every area of the law. But here, the omnipresence of sanism and pretextuality make the gap even more problematic."

44 Bay, "Making the Law," 4.

45 Patton, "These Regulations," 29: "The law becomes what is practiced, what is allowed to occur and what goes without remedy."

46 *Smith (Re)*, 2013 CanLII 92762 (ON OCCO), https://canlii.ca/t/g7cqv [Verdict], at Recommendation 101: "That the Auditor General of Canada

conduct a comprehensive audit of the jury's recommendations and that the
results of such audit be released publicly in 2019–2020."

47 Wingrove, "Ottawa to Respond"; Kane, "Thousands of Inquest
Recommendations."

48 Stone, "December?"

49 Correctional Services Canada, "Response."

50 Bromwich, "Eight Years."

51 Fine and White, "Trudeau Calls for Ban."

52 Arbour, "Commission of Inquiry"; Moore, "Ashley Smith."

53 Webster, "Controls over Solitary Confinement Needed," E4. In his article,
Webster describes Bobby Lee Worm's mistreatment: "[holding] Bobby
Lee Worm, a 26-year-old Aboriginal woman from Saskatchewan who was
held in solitary confinement for more than three and a half years while in
federal prison, was illegal and inhumane. Worm was a first-time offender
and only 19 years old when she entered prison. Under the existing CSC
management program during her years in solitary confinement, she spent
up to 23 hours a day in a 10-by-8-foot cell. Prison officials released Worm
from the program two days after the BC Civil Liberties Association filed
her lawsuit" (109).

54 Moore, "Ashley Smith."

55 Mack, "Psychiatric Survivorst," 36.

56 Kane, "Thousands."

57 Mack, "Psychiatric Survivors," 60.

58 Ibid.

59 Mack, "The Mad and the Bad," 7: "As my discussion of the nine police
killings of Mad people following that of Yu will show, this tragedy is
ongoing, as many of the social policy and police training and conduct-
focused recommendations arising from the killing of Yu have also gone
unimplemented, and police have not been held accountable for their
violent and rights-depriving actions toward Mad people."

60 Pollack, "An Imprisoning Gaze."

61 Ibid., 111.

62 Ibid., 107: "The orthodoxy of evidence-based perspectives permeates
correctionalist approaches and proclaims one story of 'who' criminalized
women are and what they need to stop offending."

63 Ibid.

64 Liegghio, "Denial of Being," 124.

65 *Smith (Re)*, 2012 CanLII 101203 (ON OCCO), https://canlii.ca/t/ghfw7
(Standing Decision, September 24 2012) at 11 [emphasis added].

66 *Smith (Re)*, 2013 (ON OCCO), September 10, 2013: "I have not been given
anything to establish her formal expertise nor does the proposed evidence

seem to be more than the non-expert opinion of an advocate that the mental health system has problems."

67 *Smith (Re)*, 2013 (ON OCCO), September 10, 2013.

68 *Chief Coroner's Rules*, Rule 6.7(c).

69 *R v Mohan*, [1994] 2 SCR 9 at para. 17.

70 *Mohan*, at para. 22.

71 *Mohan*, at para. 27: "Finally the evidence must be given by a witness who is shown to have acquired special or peculiar knowledge through study or experience in respect of the matters on which he or she undertakes to testify."

72 *Dulong v Merrill Lynch Canada Inc.* 2006 CanLII 9146 (ON SC), (2006) 80 OR (3d) 378, [2006] OJ No 1146 at paras. 20 and 21 [emphasis added].

73 *Dulong*, at paras. 21–2. [emphasis added] citing *Rice v Sockett*, [1912] OJ No. 49, 27 OLR 410 (CA) at paras. 21–2.

74 *Lane v Adga Group Consultants Inc.*, 2007 HRTO 34 (CanLII).

75 *R v RDS*, [1997] 3 SCR 484 at para. 44: "This process of enlargement is not only consistent with impartiality, it may also be seen as its essential pre-condition."

76 *Reid (Re)*, 2010 CanLII 99953 (ON OCCO); See also *Youth (Re)*, 2011 CanLII 99634 (ON OCCO).

77 Ibid.

78 *Smith (Re)*, 2013 (ON OCCO), October 4, 2013: "Since I find that the evidence proposed is not relevant and thus not admissible, it is unnecessary to decide whether the "lived experience' does or can establish the proposed witness as an expert."

79 Abrams, "Feminist Lawyering," 378: "Women discovered that they were not alone in their feelings and that they were not crazy; but they also came to view their lived experience as a source of knowledge about the world."

80 Suchman and Mertz, "Toward a New Legal Empiricism," 555.

81 Garland-Thomson, "Feminist Disability Studies," 1557; Garland-Thomson, "Integrating Disability."

82 Scully, "Review," 171: "Disability, in all its complexity, is generated through the interaction of a biological body with its social and physical context."

83 Borg, Karlsson, and Kim, "User Involvement," 285.

84 Davidow, "Cheers for Peers": "If all so many of us have been advocating for all these years was simply to develop a new title in the mental health system where someone would openly acknowledge their psychiatric history but still do the same old things, what would really be the point?"

85 Pollack, "An Imprisoning Gaze," 105.

86 See for example, Kelly, "Structural Violence," 721.

87 Stuart, "Violence and Mental Illness," 123: "too much past research has focused on the person with the mental illness, rather than the nature of

the social interchange that led up to the violence. Consequently, we know much less than we should about the nature of these relationships and the *contextual determinants of violence."* [emphasis added].

88 Pollack, "An Imprisoning Gaze," 110: "By limiting our outrage to individual and extraordinary examples of state-perpetuated violence and neglect, we evade a central conundrum; we are all complicit in the death of Ms Smith and the death and injuries suffered by prisoners everywhere."

89 Ibid.

90 DiManno, "Square Peg."

91 Perkel, "Mental Health."

92 Ring, "Incorrigible while Incarcerated," 47: "By writing that Ashley Smith was not officially labelled mentally ill prior to or while incarcerated, journalists from these newspapers problematize the assumption that Ashley's mistreatment was because she was mentally ill."

93 Ibid., 47.

94 Ibid., 48: "This alternative depiction of Ashley as resistant supports the analysis that labelling her 'disturbed' is subjective and rooted in medicalization and patriarchal understandings. Although this 'alternative' story is only published once and only appears in the Toronto Star, the fact that it exists signals that Ashley's story may be more complex than was presented in the other news articles. This alternative story that introduced Ashley as intentionally resistant prods readers to consider the repercussions of resistance for women in carceral spaces."

95 Moore, "Ashley Smith."

96 Canadian Civil Liberties Association, "Solitary Confinement"; British Columbia Civil Liberties Association, "Justice, Not Torture."

97 This is important because Ministry of Community Safety and Correctional Services governs both the Coroner's Office and provincial correctional facilities.

BIBLIOGRAPHY

Legislation

Chief Coroner's Rules of Procedure for Inquests, Rule 6.7(c).

Jurisprudence

Dulong v Merrill Lynch Canada Inc. 2006 CanLII 9146 (ON SC), (2006) 80 OR (3d) 378, [2006] OJ No 1146.

Lane v Adga Group Consultants Inc., 2007 HRTO 34 (CanLII).

James (Re): 2008 CanLII 89705.

R v Mohan, [1994] 2 SCR 9.

R v RDS, [1997] 3 SCR 484 at para. 44.

Reid (Re), 2010 CanLII 99953 (ON OCCO)

Rice v Sockett, [1912] OJ No. 49, 27 OLR 410 (C.A.)

Smith (Re), 2012 CanLII 101203 (ON OCCO) (September 24 2012).

Smith (Re), 2013 (ON OCCO) (September 10 2013) [unreported].

Smith (Re), 2013 (ON OCCO), dated 4 October2013.

Smith (Re), 2013 CanLII 92762 (ON OCCO) (December 19 2013).

Youth (Re), 2011 CanLII 99634 (ON OCCO).

Secondary Sources

Abrams, Kathryn. "Feminist Lawyering and Legal Method," *Law and Society Inquiry* 16 (1991): 373.

Arbour, Louise. *Commission of Inquiry into Certain Events at the Prison for Women in Kingston.* Ottawa, ON: Public Works and Government Services Canada, 1996. http:// www.justicebehindthewalls.net/resources/arbour_report/arbour_rpt.htm.

"Ashley Smith's Sedations in Custody Unwarranted: Report." *CBC News,* November 1, 2010. http://www.cbc.ca/news/canada/ashley-smith-s-sedations-in-custody-unwarranted-report-1.928740.

Bay, Michael. "Making the Law Match the Reality: Making the Reality Match the Law." *Journal of Ethics in Mental Health* 1, no. 1 (2006): 1–4.

Borg, M., B. Karlsson, and H. S. Kim. "User Involvement in Community Mental Health Services: Principles and Practices." *Journal of Psychiatric Mental Health Nursing* 16, no. 3 (2009): 285–92.

British Columbia Civil Liberties Association. "Justice, Not Torture: Challenging Solitary Confinement in Canadian Prisons." Accessed February 27, 2017. https://bccla.org/our-work/solitary-confinement/.

British Columbia Civil Liberties Association. "Solitary Confinement Backgrounder." January 2015. https://bccla.org/wp-content/uploads/2015/01/Solitary-Confinement-Backgrounder-FINAL1.pdf.

Bromwich, Rebecca. "Eight Years after Ashley Smith's Death, Prison Condition Remain Abhorrent." *Ottawa Citizen*, October 13, 2015. https://ottawacitizen.com/news/politics/bromwich-eight-years-after-smiths-death-prison-conditions-remain-abhorrent.

Canadian Civil Liberties Association. "Solitary Confinement." https://ccla.org/solitary-confinement/.

Chambers, Jennifer. "Addressing Trauma Is Part of Recovery." Centre for Addiction and Mental Health. December 5 2013. http://www.camhblog .com/2013/12/05/addressing-trauma-is-part-of-recovery/.

Chambers, Jennifer. "What Do Client Rights Have to Do with Trauma Informed Care?" In *Becoming Trauma Informed*, edited by Nancy Poole and Lorraine Greaves, 311–17. Toronto, ON: Centre for Addiction and Mental Health, 2012.

Correctional Services Canada. *Response to the Inquest Touching the Death of Ashley Smith*. December 2014. Accessed February 27, 2017. http://www .csc-scc.gc.ca/publications/005007-9011-eng.shtml.

Davidow, Sera. "Cheers for Peers." *Mad in America*, July 4, 2013. Accessed February 27, 2017. https://www.madinamerica.com/2013/07/cheers -for-peers/.

DiManno, Rosie. "Square Peg Beaten Down by System." *Toronto Star*, March 9, 2009.

Dykeman, Mary Jane. "Search and Seizure in Mental Health Settings." Paper presented to Ontario Bar Association, Mental Health Law in Ontario: Critical Updates, Toronto ON, April 12, 2011.

Empowerment Council. "In the Matter of the Inquest Touching the Death of Ashley Smith and in The Matter of an Application by the Empowerment Council, a Party with Standing, to Call Witnesses." Written Submission of the Empowerment Council, September 18, 2013.

Fine, Sean, and Patrick White. "Trudeau Calls for Ban on Long-term Solitary Confinement in Federal Prisons." *Globe and Mail*, November 13, 2015. https://www.theglobeandmail.com/news/national/trudeau -calls-for-implementation-of-ashley-smith-inquest-recommendations/ article27256251/.

Garland-Thomson, Rosemarie. "Feminist Disability Studies." *Signs* 30, no. 2 (2005): 1557–87.

Garland-Thomson, Rosemarie. "Integrating Disability, Transforming Feminist Theory." *NWSA Journal* 14, no. 3 (2002): 1–33.

Grassian, Stuart. "Psychiatric Effects of Solitary Confinement." *Washington University Journal of Law and Policy* 22 (2006): 325–83.

Kane, Laura. "Thousands of Inquest Recommendations Never Carried Out." *Toronto Star*. February 15, 2014. https:// www.thestar.com/news/ gta/2014/02/15/thousands_of_inquest_recommendations_never_carried_ out.html.

Kelly, B. D. "Structural Violence and Schizophrenia." *Social Science and Medicine* 61, no. 3 (2005): 721–30.

Law Commission of Ontario. *Framework for the Law as it Affects Persons with Disabilities.* Toronto, ON: Law Commission of Ontario, 2012. http://www.lco-cdo.org/en/our-current-projects/the-law-and-persons-with-disabilities/persons-with-disabilities-final-report-september-2012/a-framework-for-the-law-as-it-affects-persons-with-disabilities/.

Liegghio, Maria. "Denial of Being." In *Mad Matters: A Critical Reader in Canadian Mad Studies,* edited by Brenda Lefrançois, Robert Menzies, and Geoffrey Reaume, 122–9. Toronto, ON: Canadian Scholars' Press, 2013.

Mack, Tracy. "The Mad and the Bad: The Lethal Use of Force against Mad People by Toronto Police." *Critical Disability Discourse* 6 (2014): 7–52.

Mack, Tracy. "Psychiatric Survivors/Consumers Die and Nothing Is Done: An Examination of the Discriminatory Nature of the Ontario's *Coroner's Act.*" *Canadian Journal of Disability Studies* 3, no. 1 (2014): 36–64. http://cjds.uwaterloo.ca/index.php/cjds/article/view/145.

McEvoy, Arthur F. "A New Realism for Legal Studies." *Wisconsin Law Review* (2005): 433–54.

Miles, Thomas J., and Cass Sunstein. "The New Legal Realism." *University of Chicago Law Review* 75 (2008): 831–51.

Mohri, Linda. "Guidelines for Searching Clients in Mental Health and Addictions Settings." Paper presented to Ontario Bar Association, Mental Health Law in Ontario: Critical Updates, Toronto, ON, April 12, 2011.

Moore, Dawn. "Ashley Smith Case: A Time to End the 'Ugly Spirit of Our Penal System.'" *Globe and Mail,* January 15, 2013. https://www.theglobeandmail.com/globe-debate/ashley-smith-case-time-to-end-the-ugly-spirit-of-our-penal-system/article7354170/.

National Film Board. "Interactive Portrait Goes inside US Prison System." February 26, 2015. https://blog.nfb.ca/blog/2015/02/26/interactive-portrait-goes-inside-us-criminal-justice-system/.

Nixon, Rob. *Slow Violence and the Environmentalism of the Poor.* Cambridge, MA: Harvard University Press, 2013.

Patton, Lora. "These Regulations Aren't Just Here to Annoy You: The Myth of Statutory Safeguards, Patient Rights and *Charter* Values in Ontario's Mental Health System." *Windsor Review of Legal and Social Issues* 25 (2008): 9–32.

Pedlar, Alison, Felice Yuen, and Daria Fortune. "Incarcerated Women and Leisure: Making Good Girls Out of Bad?" *Therapeutic Recreation Journal* 42, no. 1 (2008): 24.

Perkel, Colin. "Mental Health Act Used for Body-Cavity Searches of Teen Inmate Ashley Smith." *Globe and Mail,* January 23, 2013.

https://www.theglobeandmail.com/news/national/mental-health-act-used-for-body-cavity-searches-of-teen-inmate-ashley-smith/article7714064/.

Perlin, Michael L. "Half-Wracked Prejudice Leaped Forth: Sanism, Pretexuality, and Why and How Mental Disability Law Developed as it Did." *Journal of Contemporary Legal Issues* 10 (1999): 28–9.

Pollack, Shoshana. "An Imprisoning Gaze: Practices of Gendered, Racialized and Epistemic Violence." *International Review of Victimology* 19, no. 1 (2012): 103–14.

Psychiatric Patient Advocacy Office. *Searches: Person and Property.* Toronto, ON: PPAO, 2009.

Ring, Jessi. "Incorrigible While Incarcerated: Critically Analyzing Mainstream Canadian News Depictions of Ashley Smith." *Canadian Graduate Journal of Sociology and Criminology* 3, no. 1 (2014): 34–53.

Sapers, Howards. *A Preventable Death.* Ottawa, ON: Correctional Investigator of Canada, 2008. http:// www.oci-bec.gc.ca/cnt/rpt/pdf/oth-aut/oth-aut20080620-eng.pdf.

Scully, Jackie Leach. Review of *Feminist Disability Studies,* edited by Kim Q. Hall. *International Journal of Feminist Approaches to Bioethics* 6, no. 1 (2013): 166–72.

Silbey, Susan S. "After Legal Consciousness." *Annual Review of Law and Social Science* 1 (2005): 323–68.

Stone, Laura. "December? Later? Tories Won't Say When They Will Respond to Ashley Smith Recommendations." *Global, News,* September 3, 2014. https://globalnews.ca/news/1542295/december-later-tories-wont-say-when-theyll-respond-to-ashley-smith-recommendations/.

Stuart, Heather. "Violence and Mental Illness: An Overview." *World Psychiatry* 2, no. 2 (2003): 121–4.

Suchman, Mark, and Elizabeth Mertz. "Toward a New Legal Empiricism: Empirical Legal Studies and New Legal Realism." *Annual Review of Law and Social Science* 6, no 1 (2010): 555–79.

UN Committee against Torture. *Consideration of Reports Submitted by States Parties under Article 19 of the Convention: Concluding Observations of the Committee Against Torture: Canada.* Doc No. CAT/C/CAN/CO/6. Geneva: UN Committee against Torture, 2012.

Webster, Paul. "Controls over Solitary Confinement Needed." *Canadian Medical Association Journal* 187, no. 1 (2015): E3–E4.

Wingrove, John. "Ottawa to Respond to Details of Ashley Smith Inquest on Federal Prisons." *Globe and Mail,* December 10, 2014. https://www.theglobeandmail.com/news/national/ottawa-to-respond-to-details-of-ashley-smith-inquest-on-federal-prisons/article22036626/.

14 Recounting Huronia: A Reflection on Legal Discourse and the Weight of Injustice

JEN RINALDI AND KATE ROSSITER

Introduction

The Huronia Regional Centre (HRC) was a total institution[1] built and run by the province of Ontario, Canada, to warehouse people diagnosed with intellectual disabilities.[2] Opened in 1876, Huronia's reputation as a site of ongoing and often horrific abuse and neglect emerged over the latter half of the twentieth century, yet the institution remained open until 2009. In 2010, a landmark class action lawsuit was brought by survivors against the Government of Ontario for failing in its fiduciary duty[3] in relation to the mistreatment residents experienced while institutionalized. Plaintiffs Patricia Seth and Marie Slark and their litigation guardians Marilyn and Jim Dolmage insisted on legal recognition of and compensation for the intense suffering of residents who lived in the Centre between 1945 and 2009. A settlement was reached out of court in 2013 for $35 million.

While the settlement in many ways marks a victory, and despite best efforts to simplify forms and instructions,[4] the claims process has been marked by a sustained lack of attention to the engagement of legal discourse with notions of and assumptions around ability and may leave out a great deal of what was experienced at HRC. We approach this work as two members of a research project called Recounting Huronia, funded by the Social Sciences and Humanities Research Council. This project has engaged scholars, artists, allies, and Huronia survivors in order to explore lived histories of institutionalization. The authors of this chapter are both scholars who have worked with the Recounting Huronia project for several years. Attenuated to the incalculability of injustice, Recounting Huronia[5] has just begun to explore and story survivors' experiences of the HRC and confronts the impossibility of ever finding comprehensive frames for those experiences. This work is taken on by our collective in response to a concern unpacked here: that our commitment to justice for survivors, to the recounting of Huronia's past, extends beyond the parameters of the settlement and, indeed, challenges the limited and often harmful terms of the settlement itself.

We intend here to identify the shortcomings found in the language and terms of the settlement to lay the groundwork for alternative methods of raising consciousness and seeking reparation. In this work we endeavour to describe the settlement language not as a victory but rather as an extension of the failure of justice that marks Huronia's very fraught history. This history is violent, for the settlement directly addresses forms of physical and sexual abuse, but we claim that practices of institutionalization are inherently and systemically violent, and that the legal processes by which those practices are discursively framed – or even left out of analysis – themselves commit acts of violence in the particular ways they fail and disempower claimants. We ask, how does the language of the claims process work to re-inscribe systemic forms of injustice? To do so we look first at the structure and language of the settlement and address ways in which the discourse employed may further marginalize the most vulnerable within the class and inadvertently retrench forms of trauma. Second, we explore how the language of the settlement extends harmful discursive institutional practices and may in fact leave open space for institutionalization to reoccur.

Understanding the Language of the Settlement

As noted in the Ontario Superior Court hearing during which the aggrieved parties were certified as a class,[6] the HRC (originally named the Orillia Asylum for Idiots) was opened under provincial statutory law, the 1839 Act to authorize the erection of an Asylum within this Province for the reception of Insane and Lunatic persons, and was sustained under subsequent statutes.[7] Over its 133 year history, the HRC housed a wide variety of marginalized peoples, including teenaged mothers, people labelled indigents for their reliance on social welfare programs, and those with what might now be qualified as psychiatric disabilities. However, its primary goal was to contain individuals who fit within newly emerging (and eugenically informed) diagnostic criteria for what has been termed idiocy, mental retardation, and developmental and intellectual disability.

At its height in the mid-twentieth century, Huronia's major focus was housing and remediating children with intellectual disabilities. While there is little evidence regarding the class and racial makeup of HRC residents, anecdotal evidence suggests that a large proportion came from impoverished backgrounds, including those who suffered extreme and debilitating forms of deprivation in infancy. However, this is not the entire residential picture: many came from middle- and upper-middle-class homes, placed into care by parents who were ashamed of their offspring or convinced the institution, informed by medical science, would do a better job of caring for their children than they could at home.

During the institution's tenure, as cited through the class certification process, the Crown received a 1971 report wherein Walton B. Williston identified staff shortages, overcrowding, outdated living residences, and coerced labour for little or no pay.[8] In the suit, plaintiffs alleged the Crown failed in its duties to residents by ignoring report findings and keeping Huronia open for decades thereafter. This breach resulted, they claimed, in emotional, physical, and psychological abuse.[9] By 2013, allegations of a breach entailed more specifically the Crown's "funding, operation, management, administration, supervision and control of the Huronia Regional Centre."[10] The class alleged that the Crown failed to enact prevention policies or improve quality of care notwithstanding reports like Williston's of overcrowding and understaffing, and recommendations for improvement.

Such were the arguments raised before a settlement was reached. The terms of the settlement were developed in consultation with disability advocacy groups and were heralded for reflecting "the sensitive nature of this litigation and the unique circumstances of the class members."[11] This was accomplished, in part, by providing non-monetary benefits: a formal apology; the production of case documents for scholarly research; and a number of commemorative initiatives, including a plaque, a registry, appropriate signage on the cemetery grounds, scheduled access to Huronia grounds, and an opportunity for scholars to archive artefacts.[12] Further, a settlement fund was established that amounted to $35 million, in addition to costs to the Crown for administering the claims process, and the promise that compensation awards would not be subject to taxation or claw-backs.[13]

The settlement agreement entailed a system for determining eligibility for funds, demarcated by two claim forms. Section A claims required only a solemn declaration of harm while institutionalized at Huronia without need of evidence or an accounting, for up to $2000. Claimants were directed to check a box indicating "I was harmed or hurt when I lived at Huronia or at a place where Huronia put me."[14] Section B claims required details of harm or abuse in writing and the amount of financial compensation awarded was based on the allocation of points for the kind, intensity, and frequency of harm incurred at the institution. Within this document, claimants were instructed to identify harm or abuse, and were provided with a series of examples of actionable physical harms, including "calling you names, insulting or yelling at you"; "giving you scars, bruises, broken bones, broken teeth or any other injury to your body or how you look"; "giving you too much or too little, or the wrong medication."[15] Examples of sexual abuse included "touching or making you touch someone else in a sexual way when you did not want to"; "making you watch, listen or talk about sexual things when you did not want to"; "making you stand or walk around naked"; "putting or trying to put something in your mouth, vagina or anus when you did not want them to."[16] The document stated after these lists, "there are many other things that are abuse," and directed claimants to "write down anything that harmed you."[17]

As established in the compensation scheme, Justice Ian Binnie was tasked with overseeing the claims administration process, and alongside Crawford Class Action Services evaluated Section B claim forms, assigning points according to the settlement agreement's point allocation system.[18] Under the point allocation system, there were six possible categories of abuse. Under physical assault, level one for 100 points consisted of repeated, persistent, and excessive wrongful acts – demeaning behaviour, humiliation, or physical punishment; level two for 200 points entailed assaults not resulting in serious physical injury; and level three for 400 points required that acts resulted in serious physical injury, such as a bruise or laceration. Level one sexual assaults – nonconsensual behaviour or contact – constituted 200 points; level two, repeated non-consensual sexual behaviour, was worth 400 points; and level three, or repeated incidents of serious sexual assault, amounted to 600 points. The number of points tallied on claims determined the amount of compensation awarded, up to $35,000 per Section B claimant (a maximum limit that could increase to $42,000 if Section B claims did not exhaust the net settlement fund).[19]

Quantifying Injustice: A Critique of Terminology and Process

While the examples offered in the Section B claim form and the typology of abuse outlined in the point allocation system sound like adequate – indeed, striking – illustrations of violence, and certainly should be catalogued and accounted for, there is also much to critique about both the language and process of these claims. First, what is clear from the identified examples is an emphasis on *active* language. Throughout the proceedings members of the judiciary cited the plaintiffs' allegations that the Crown was in breach of a duty of care resulting in HRC residents being actively harmed, as well as neglected to the point of harm.[20] But settling out of court has meant that the most definitive and precise declaration that the Crown committed wrongdoing can be found in then Ontario premier Kathleen Wynne's public apology, which directly addressed neglect as a form of harm;[21] and as the claims process unfolded, the Crown was not held accountable or required to compensate for harm born of institutional neglect, often resulting in grievous forms of abuse and mistreatment.

In settlement documents, particularly the claim forms themselves, neglect was left absent from claimable items. While the term *neglect* might signal a range of possible scenarios that illustrates systemic issues within the institution – overcrowding, understaffing, lack of resources, lack of adequate training – the move to *abuse* in the claim form denotes a much more active relationship to harm, that is, the wilful and conscious inflicting of pain or suffering on another. Given this linguistic shift, some of the nuance to the harms experienced is lost, like when children spent the better part of their days in diapers and caged cribs because not enough staff was available to tend to them, or residents had their teeth surgically removed after years of inadequate dental care. How does one account for regimens of approved medications that came with severe and lasting side effects; the instances where residents were seen nude simply because they lacked clean clothes or their bathroom stalls lacked doors; the number of years spent uneducated because education cost money and was thought wasted on the intellectually disabled; the exploited labour residents had to invest to maintain their own prison because work cultivated moral character?

This is deeply problematic, especially for survivors at a significant disadvantage in terms of making or substantiating claims. First, survivors who are able to talk struggle to define normal daily living practices *as forms of abuse.* Second, and perhaps more problematically, non-verbal survivors, survivors who cannot revisit their memories of violence without experiencing profound re-traumatization, and the dead (many of whom are buried in unmarked graves, their original tombstones dug up and repurposed for sidewalks on the HRC grounds)[22] are left at a disadvantage because they cannot adequately or at all describe whether and how injuries or mistreatment occurred. Caregivers, support workers, and loved ones have been tasked with cobbling together reasonable explanations for possible harm relying on institutional and medical records, resultant behaviours (phobias, compulsions, often-repeated phrases, etc.), and accounts of other, verbal survivors who were residents at the same time. Given that instances of institutional abuse were rarely included as such within residents' files, much of the content of these claims is based on informed guesswork. And there are survivors who simply lack family support altogether when making claims. This means that the most egregious examples of violence may be identified, but more complicated instances of structural violence, even the structural conditions that make possible or exacerbate violence, are much more difficult to account for.

The harmful use of passive language and limiting survivors' capacity to articulate abuse and neglect is not novel to the claims process; indeed, these practices extend subtle but oppressive protocols which have roots within institutional histories. In her analysis of the oral history of Michener, a still-open institution for intellectually disabled people in the province of Alberta (an institution parents and the state insist is humane to leave open notwithstanding),[23] Malacrida describes institutional case files as using passive language to account for injury, without attributing injury to cause; and records of injury tend to appear only after family members visited and lodged complaints upon speaking with residents or witnessing bodily evidence of violence. She quotes case files: "The files where evidence of violence was discussed are riddled with passive voice. For example, a resident injured by rough handling was described in language that almost sounds as if she injured herself: '[X] hit right eyebrow on bed rail while being put to bed sustaining a laceration.'"[24] Malacrida also discusses at length institutional strategies around isolating residents from the outside world by discouraging family from visiting, for the sake of facilitating adjustment; this would surely result in fewer complaints on record in the absence of advocates.[25]

It is not unreasonable to assume similar practices were carried out at Huronia. The 1960 informational video about provincial institutions

One on Every Street noted that family members of Huronia residents were advised not to visit when visits negatively impacted residents' adjustment to institutional life.[26] Located far from urban centres such as Toronto, Huronia was difficult to access and family members were permitted to visit with residents only in public spaces (i.e., common rooms) and for limited amounts of time. Parental access to spaces of deep neglect – overcrowded wards, for example – was not permitted. Thus, in the face of scant evidence, some HRC claimants were only capable of submitting Section A claim forms when they could have qualified for much more compensation than Section A claims can merit; and some claimants who submitted Section B claims were able only to supply limited testimony and have had their claims either downgraded to an A claim, or have received fewer points based on lack of clear evidence of active harm. This is particularly egregious with respect to highly impaired, non-verbal survivors who often had much longer institutional stays than more verbal survivors and who would thus have undoubtedly witnessed and endured abuse and neglect for sustained periods of time – entire lifetimes in some cases.

The Logic of "A Few Bad Apples": Leaving Space for Institutionalization

As we have discussed, the work to recount Huronia has begun in the courtroom. To quote Justice Barbara A. Conway's 2014 decision to approve class counsel's fees: "These class actions provided a means for [survivors] to ... create public awareness of the history of these institutions and the alleged experiences of the residents there."[27] And certainly, HRC survivors should be heralded as legal trailblazers. Survivors from two now closed Ontario institutions for persons with intellectual disabilities have successfully settled class action suits: Rideau Regional Centre, near Ottawa, Ontario; and Southwestern Regional Centre, located near Chatham, Ontario.[28] Further, suits regarding the institutionalization of persons with physical disabilities, at the Nova Scotia Home for Coloured Children in Westphal Nova Scotia and the W. Ross MacDonald School for the visually impaired (formerly the Ontario School of the Blind) in Brantford, Ontario, are underway.[29] Directly inspired by the HRC settlement, a class of 8800 persons labelled intellectually disabled settled a $36 million class action suit against Ontario for the harm and neglect they experienced in 12 institutions across the province.[30]

However, legal victory has not meant justice – or rather, to equate *legal victory* with *justice* in this circumstance may mean that the conditions for institutional violence are not adequately challenged. Rather, given the limits of what tort law can accomplish,[31] this legal victory has involved the hierarchicalization and monetization of trauma, a weighing of the worth of trauma. Lost in the quantification of harm are the institutional dynamics and conditions that caused such harm, which cannot be quantified or even reasonably captured in the framework of legal storytelling. In leaving absent these conditions, the settlement problematically leaves open the possibility for institutionalization to reoccur.

A 2000 Law Commission of Canada report on physical and sexual child abuse in Canadian institutional settings, including training schools for intellectually disabled youth, long-term mental health care facilities, and sanatoria,[32] notes that turning to legal recourses for the purpose of redress – looking to the criminal justice system and pursuing lawsuits in civil court to hold people and government bodies responsible – reveals the limits to these systems to address systemic oppression. The report indicates in its analysis of criminal proceedings, and by extension civil proceedings[33] that "the criminal justice system is well-suited to identifying individual perpetrators of abuse and holding them liable. It is, however, less effective in shedding light on the systemic problems that may have allowed the abuse to occur in the first place."[34] Ben-Moshe seems to agree with this assessment, arguing that justice frameworks of this sort fail to "address the structural inequalities that lead to injustice in the first place [or to] question the basic assumptions of the system."[35] Her recommendation is not reform but abolition of disability incarceration in all its manifestations, to go "beyond protesting the current circumstances, to creating new conditions of possibility by collectively contesting the status quo."[36] This call for abolition is especially resonant given that despite the rash of lawsuits following the HRC settlement, Alberta's Michener – the same Michener whose history is laid bare in Malacrida's work – remains open.

Thus, Huronia's history as recounted within the existing legal framework is fragmented, formal, and missing accounts from the most vulnerable and least able to self-advocate and may well be losing track of the experience of injustice through efforts to articulate it. The implications are enormous, even beyond the problems around ensuring those wronged are compensated: that only abuse is acknowledged in the HRC claims process might imply that institutionalization can still be done right, with enough sensitivity, training, oversight, and so on, that is, that the problem lies with a few abusive "bad apple" staff. The settlement language, with its emphasis on abuse rather than neglect, obfuscates institutional practices and dehumanizing forms of structural oppression inherent to institutionalization itself.

Given that institutional practices have since their origins created and perpetuated systemic violence, it is difficult to imagine what institutionalization done right would entail. Asylums marked for treating mental retardation first established under the 1839 provincial legislation were justified through segregationist, custodial policies and practices designed for the dual purpose of caring for people believed incapable of social integration and protecting communities from the multiple threats disability might pose – to safety, to reproduction, to social order. Rossiter and Clarkson claim in their socio-historical accounting of the HRC that "from their inception, life within Canadian institutions was unrelentingly oppressive [and] after many years of financial strain, provincial neglect, chronic overcrowding and prevailing cultural attitudes of fear, abjection and the need for social isolation left people with [intellectual disability diagnoses] in institutions vulnerable to widespread abuse."[37] That is, abuse was made possible and routinized through systemic conditions. Stenfert Kroese and Holmes elaborate on these conditions, focusing on an historical trend to medicalize disability or to categorize disability as a condition in need of fixing or curing to restore a person's health or species-typical status. The implications for persons labelled with "incurable" disabilities entail indefinite confinement and a social stigma impossible to overcome: "as there are no cures for learning disabilities,[38] patients were destined to stay in hospital until death. They were at the mercy of strict rules, regulations and routines whereby other people decided when they were to get up, when to wash, when to eat, what to wear, and who to befriend."[39] Stenfert Kroese and Holmes go on to argue that extreme conditions of isolation, control, and deprivation have their impact upon persons, creating resistant behaviours, what the authors call severe psychological disturbances, and learned helplessness that through cyclical logic only serve to reinforce the call to keep those institutionalized out of communities and within carceral spaces.[40]

Canadian self-/advocacy organizations have for these reasons supported deinstitutionalization. Adopted by the Canadian Association for Community Living, People First Canada, and Community Living Ontario in 2013, and endorsed by organizations across Canada, a document entitled "Common Principles on the Inclusion of People with Disabilities in Their Communities" uses United Nations language to acknowledge "the physical, psychological and emotional harm people with disabilities have had to endure as a direct result of having been confined or forced to live in institutional settings."[41] The principles endorsed in this document hold that institutions deny full citizenship and community inclusion, and *"do not and cannot* contribute to the health and well-being of persons with disabilities."[42] People First Canada and the Canadian Association for Community Living have endeavoured to realize these principles by monitoring progress towards deinstitutionalization in *Institution Watch*, a regular newsletter dedicated to the idea that "as a society, we have long ago recognized that institutions are just not good for people."[43]

Conclusion: Remembering Injustice, Imagining a Future without Institutional Violence

Huronia's is a long yet living history that has yet to be responsibly documented. Persons housed there were relegated to a geographical and sociopolitical periphery, sometimes forgotten by loved ones, surely ignored by the state even when reports like Williston's surfaced. Their fiduciaries managed their stories – for, persons diagnosed with intellectual disabilities are not always trusted to be authorities over their own experience. And in institutional spaces like the HRC, acts of defiance, even the identification of wrongdoing, could result in punishment and medication. This is a reality that Seth and Slark experienced and related in their statements of claim:[44] Slark was medicated for "acting out," Seth for "speaking out."[45] That this history lives on in now-aging survivors makes the task of recounting a history of injustice all the more pressing.

So what is to be done about bearing witness to the suffering endured at the HRC? How do we account for histories that cannot be verbalized, trauma that cannot (and should not) be weighed through a system of points? We suggest that the settlement is best viewed as a starting point rather than a final victory. After all, to quote Urban Walker: "reparations can only ever be an act or process at one time; the reciprocal accountability they token must be secured and shown real over time."[46] That time, we argue, is just beginning for Huronia survivors, and the legal settlement offers an opportunity for reflection to better grasp the enormity of suffering, and to act on the knowledge that institutionalization is inherently violent. While we cannot predict where such reflection might lead, nor can we prescribe a remedy for those who must live with the ongoing consequence of institutional trauma, we can offer suggestions from our own experience regarding the potential role of the legal system as responsible parties in the work of collective memory-making around and beyond the HRC settlement.

The Law Commission of Canada (LCC) report earlier cited offers legally entrenched recommendations beyond civil proceedings. These include petitioning to Ombudsman offices, which are independent, impartial bodies appointed in their jurisdictions to investigate complaints and publicly report their policy recommendations to government.[47] Similarly, public inquiries can offer recommendations for corrective action and are, according to the LCC, report "most effective in holding organizations and governments, not individuals, accountable for their actions."[48] Truth and reconciliation commissions, like that organized for Indigenous populations subjected to residential schooling, are effective in cases of intergenerational injury that reverberate through communities.[49] Beyond these recourses, the report recommends community initiatives for meeting "the most compelling needs of survivors by involving them directly in the design and delivery of helping and healing";[50] and redress programs designed to meet survivors' needs through financial compensation and support.[51]

Community initiatives have already developed around political action and community arts praxis. The organization Remember Every Name is known for its political activism related to the HRC cemetery, insofar as self-advocates and allies have been painstakingly working to document who is buried where.[52] Tangled Art + Disability has hosted an art show, *Surviving Huronia*, where Seth and Slark told stories in their opening address and art featuring themes of institutional life and violence were exhibited.[53] And the participatory arts-based research project Recounting Huronia has been working with survivors to story their experiences of institutionalization, which will culminate in a digital archive, a speakers bureau, and a cabaret. These collectives have sought to honour the polyvocality of the survivor community, to respect and witness a wide variety of institutional experiences (however these may be expressed), and to build community around, among, and with survivors, where social memory may be woven together, may come to be embodied and enfleshed, and may be shared in ways that are not easily ignored, dismissed, or forgotten. We believe these more flexible and nimble approaches may be better suited to the healing and activism vital in the search for justice for the Huronia survivor community.

NOTES

1 A *total institution* is a residential facility separated out from community, where persons committed live, sleep, and perform all daily activities including work and school. Residents of total institutions are often subjected to around the clock surveillance and may live in such an institution for a prolonged period of time – months, years, and even lifetimes.

2 In our research collective, there are survivors who feel strongly about not identifying with a disability label at all, others who are affected by disability language and its associated stigma, others still who even embrace words like *retarded* in acts of reclamation. Though their range is vast, each reaction entails resisting the diagnoses once deployed to institutionalize them.

3 A fiduciary duty is a legal term denoting an important relationship involving trust, where one party has power and the other party is vulnerable. Canadian law has marked physician/patient relationships as fiduciary in nature, for instance.

4 Retired Supreme Court Justice Ian Binnie and the Koskie Minsky law firm oversaw the claims process, and following a court mandate ensured forms were in plain language. Slark and Seth also participated in efforts to tour Ontario community living centres, to teach survivors how to submit claims. The process was simplified to ensure persons with intellectual disabilities would not struggle with accessing compensation.

5 This project is funded by Canada's Social Science of Humanities and Research Council, a member of the federal Tri-Council funding body.

6 Class certification is a process according to which a group of people is found to share similar legal issues, so determination of the issues individuals raise is binding for the group. Class action lawsuits are brought under civil law, where an aggrieved party – in this case a class of persons – can seek compensation from another party accused of committing wrongdoing that caused harm.

7 *An Act to authorise the erection of an Asylum within this Province for the reception of Insane and Lunatic Persons*, Statutes of Upper Canada 1839, 2 Vic., Cap. XI; cited in *Dolmage v Ontario* (2010), ONSC 1726, at para. 5.

8 *Dolmage v Ontario* (2010), ONSC 1726, at paras. 15–16. [*Dolmage v Ontario*]

9 Ibid., at para. 23.

10 *Dolmage v Ontario* (2010), ONSC 6131, at para. 29. [*Dolmage v Ontario*]

11 *Dolmage v HMQ* (2013), ONSC 6686, at para. 23. [*Dolmage v HMQ*]

12 Ibid., at paras. 12–13.

13 Ibid., at para. 13.

14 Koskie Minsky Law, "Huronia Regional Centre," 7.
15 Ibid., 9–10.
16 Ibid., 11.
17 Ibid., 12.
18 *Dolmage v HMQ*, at para. 17.
19 *Dolmage v HMQ*, at para. 6.
20 E.g., *Dolmage v Ontario, supra* note 8, at para. 2.
21 Wynne, "Ontario's Apology": "In the case of Huronia, some residents suffered neglect and abuse within the very system that was meant to provide them care," at para. 5.
22 Alamenciak, "Remembering the Dead."
23 "Michener Centre Closure."
24 Malacrida, *A Special Hell*, 94.
25 Ibid.
26 Ontario Government Department of Health, *One on Every Street*.
27 *Dolmage, McKillop and Bechard v HMQ* (2014), ONSC 1283, at para. 10.
28 *Bechard v Ontario* (Court File No CV-10–411191); *McKillop v Ontario* (Court File No CV-10–417343).
29 *Elwin v Nova Scotia Home for Coloured Children* (2014), ONSC 1282; *Seed v Ontario* (2012), ONSC 4588.
30 Leslie, "Former Residents"; Chown Oved, "$1 Billion Class-Action."
31 Tort law is an area of civil law where plaintiffs may sue for injuries or harms sustained due to some breach in duties owed.
32 Law Commission of Canada Executive Summary, *Restoring Dignity*, 1.
33 Granted, civil proceedings include the mechanisms to solidify those wronged as a class, as well as the means to hold larger bodies – not just singular persons – accountable for wrongdoing. Nevertheless, as is the case in criminal proceedings, fault for active, overt instances of wrongdoing is certainly easier to find than systemic or structural oppression that is diffuse, generational, and woven into social fabrics.
34 Law Commission of Canada Executive Summary, *Restoring Dignity*, 5.
35 Ben-Moshe, "Alternatives to (Disability) Incarceration," 260.
36 Ibid., at 256.
37 Rossiter and Clarkson, "Opening Ontario's," 12.
38 Stenfert Kroese and Holmes are discussing institutionalization in the UK context, where the term learning disability is equivalent to the North American term intellectual or developmental disability.
39 Stenfert Kroese Holmes, "'I've Never Said," 71.
40 Ibid.
41 Baker Law, "Common Principles."

42 Ibid., emphasis our own.
43 Larson Haddad, "A Message," 1.
44 Plaintiffs begin civil proceedings by filing statements of claim that outline the reasons for pursuing a lawsuit. Defendants receive statements of claim to prepare their response, and courts refer to these documents when determining whether the case should proceed.
45 *Dolmage v Ontario, supra* note 8, at paras. 29, 31.
46 Urban Walker, "Vulnerability," 129.
47 Law Commission of Canada Executive Summary, *Restoring Dignity,* 1.
48 Ibid., 7.
49 Ibid.
50 Ibid., 8.
51 Ibid.
52 Alamenciak, "Remembering the Dead."
53 Tangled, "Surviving Huronia."

BIBLIOGRAPHY

Legislation

An Act to authorise the erection of an Asylum within this Province for the reception of Insane and Lunatic Persons. Statutes of Upper Canada 1839, 2 Vic., Cap. XI.

Jurisprudence

Bechard v Ontario (Court File No CV-10–411191).
Dolmage v Ontario (2010), ONSC 1726.
Dolmage v Ontario (2010), ONSC 6131.
Dolmage v HMQ (2013), ONSC 6686.
Dolmage, McKillop and Bechard v HMQ (2014), ONSC 1283.
Elwin v Nova Scotia Home for Coloured Children (2014), ONSC 1282.
McKillop v Ontario (Court File No CV-10–417343).
Seed v Ontario (2012), ONSC 4588.

Secondary Materials

Alamenciak, Tim. "Remembering the Dead at Huronia Regional Centre." *Toronto Star,* December 29, 2014. https://www.thestar.com/news/gta/2014 /12/29/remembering_the_dead_at_huronia_regional_centre.html.

Bakers Law. "Common Principles on the Inclusion of People with Disabilities in their Communities: Institutionalization as a Form of Discrimination." September 24, 2014. https://www.bakerlaw.ca/blog/institutionalization-form-discrimination.

Ben-Moshe, Liat. "Alternatives to (Disability) Incarceration." In *Disability Incarcerated: Imprisonment and Disability in the United States and Canada*, edited by Liat Ben-Moshe, Chris Chapman, and Allison C. Carey, 255–72. New York: Palgrave Macmillan, 2014.

Chown Oved, Marco. "$1-Billion Class-Action Suit Claims Residential Hospital Abuse." *Toronto Star*, August 27, 2015. https://www.thestar.com/news/gta/2015/08/27/1-billion-class-action-suit-claims-residential-hospital-abuse.html.

Koskie Minsky Law. "Huronia Regional Centre Claims Process Materials (2015)." http://kmlaw.ca/cases/huronia-regional-centre/.

Larson, Laurie, and Shane Haddad. "A Message from the Task Force." Institution Watch 10, no 1 (Spring 2016): 1–2.

Law Commission of Canada Executive Summary. *Restoring Dignity: Responding to Child Abuse in Canadian Institutions*. Minister of Public Works and Government Services, 2000.

Leslie, Keith. "Former Residents of 12 Ontario Institutions for Developmentally Disabled Win $36-Million Lawsuit." *National Post*, April 27, 2016. http://www.nationalpost.com/m/wp/blog.html?b=news.nationalpost.com/news/canada/former-residents-of-12-ontario-institutions-for-developmentally-disabled-win-36-million-lawsuit.

Malacrida, Claudia. *A Special Hell: Institutional Life in Alberta's Eugenic Years*. Toronto, ON: University of Toronto Press, 2015.

"Michener Centre Closure Halted, Residents Allowed to Return." *CBC News*, September 19, 2014. http://www.cbc.ca/news/canada/edmonton/michener-centre-closure-halted-residents-allowed-to-return-1.2771739.

Ontario Government Department of Health. *One on Every Street*. Ottawa, ON: Fletcher Film Productions, 1960.

Rossiter, Kate, and Annalise Clarkson. "Opening Ontario's 'Saddest Chapter': A Social History of Huronia Regional Centre." *Canadian Journal of Disability Studies* 2, no. 3 (2013): 1.

Simmons, Harvey G. *From Asylums to Welfare*. Toronto National Institute on Mental Retardation, 1982.

Stenfert Kroese, Biza, and Guy Holmes. "'I've Never Said "No" to Anything in My Life': Helping People with Learning Disabilities Who Experience Psychological Problems." In *This Is Madness Too: Critical Perspectives on Mental Health Issues*, edited by Craig Newnes, Guy Holmes, and Cailzie Dunn. Ross-on-Wye, UK: PCCS Books, 2013.

Tangled Art + Disability. "Surviving Huronia," 2014. http://tangledarts.org/
    events/surviving-huronia/.
Urban Walker, Margaret. "Vulnerability and the Task of Reparations."
    In *Vulnerability: New Essays in Ethics and Feminist Philosophy*, edited by
    Catriona Mackenzie, Wendy Rogers, and Susan Dodds. New York: Oxford,
    2014.
Wynne, Kathleen. "Ontario's Apology to Former Residents of Regional
    Centres for People with Developmental Disabilities," 2013. https://www
    .mcss.gov.on.ca/en/mcss/programs/developmental/Premier_Apology.aspx.

15 Madding the Muslim Terrorist: Orientalist Psychology in Canada's "War on Terror"

AZEEZAH KANJI

Psychology has a long and intimate entanglement with projects of race and empire. From British psychiatrist J.C. Carothers' studies on Kikuyu brains demonstrating that the Mau uprising was "not political but psycho-pathological,"[1] to analyses of the disfiguring effects of Islam on North Africans' brains by the French colonial psychiatrists of the School of Algiers,[2] to the diagnoses of activists involved in the American Civil Rights Movement as schizophrenic by government authorities and psychiatrists:[3] the psy-disciplines (psychology, psychiatry, psychoanalysis) have been instrumental in pathologizing racialized subjects, normalizing racial systems of rule, and de-rationalizing and delegitimizing resistance to these systems. This chapter focuses on the intersection of discourses of race and madness in the construction of the post-2001 war on terror's figure of the "mad Muslim terrorist": a figure whose violence, or potential violence, is represented as simultaneously evil and irrational. Through analysis of a complex of sites where psy-disciplines and discourses are yoked to the project of national security – judicial depictions of terrorist psychologies in terrorism prosecutions, psychological risk-assessment tools used in terrorism sentencing, and psychological theories of pre-criminal radicalization applied to the general Muslim population – I consider how pathologizing portrayals of Muslim minds rationalize Canadian counter-terrorism's exercises of exceptional state violence against, and control over, domestic Muslim populations.

In his foundational text *Orientalism*, Edward Said analysed the constellation of representations that made the Middle East into an object for European colonial rule, including lucubrations on the particular deficiencies and inferiorities of the Oriental mind.[4] British colonial administrator Lord Cromer, for instance, explained in his 1908 two-volume opus on *Modern Egypt* that while "the European is a close reasoner" and "a natural logician," "the mind of the Oriental, on the other hand, like his picturesque streets, is eminently wanting in symmetry ... Although the ancient Arabs acquired in a somewhat higher degree the science of dialectics, their descendants are singularly deficient in the logical faculty."[5] The global war on terror has breathed new life into Orientalist fascinations with the peculiarities of the "Muslim mind," and what Princeton professor of Near Eastern Studies Bernard Lewis called the "roots of Muslim rage" planted deep within it.[6] Muslim violence is attributed to irascible and fanatic psychologies rather than real political grievances, and so rendered inherently illegitimate; the mind of the Muslim "terrorist" is depicted not as picturesquely asymmetrical (à la Lord Cromer) but as perversely twisted.

In *Disciplining Terror: How Experts Invented "Terrorism,"* Lisa Stampnitzky charts a shift that has occurred in the way the term "terrorism" is applied: while originally conceptualized as a *tactic* or a *tool* used by a wide variety of political actors,

> as the problem of terrorism took shape over the course of the 1970s, 1980s, and 1990s, it came to be understood as rooted to a terrorist identity, rather than as a tactic that any group might adopt. This led to the proposition that terrorists commit terrorism because they are terrorists. The identity contains its own explanation: "terrorists' are evil, irrational actors whose action is driven not by normal interests or political motives but, instead, by their very nature as terrorists."[7]

This terrorist identity is deeply racialized in the age of the war on terror: in Canada, the term *terrorism* serves in government policy documents and in mainstream media reports as a "seemingly [racially] neutral synonym"[8] for violence, or the threat of violence, emanating from Muslims.[9]

Representations of "Islamic extremism" and "radical Islam" as forms of collective psychopathology afflicting Muslim populations project danger and violence onto Muslim bodies, marking them for neutralization and pacification by pre-emptive military invasion and counter-insurgency abroad, and criminalization and surveillance at home. Theories of radicalization – which draw a determinate path from possession of certain ideologies and beliefs labelled extreme, to participation in violence – attempt to render the threat of Muslim violence simultaneously intelligible and irrational, and justify coercive interventions to correct Muslim propensities for violent extremism. Despite the repeated and rigorous debunking that the theory of radicalization has received – in the words of John Horgan, "the idea that radicalization causes terrorism is perhaps the greatest myth alive today ... the overwhelming majority of people who hold radical beliefs do not engage in violence [and] there is increasing evidence that people who engage in terrorism don't necessarily hold radical beliefs"[10] – the discovery of the mechanisms of radicalization remains a holy grail for security agencies. The Canadian Security Intelligence Service (CSIS), for example, has been recruiting psychologists "to assist the Service in better understanding radicalization and terrorism."[11] Given CSIS's almost-exclusive preoccupation with Muslims as the source of terrorism,[12] the service's explorations into the psychology of radicalization are likely to be similarly focused predominantly on Muslim minds. Psychology becomes a continuation of war by other means (to adapt the well-known Foucauldian aphorism).[13]

Alison Howell has observed that "the psy disciplines are ... governmental technologies that act as authoritative sets of knowledge that divide up populations of those who self-govern, from those who need assistance to self-govern, to those who are irredeemable or incurable, and thus subject to authoritarian measures."[14] In the field of counter-terrorism, supposedly "authoritative sets of knowledge" about Muslim extremism inform the sorting out of the Muslim population into those who are to be punished by authoritarian measures for being terrorists (irredeemably and incurably); those who are to be prevented from becoming terrorists, by provision of assistance to self-govern; and those who are to be recruited as "community partners" into these projects of punishment and prevention (which often bleed into one another, so that punishment is increasingly preventive, and prevention looks increasingly like punishment).

On Punishment

Terrorism was defined in Canadian law for the first time in post-9/11 amendments to the Criminal Code (the 2001 Anti-terrorism Act), as violence to people or property

> that is committed in whole or in part for a political, religious or ideological
> purpose ... with the intention of intimidating the public, or a segment

of the public, with regard to its security ... or compelling a person, a government or a domestic or an international organization to do or refrain from doing any act.[15]

There are two particularly salient features of Canada's legal counter-terrorism framework to note:

1. It is especially oriented towards pre-emptive criminalization, so that a wide range of actions only remotely and tangentially connected to violence have now been criminalized as "terrorism offences," such as "entering or remaining in any country for the benefit of, at the direction of or in association with a terrorist group";[16] "leaving [or attempting to leave] Canada to participate in [the] activity of a terrorist group" or to "facilitate terrorist activity";[17] "providing," "collecting," or "making available" property or services for "terrorist purposes";[18] and, since the passage of Bill C-51, the Anti-terrorism Act, 2015, "the "promotion or advocacy of terrorism offences in general."[19] This unusually pre-emptive orientation arises from legislators' understanding that the task of counter-terrorism is not simply the punishment of guilt, but rather the management of risk. Appearing before the Special Senate Committee to discuss Bill C-36 (which would be enacted as the 2001 Anti-terrorism Act), then minister of justice Anne McLellan asserted: "It has become clear that the scope of the threat that terror poses to our way of life has no parallel ... [P]unishing terrorists for crimes after they occur is simply not enough ... We cannot wait for terrorists to strike before we begin investigations and make arrests where there is a reasonable suspicion that a terrorist act will take place. To wait would be irresponsible."[20]

2. Unlike in some other legal systems (including the US one), *terrorism* is explicitly defined in Canadian law by the presence of a political, religious, or ideological motive – which has the alchemical effect of supposedly transforming actions that might otherwise be innocuous (like planning to travel) into sources of exceptional danger to society. The extremely capacious scope of terrorism offences is, however, effectively restricted by implicit racial ideas about whose violence constitutes terrorism, and what types of motives constitute terrorist motives; by the never explicitly articulated (at least outside of ostentatiously Islamophobic right-wing publications) but pervasive "common sense" that the paradigmatic terrorist is a Muslim driven by so-called Islamic extremism.

There have been 26 completed prosecutions under these anti-terrorism provisions, with a 95% conviction rate for cases brought to trial,[21] and all but one have involved Muslims or people linked to Muslim groups (see Table 15.1). (At least 14 people have been killed in white supremacist or right-wing attacks in Canada since 2001,[22] but none of the attackers have been charged with terrorism – see the discussion of the Justin Bourque case below.) None of the Canadian terrorism convictions have been for acts of violence actually executed, but for plots and plans, frequently developed with significant input and encouragement from state informants.[23] And yet, judges treat those accused of terrorism as exceptionally heinous offenders, who are deserving of exceptionally harsh sentences (imprisonment for terms often exceeding ten years, even for peripheral involvement in plots) – not so much because of what they have already done, but because of the immanent dangerousness and evil encoded in the ideas held to be inside of them. As Justice Durno of the Ontario Superior Court proclaimed in *R v Khalid* (one of the prosecutions involving the "Toronto 18," a group of young Muslim men who planned attacks on several targets in Toronto): "Terrorist offences are a most vile form of criminal conduct ... They attack the very fabric of Canada's democratic ideals. Those involved live by a philosophy that rejects the democratic process. Their motivation is unique and fundamentally at odds with the rule of law."[24] And in *R v Gaya* (another Toronto 18 prosecution), Justice Hill of the same court proclaimed that the "evil of terrorism" is anathema in "civilized societies committed to the rule of law, [where] it is freedom of expression and democratic processes which advance public debate relating to political, religious, economic and social issues."[25] Almost all terrorism sentencing decisions contain language in this vein. Violent terrorism is projected as something external to Canadian values and society, obscuring Canada's own foundational structures of violence: most importantly, the white supremacy and patriarchy that undergird the settler colonial state.[26]

The work that racial logic does in terrorism cases is highlighted through contrast with cases involving white defendants, charged with acts of violence that would likely be called *terrorism* if performed by a Muslim. Justin Bourque, for example, pled guilty to killing three Royal Canadian Mounted Police (RCMP) officers and wounding two in a targeted shooting spree in 2014, and was sentenced to life in prison for murder and attempted murder; he was not prosecuted for terrorism.[27] While Bourque's own lawyer characterized him as "dedicat[ed]

Table 15.1. Post-9/11 terrorism prosecutions in Canada

Defendant	Outcome	Sentence
Project Awaken		
Momin Khawaja	Guilty	Life
Project O-Sage (the "Toronto 18")		
Ibrahim Alkalel Mohammed Aboud	Charges stayed	Peace bond
Shareef Adelhaleem	Guilty	Life plus 5 years
Fahim Ahmad	Pled guilty	16 years
Zakaria Amara	Pled guilty	Life
Asad Ansari	Guilty	6 years, 5 months (less time served), 3 years' probation
Steven Vikash Chand	Guilty	10 years
Mohammed Ali Dirie	Pled guilty	7 years, peace bond on release
Amin Mohamed Durrani	Pled guilty	7.5 years, 3 years' probation
Saad Gaya	Pled guilty	18 years
Ahmad Mustafa Ghany	Charges stayed	Peace bond
Jahmaal James	Pled guilty	7 years
Saad Khalid	Pled guilty	20 years
Yasim Abdi Mohamed	Charges stayed	
Nishanthan Yogakrishnan	Guilty	2.5 years, 3 years' probation
Youth	Charges stayed	Peace bond
Youth	Charges stayed	Peace bond
Youth	Charges dropped	
Project Summum		
Said Namouh	Guilty	Life plus 20 years
Project Severe		
Mohamed Hassan Hersi	Guilty	10 years
Project Samosa		
Hiva Alizadeh Mohammad	Pled guilty	24 years
Misbahuddin Ahmed	Guilty	12 years
Khurram Syed Sher	Acquitted	
Project Sagittaire		
Mouna Diab	Charges dropped	

Defendant	Outcome	Sentence
Project Smooth (the "Via Rail Plot")		
Chiheb Esseghaier	Guilty	Life, with concurrent sentence of 14 years, 4 months
Raed Jaser	Guilty	Life, with concurrent sentence of 8 years, 4 months
Project Souvenir (the "Canada Day Plot")		
John Stuart Nuttal	Guilty, but no conviction entered because defendant was entrapped	
Amanda Korody	Guilty, but no conviction entered because defendant was entrapped	
Project Slipstream		
Ashton Larmond	Pled guilty	17 years
Carlos Larmond	Pled guilty	7 years
Suliman Mohamed	Pled guilty	7 years
Other Cases		
Prapaharan Thambithurai	Pled guilty	6 months
Youth	Guilty	2-year custody supervision, 12 months' probation
Youth	Pled guilty	TBD

Source: Adapted from Craig Forcese, "Informal Tabulation of Completed Terrorism Prosecutions in Canada Involving Incidents Occurring After the Enactment of the 2001 *Anti-Terrorism Act*," September 14, 2016, http://static1.1.sqspcdn.com/stati c/f/842287/27246552/1473886808017/Terrorism+Prosecutions+Table.pdf?token=io6%2 BS4T7t2EYBV3Wpki%2FcX%2BpQx4%3D.

to 'right wing' gun nut culture,"[28] the ideological underpinnings for his rampage received comparatively minimal attention in the judicial process – which elaborated on Bourque's fondness for violent video games, his residual frustrations from being home-schooled, and his emotional turmoil at the time of the shooting from sleep and marijuana deprivation.[29] In his sentencing, the judge described Bourque as the perpetrator of "one of the worst [crimes] in Canadian history,"[30] but never as a "terrorist" (although he did "terrorize" the community).[31] Bourque's actions were decried as "horrific" and "heinous,"[32] but not as fundamentally antithetical to "civilized societies committed to the rule of law" or as existentially threatening to "the very fabric of Canadian democratic ideals." Such Manichaean language seems reserved for those assumed to be animated by "Muslim rage." Bourque was not painted as an enemy outsider, but as an insider gone horribly astray, in stark contrast to the law's phantasm of the radical Muslim terrorist.

The differential treatment of Muslim "terrorists" as compared to white supremacist and right-wing perpetrators of mass violence is evident in the prevailing inclination to depoliticize white actors' violence, by explaining it as a product of individual "mental illness" as opposed to racist ideology. For example, Anders Breivik, the Norwegian far-right ideologue who killed 77 people in 2011 as a protest against Muslim immigration and policies of multiculturalism, was represented as paranoid schizophrenic at his trial by both the prosecution and his defence: a diagnosis that Breivik himself repudiated as an effort to delegitimize his ideology by ascribing it to "insanity."[33] In such cases, "mental illness labelling ... disqualif[ies] an ideology by insisting on the individual illness of a person ... Their ideologies are pictured as the rotten fruits of disturbed individual minds, and certainly not the results of broader social interactions."[34] In cases involving Muslims charged with terrorism offences, in contrast, Canadian courts have rejected claims of mental illness that might mitigate the culpability of the accused.[35] Instead, it is maintained that "the underlying motivation renders [terrorism and violent extremism] significantly different from other criminal violence" because "there is consensus that terrorists do not act out of mental imbalance, psychopathology or psychopathy," but are rather driven by "large ideological issues";[36] in the case of *R v Gaya*, for instance, his "sense of religiously motivated moral outrage" stemming from "his religious beliefs, his sympathy towards the suffering 'limbs' of the Muslim Nation, and his perceived sense of duty to stand up to the Canadian Government towards change in foreign policy."[37]

While responsibility for the violence of white killers is individualized (assigned to the particular psychology or circumstances of the perpetrator), responsibility for the planned violence of Muslim terrorists is collectivized (assigned to a complex of theological and political beliefs associated with Muslims and Islam). While whiteness is exonerated by severing individual psychopathology from the collective, Muslimness is condemned by its suturing to collective madness.

Because Muslims convicted of terrorism, unlike other offenders, are imagined to be inexorably impelled towards violence by their infection with radical religious ideology, the tests normally used to assess risk of recidivism and potential for rehabilitation have been deemed inadequate in terrorism cases. And so, in *R v Ahmed* a special Assessment and Treatment of Radicalization Scale (ATRS) was administered to the convicted.[38] Despite the superficially race- and religion-neutral name of the scale, its Muslim-centric formulation is evident from the six dimensions measured:

> The first subscale reflects Negative Attitudes Towards Israel, because the Israeli-Palestinian conflict is considered as one of the central sources of grievance promoted by many extremists. The second subscale is Political Views, which measures the important political views that are advocated by Middle Eastern extremists such as opposing secular laws and governments, and advocating the implementation of Sharia Law. The third subscale assesses participants' Attitudes Toward Women. Middle Eastern extremists believe women are inferior to men. The fourth subscale measures Negative Attitudes Towards Western Culture. Middle Eastern extremists have been vocal in their rejection of Western culture claiming that Western civilization is corrupt and that the West is trying to undermine their religion. Extremists generally emphasize the prevalence of negative attitudes in Muslim countries towards non-Muslim cultures. The fifth subscale, Religiosity, assesses respondents' commitment to their religion. Extremists use religion to advocate for their cause and to recruit new pools of extremists. Some questions in this subscale tap into extreme religious views that are common in the Middle East. The sixth subscale, Condoning Fighting, measures views that condone fighting and promote acts of violence as a means for the revival of religion with the goal of destroying infidels and achieving one world under the Islamic religion.[39]

This test was developed by a former chief psychologist at Correctional Service of Canada, Dr Wagdy Loza, specifically to measure what he has named Middle Eastern Extremist Ideologies: "extreme religious ideologies that a few years ago were not known to the average Canadian citizen."[40] Loza himself has acknowledged that there is no way of assessing the predictive value of his scale, to determine whether possession of such purportedly Extremist Ideologies actually correlates with engagement in future acts of violence; as he puts it, "using the current data for future predictive studies (i.e., test if highly extremist responses will result in terroristic acts) is not possible."[41] In short, there is no independent empirical basis for using the ATRS to assess risk of future participation in violence, other than its correspondence with stereotypical preconceptions about what makes Muslims dangerous. The scale knits together racializing representations of Muslim masculinity as exceptionally misogynistic ("Middle Eastern extremists believe women are inferior to men") and exceptionally terroristic. This reinforces the gendered logic of the war on terror, in which Western democracies (and their militaries) have pitched themselves as the saviours of "imperilled Muslim women" from "dangerous Muslim men"[42] – rationalizing violence against Muslim women as well as Muslim men both at home (in the form of oppressive national security measures[43]) and abroad (in the form of war).

However, even the profoundly Orientalist way of thinking about rehabilitation articulated through the ATRS has been marginalized in favour of a more punitive response to terrorism cases, based on a presumption that many of those convicted of terrorism are irredeemably terroristic. According to the Ontario Superior Court in *R v Esseghaier*, "the rigid ideological belief systems that often motivate terrorist offences can give rise to an inference of ongoing dangerousness."[44] The asserted uniqueness of terrorism is expressed in a severe approach to punishment, at all stages of the legal process:[45] a "reverse onus" to prove eligibility for pre-trial bail is imposed on those accused of terrorism;[46] the main purposes in sentencing are said to be denunciation and deterrence, rather than rehabilitation, leading to very long sentences even when no act of violence has actually been executed;[47] "terrorist motive" can be considered an aggravating factor at sentencing, further increasing terms of imprisonment;[48] the option for sentences to run concurrently is removed – all sentences for terrorism (except for life sentences) must be served consecutively;[49] and a greater portion of the sentence than usual must presumptively be served before the convicted is eligible for parole.[50] In 2010, the Custody Rating Scale – which Correctional Services uses to determine whether prisoners will be incarcerated in minimum-security, medium-security, or maximum-security conditions – was amended to virtually ensure that those convicted of terrorism offences would receive a high level of security classification, subjecting them to greater amounts of surveillance and control.[51] The threat of prison "radicalization" has been used to justify increasing surveillance of Muslim terrorism convicts and depriving them of access to religious literature and services.[52] "[R]egardless of the actual threat of convicted terrorists, these Muslim men are considered among the most violent and dangerous individuals within the Canadian penal system, despite not having committed any acts of violence or terrorism," Jeffrey Monaghan remarks. "Their containment and constant monitoring is governed by rationalities that code these individuals as extremely dangerous subjects and, additionally, as threats to liberal democracy in general."[53]

While analyses of the relationship between race, law, and counter-terrorism have often focused on "spaces of exception" – spaces like Guantanamo Bay, where the normal rule of law is said to be suspended[54] – representations of Muslim terrorists as bearers of exceptional psychological profiles have inscribed and institutionalized exceptional treatment for those convicted of terrorism in the normal Canadian criminal justice system (which was already a system of settler colonial carceral violence, built around the construction of racialized threats[55]). The pathologization and criminalization of religious and political beliefs connected to Muslim identity also rationalizes exercises of exceptional surveillance and securitization of the general Muslim population, in the name of preventive counter-radicalization. In the framework of counter-radicalization/countering violent extremism (CVE), "nonviolent political activity by Muslim groups that are thought to share an ideology with terrorists is seen as another manifestation of the same radicalization process," notes Arun Kundnani. "It is thereby depoliticized and seen as complicit with religiously inspired terrorism."[56]

On Prevention

Counter-radicalization and CVE programs are frequently pitched as a gentler alternative to carceral counter-terrorism, as a means of proactively intercepting people on the path of violent extremism before they engage in criminalized activity. In 2016 the federal government announced that it would be devoting $35 million over the next five years to the development of an Office of Community Outreach and Counter-Radicalization.[57] A background guide produced by the government to inform recent community consultations on Canada's national security framework emphasizes the necessity of "steer[ing] at-risk individuals away from radicalization to violence," by "support[ing] local communities to address this issue"[58] – in other words, by inculcating modes of self-policing in particular communities understood to be incubators of terrorism. Municipal counter-radicalization initiatives have been operating in Calgary, Montreal, and Toronto for the last few years.[59]

In the Toronto program, people thought to be at risk of "extremism" are referred to hubs of service providers – medical and psychological professionals, the school board, community housing – that will formulate an intervention.[60] The program has apparently distilled more than one hundred factors to determine whether someone is on the path to radicalization, but this expansive list of risk factors has not been disclosed for public scrutiny.[61] This inspires particular concern because counter-radicalization initiatives in other jurisdictions have drawn on dubious "science" to stigmatize particular opinions and behaviours as harbingers of violence. As the Open Society Justice Initiative found in its October 2016 study of Prevent, the United Kingdom's counter-radicalization strategy, for instance, "Prevent's targeting of non-violent extremism and 'indicators' of risk of being drawn into terrorism lack a scientific basis. Indeed, the claim that non-violent extremism – including 'radical' or religious ideology – is the precursor to terrorism has been widely discredited by the British government itself, as well as numerous reputable scholars."[62] In a report released last February, United Nations Special Rapporteur on Counter-Terrorism and Human Rights Ben Emmerson criticized prevailing approaches to countering radicalization as conceptually flawed and ineffective. "Many programmes directed at radicalization are based on a simplistic understanding of the process as a fixed trajectory to violent extremism with identifiable markers along the way," Emmerson concluded. "States have tended to focus on those that are most appealing to them, shying away from the more complex issues, including political issues such as foreign policy and transnational conflicts" – preferring to instead emphasize "religious ideology as the driver of terrorism and extremism."[63]

Analyses of the causes and dynamics of radicalization produced by Canadian security agencies fixate on the role of "extremist narratives" as motivators of violence. In a study by the RCMP entitled *Words Make Worlds: Terrorism and Language*, extremism is characterized as a "cultural and emotional phenomenon"[64] rooted in a "strong sense" of "perceived oppression" and "a spirit of specifically Islamic activism and mobilization that is often in conflict with Western social and political norms."[65] Muslims' experiences of oppression are relativized and minimized as *perceptions*, and pathologized as sources of potential violence,

while the actualized violence of structures of Islamophobia that subject Muslims to war and torture and surveillance remains hidden from
view. And so, the nostrum that is prescribed for this "cultural and emotional phenomenon" is reprogramming of Muslims with "alternative
narratives"[66] ("we need to find ways of counterbalancing the culture of
death and martyrdom with a culture that celebrates the value of life"[67]),
rather than political transformation to address systemic racism. And
indeed, the development of counter-radicalization programs in Canada
has coincided with the constriction of political space to work for such
anti-Islamophobic transformation non-violently, with the introduction
of increasingly draconian counter-terrorism laws that potentially crimi-
nalize and securitize forms of political advocacy and activism (like Bill
C-51, the Anti-terrorism Act, 2015).[68]

In *Madness and Civilization*, Michel Foucault critiqued the popular
understanding that Philippe Pinel's unchaining of those labelled *mad*
in French hospices constituted liberation, rather than subjection to new
forms of normalizing power (through techniques such as close observation): "the absence of constraint in the nineteenth-century asylum is
not unreason liberated, but madness long since mastered."[69] Likewise,
the absence of physical constraints and formal criminal penalization
does not render counter-radicalization a non-coercive enterprise. With
counter-radicalization, the concentrated state violence of criminalization is supplemented with more diffuse operations of power, circulated
through the capillaries of everyday social life. Mosques and schools
become sites where individuals are surveilled and disciplined for signs
of radicalization; provision of services like housing and health care
become part of national security strategy. As the American Civil Liberties Union, Article 19, and the Brennan Center for Justice at New York
University pointed out in a joint letter to Ben Emmerson: "CVE initiatives in the United States and Europe focus overwhelmingly on Muslim
communities, with the discriminatory impact of stigmatizing them as
inherently suspicious and in need of special monitoring. They transform the relationship between Muslims and schools and social service
providers into security-based engagements."[70] Moreover, as Amna
Akbar has documented in the American context, counter-radicalization
and other projects portrayed as collaborations with Muslim communities are frequently continuous with more obviously coercive exercises
of state security and police power.[71] Innocuous-sounding "community
engagement" initiatives, for example, have served as opportunities for
police to collect "intelligence" on Muslims' opinions and activities.[72]

While Canadian security agencies' public reports on radicalization are careful to distinguish Islam in general from variants deemed to be extreme,[73] their "findings" that terrorists often appear to be ordinary and well-integrated,[74] and that "Sunni Islamist radicalization" can occur "just about anywhere ... these people gather,"[75] ensure that in practice large segments of the Muslim population will be placed under scrutiny. When "home-grown terrorists" are characterized, in the words of one Ontario Superior Court judge, as a "particularly virulent form of cancer that must be aggressively eradicated,"[76] the entire body imagined to be susceptible to sickness is targeted for treatment.

Conclusion: On Resistance

One type of resistance to the collective securitization of Muslims in the domestic War on Terror has been the recasting of Muslims framed as *terrorists* as sufferers of *mental illness* instead[77] – mimicking the preservation of the innocence of whiteness through the individualizing psychopathologization of white mass killers. However, such responses reproduce the reification of mental illness as a category separate from mental health, and reinforce the stigmatizing and criminalizing association of mental illness with violence. At the same time, they perpetuate the de-rationalization of the political grievances that lie behind what is dismissed as "Muslim rage," reducing them to figments of mad Muslim minds: problems to be solved by medical and penal intervention, rather than the real possibility of non-violent political transformation. Individual Muslims are pathologized, while the systemic pathologies of structural Islamophobia made manifest in the War on Terror continue to escape examination. Muslims are represented as being in need of better adjustment to a world that enacts violence on them, while the world itself stays on course. But as Martin Luther King Jr said, "there are some things in our social order to which I'm proud to be maladjusted ... It may well be that the salvation of our world lies in the hands of the maladjusted."[78] Instead of fixating on the madness of Muslims, let us heal the social order that makes Muslims mad.

NOTES

1 Carothers, *The Psychology of Mau Mau.*
2 Keller, "Taking Science."

3 Metzl, *The Protest Psychosis*.

4 Said, *Orientalism*.

5 Said, *Orientalism*, 38.

6 Lewis, "The Roots."

7 Stampnitzky, *Disciplining Terror*, 179–80.

8 Haney Lopez, *White by Law*, 91.

9 See for example Public Safety Canada, "Building Resilience"; Public Safety Canada, "2013 Public Report"; Public Safety Canada, "2014 Public Report"; Public Safety Canada, "2016 Public Report."

10 Knefel, "Everything You've Been Told."

11 Ling, "Canada's Spy Agency."

12 Canadian Security Intelligence Service, "Public Report."

13 Foucault, *"Society Must Be Defended,"* 15.

14 Howell, "Victims or Madmen?", 44.

15 *Criminal Code*, RSC 1985, c C-46, s 83.01(1)(b). The *Code* also lists specific acts that constitute terrorism, derived from international counter-terrorism conventions.

16 Ibid., s 83.18(3)(d).

17 Ibid., ss 83.181 and 83,191.

18 Ibid., ss 83.02 and 83.03.

19 Ibid., s 83.221.

20 Senate of Canada, "Proceedings."

21 Forcese and Roach, *False Security*, 278; Forcese, "Informal Tabulation."

22 Solyom, "The Trump Effect"; Solyom, "Quebec Mosque Shooting."

23 Roach, "Be Careful."

24 *R v Khalid*, 2009 OJ 6414 (ONSC), para. 108.

25 *R v Gaya*, 2008 CanLII 24539 (ONSC), para. 161.

26 Thobani, *Exalted Subjects*.

27 *R v Bourque*, 2014 NBQB 237.

28 "Justin Bourque's Lawyer."

29 *R v Bourque*.

30 Ibid, para. 38.

31 Ibid, para. 15.

32 Ibid, paras. 2 and 48.

33 Baele, "Are Terrorists Insane?"

34 Ibid, 266.

35 *R v Esseghaier*, 2015 ONSC 5855, paras. 74–86.

36 *R v Amara*, 2010 ONSC 251, para. 47.

37 *R v Gaya*, 2010 ONSC 434, para. 43.

38 *R v Ahmed*, 2014 ONSC 6153.

39 Ibid., para. 30.
40 Loza, "The Prevalence," 925.
41 Ibid., 926.
42 Razack, "Imperilled Muslim Women."
43 Harkat, "Sophie Harkat's Husband."
44 *R v Esseghaier,* para. 97.
45 See, generally, Public Prosecution Service of Canada, "National Security."
46 Roach, "Be Careful," 105–13.
47 See for example *R v Khawaja,* 2012 SCC 69, paras. 126 and 130.
48 *Criminal Code,* s 718.2.
49 Ibid., s 83.26.
50 Ibid., s 743.6(1).
51 Monaghan, "Terror Carceralism."
52 Monaghan, "Criminal Justice Policy."
53 Monaghan, "Terror Carceralism," 8.
54 Gregory, "The Black Flag."
55 Nichols, "The Colonialism of Incarceration."
56 Kundnani, *The Muslims Are Coming!,* 118
57 Zillo, "Canada Committed."
58 Government of Canada, "Our Security, Our Rights," 16.
59 "Anti-Radicalization Program"; "Montreal Anti-Radicalization Centre Officially Launches"; Nasser, "Toronto Lifts Curtain."
60 Nasser, "Toronto Lifts Curtain."
61 Ibid.
62 Open Society Justice Initiative, "Eroding Trust," 16.
63 Emmerson, "Report of the Special Rapporteur," para. 15.
64 Royal Canadian Mounted Police, "Words Make Worlds," 12.
65 Ibid., 10.
66 Ibid., 13.
67 Ibid.
68 Roach and Forcese, "Bill C-51."
69 Foucault, *Madness and Civilization,* 239.
70 American Civil Liberties Union, "Article 19."
71 Akbar, "Policing 'Radicalization'"; Akbar, "National Security's Broken Windows."
72 Ibid.
73 Royal Canadian Mounted Police, "Words Make Worlds."
74 Royal Canadian Mounted Police, "Radicalization."
75 Bell, "Venues of Sunni."
76 *R v Larmond,* 2016 ONSC 5479, para. 3.

77 See for example Anderson, "The Enemy"; Heer, "The Line."
78 King Jr, "A Look."

BIBLIOGRAPHY

Legislation

Criminal Code, RSC 1985, c C-46.

Jurisprudence

R v Ahmed, 2014 ONSC 6153.
R v Amara, 2010 ONSC 251.
R v Bourque, 2014 NBQB 237.
R v Esseghaier, 2015 ONSC 5855.
R v Gaya, 2008 CanLII 24539 (ONSC).
R v Gaya, 2010 ONSC 434.
R v Khalid, 2009 OJ 6414 (ONSC).
R v Khawaja, 2012 SCC 69.
R v Larmond, 2016 ONSC 5479.

Secondary Materials

Akbar, Amna. "National Security's Broken Windows." *UCLA Law Review* 62
    (2015): 834–907.
Akbar, Amna. "Policing "Radicalization,'" *UC Irvine Law Review* 3, no. 4
    (2013): 809–83.
American Civil Liberties Union, Article 19, and Brennan Center for
    Justice. "Letter to Ben Emmerson, Special Rapporteur on the Promotion
    and Protection of Human Rights and Fundamental Freedoms While
    Countering Terrorism." December 24, 2015. https://www.brennancenter
    .org/sites/default/files/Final%20122415%20Letter%20Re%20CVE%20
    to%20SR.pdf.
Anderson, Mitchell. "The Enemy Is Neglect of Mental Illness."
    Tyee, October 25, 2014. https://thetyee.ca/Opinion/2014/10/25/Enemy
    _Is_Neglect_Of_Mental_Ilness/.
"Anti-Radicalization Program Launched in Calgary." *CBC News*,
    February 17, 2015. http://www.cbc.ca/news/canada/calgary/
    anti-radicalization-program-launched-in-calgary-1.2960192.

Baele, Stephane J. "Are Terrorists Insane? A Critical Analysis of Mental Health Categories in Lone Terrorists' Trials." *Critical Studies on Terrorism* 7, no. 2 (2014): 257–76.

Bell, Stewart. "Venues of Sunni Islamist Radicalization in Canada." *National Post*, January 3, 2013. https://news.nationalpost.com/news/canada/islamist-extremists-radicalizing-canadians-at-a-large-number-of-venues-secret-report-reveals.

Canadian Security Intelligence Service. "Public Report 2014–2016." February 28, 2017. ttps://www.canada.ca/en/security-intelligence-service/corporate/publications/public-report-2014-2016.html.

Carothers, J. C. *The Psychology of Mau Mau.* Nairobi, Kenya: Government Printer, 1955.

Emmerson, Ben. "Report of the Special Rapporteur on the Promotion and Protection of Human Rights and Fundamental Freedoms While Countering Terrorism." A/HRC/31/65. February 22, 2016. https://www.justsecurity.org/wp-content/uploads/2016/04/Emmerson-UNHRC-Report-A-HRC-31-65_UneditedVersion.pdf

Forcese, Craig, and Kent Roach. *False Security: The Radicalization of Canadian Anti-Terrorism.* Toronto, ON: Irwin Law, 2015.

Forcese, Craig. "Informal Tabulation of Completed Terrorism Prosecutions in Canada Involving Incidents Occurring After the Enactment of the 2001 Anti-Terrorism Act." September 14, 2016. http://static1.1.sqspcdn.com/static/f/842287/27246552/1473886808017/Terrorism+Prosecutions+Table.pdf?token=io6%2BS4T7t2EYBV3Wpki%2FcX%2BpQx4%3D.

Foucault, Michel. *Madness and Civilization: A History of Insanity in the Age of Reason.* Translated by Richard Howard. Oxford: Routledge, 2001.

Foucault, Michel. *"Society Must Be Defended": Lectures at the College de France, 1975–76.* Translated by David Macey. New York: Picador, 1997.

Government of Canada. "Our Security, Our Rights: National Security Green Paper, 2016: Background Document." 2016. https://www.publicsafety.gc.ca/cnt/rsrcs/pblctns/ntnl-scrt-grn-ppr-2016-bckgrndr/ntnl-scrt-grn-ppr-2016-bckgrndr-en.pdf.

Gregory, Derek. "The Black Flag: Guantanamo Bay and the Space of Exception." *Geografiska Annaler: Series B, Human Geography* 88, no. 4 (2006): 405–27.

Haney Lopez, Ian. *White by Law: The Legal Construction of Race.* New York: New York University Press, 2006.

Harkat, Sophie. "Sophie Harkat's Husband Mohamed Is Being Deported. Here's What She Has to Say." *Rabble*, October 17, 2015. http://rabble.ca/news/2015/10/sophie-harkats-husband-mohamed-being-deported-heres-what-she-has-to-say.

Heer, Jeet. "The Line Between Terrorism and Mental Illness." *New Yorker,*
   October 25, 2014. https://www.newyorker.com/news/news-desk/
   line-terrorism-mental-illness.

Howell, Alison. "Victims or Madmen? The Diagnostic Competition over
   "Terrorist' Detainees at Guantanamo Bay." *International Political Sociology* 1,
   no. 1 (2007): 29–47.

"Justin Bourque's Lawyer Slams Gun Laws." *CBC News,* October
   31, 2014. http://www.cbc.ca/news/canada/new-brunswick/justin
   -bourque-s-lawyer-slams-gun-laws-1.2820233.

Keller, Richard C. "Taking Science to the Colonies: Psychiatric Innovation
   in France and North Africa." In *Psychiatry and Empire,* edited by Sloan
   Mahone and Megan Vaughan, 17–40. Basingstoke, UK: Palgrave
   Macmillan, 2007.

King Jr, Martin Luther. "A Look to the Future." Address presented
   at Highlander Folk School, Monteagle, Tennessee, September 2, 1957.
   https://kingencyclopedia.stanford.edu/encyclopedia/
   documentsentry/a_look_to_the_future_hfs.1.html.

Knefel, John. "Everything You've Been Told About Radicalization
   is Wrong." *Rolling Stone,* May 6, 2013. https://www.rollingstone.com/
   politics/news/everything-youve-been-told-about-radicalization-is
   -wrong-20130506.

Kundnani, Arun. *The Muslims Are Coming! Islamophobia, Extremism, and the
   Domestic War on Terror.* London, UK: Verso Books, 2014.

Lewis, Bernard. "The Roots of Muslim Rage." *The Atlantic,* September 1990.

Ling, Justin. "Canada's Spy Agency Wants to Hire Shrinks to Study
   Terrorists." *Vice,* February 15, 2016. https://news.vice.com/article/
   canadas-spy-agency-wants-to-hire-shrinks-to-study-terrorists.

Loza, Wagdy. "The Prevalence of Middle Eastern Extremist Ideologies
   Among Some Canadian Offenders." *Journal of Interpersonal Violence* 25, no. 5
   (2010): 919–28.

Metzl, Jonathan. *The Protest Psychosis: How Schizophrenia Became a Black
   Disease.* Boston, MA: Beacon Press, 2010.

Monaghan, Jeffrey. "Criminal Justice Policy Transfer and Prison Counter-
   Radicalization: Examining Canadian Participation in the Roma-Lyon
   Group." *Canadian Journal of Law and Society* 30, no. 3 (2015): 381–400.

Monaghan, Jeffrey. "Terror Carceralism: Surveillance, Security Governance
   and De/Civilization." *Punishment and Society* 15, no. 1 (2012): 3–22.

"Montreal Anti-Radicalization Centre Officially Launches after Months
   in Service." *CBC News,* November 22, 2015. http://www.cbc.ca/news/
   canada/montreal/montreal-anti-radicalizaton-centre-terrorism-1.3330350.

Nasser, Shanifa. "Toronto Lifts Curtain on Extremism Prevention Plan Quietly Operating for More Than 2 Years." *CBC News*, November 26, 2016. http://www.cbc.ca/news/canada/toronto/toronto-police-deradicalization -program-1.3867442.

Nichols, Robert. "The Colonialism of Incarceration." *Radical Philosophy Review* 17, no. 2 (2014): 435–55.

Open Society Justice Initiative. "Eroding Trust: The UK's PREVENT Counter-Extremism Strategy in Health and Education." 2016. https://www .opensocietyfoundations.org/sites/default/files/eroding-trust-20161017_0 .pdf.

Public Prosecution Service of Canada. "National Security." In *Public Prosecution Service of Canada Deskbook*. Ottawa, ON: PPSC, 2016. http:// www.ppsc-sppc.gc.ca/eng/pub/fpsd-sfpg/fps-sfp/tpd/p5/ch01.html.

Public Safety Canada. "Building Resilience Against Terrorism: Canada's Counter-Terrorism Strategy." 2012. https://www.publicsafety.gc.ca/cnt/ rsrcs/pblctns/rslnc-gnst-trrrsm/index-en.aspx.

Public Safety Canada. "2013 Public Report on the Terrorist Threat to Canada." 2013. https://www.publicsafety.gc.ca/cnt/rsrcs/pblctns/trrrst-thrt-cnd/ index-en.aspx.

Public Safety Canada. "2014 Public Report on the Terrorist Threat to Canada." 2014. https://www.publicsafety.gc.ca/cnt/rsrcs/pblctns/2014-pblc-rpr -trrrst-thrt/index-en.aspx.

Public Safety Canada. "2016 Public Report on the Terrorist Threat to Canada." 2016. https://www.publicsafety.gc.ca/cnt/rsrcs/pblctns/2016-pblc-rpr-trrrst -thrt/index-en.aspx.

Razack, Sherene H. "Imperilled Muslim Women, Dangerous Muslim Men and Civilised Europeans: Legal and Social Responses to Forced Marriages." *Feminist Legal Studies* 12, no. 2 (2004): 129–74.

Roach, Kent. "Be Careful What You Wish For? Terrorism Prosecutions in Post-9/11 Canada." *Queen's Law Journal* 40, no. 1 (2014): 99–140.

Roach, Kent, and Craig Forcese. "Bill C-51 Backgrounder #1: The New Advocating or Promoting Terrorism Offence." February 3, 2015. https:// papers.ssrn.com/sol3/papers.cfm?abstract_id=2560006.

Royal Canadian Mounted Police. "Radicalization: A Guide for the Perplexed." June 2009. http://publications.gc.ca/site/archivee-archived .html?url=http://publications.gc.ca/collections/collection_2012/grc-rcmp/ PS64-102-2009-eng.pdf.

Royal Canadian Mounted Police. "Words Make Worlds: Terrorism and Language." https://shawglobalnews.files.wordpress.com/2015/07/ ps64-98-2007-eng.pdf.

Said, Edward W. *Orientalism*. New York: Random House, 1979.

Senate of Canada. "Proceedings of the Special Senate Committee on the Subject Matter of Bill C-36." October 22, 2001. https://sencanada.ca/en/Content/Sen/committee/371/sm36/01evb-e.

Solyom, Catherine. "Quebec Mosque Shooting: What Happened to Alexandre Bissonette?" *Montreal Gazette*, February 1, 2017. https://montrealgazette.com/news/local-news/quebec-mosque-shooting-what-happened-to-alexandre-bissonnette.

Solyom, Catherine. "The Trump Effect and the Normalization of Hate in Quebec." *Montreal Gazette*, November 15, 2016. https://montrealgazette.com/news/quebec/the-trump-effect-and-the-normalization-of-hate.

Stampnitzky, Lisa. *Disciplining Terror: How Experts Invented "Terrorism."* Cambridge, UK: Cambridge University Press, 2013.

Thobani, Sunera. *Exalted Subjects: Studies in the Making of Race and Nation.* Toronto, ON: University of Toronto Press, 2007.

Zillo, Michelle. "Canada Committed to Becoming World Leader in Counter-Radicalization: Freeland." *Globe and Mail*, April 24, 2017. https://www.theglobeandmail.com/news/politics/canada-committed-to-becoming-world-leader-in-counter-radicalization-freeland/article34799855/.

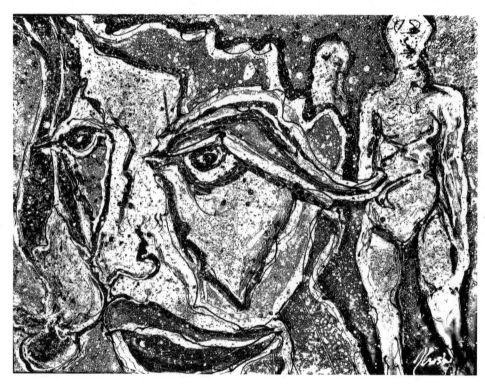

The Divide, painting by Jennifer Crosby

PART IV

Geographies of Violence

The five contributions in Part IV attend to the practices of institutions and the institutionalization of practices that are implicated in the enactment of violence upon people with psychosocial disabilities. Three chapters focus exclusively on the psychiatric institution and the institution of psychiatry, one travels away from the psychiatric institution to consider the violence of carceral segregation practices, and one considers the direct and indirect violence done to marginalized Mad community members through gentrification.

Chapter 16 is authored by Mick McKeown, Amy Scholes, Fiona Jones, and Will Aindow, self-described as "people with quite different experiences of violence in relation to the practice and organization of psychiatric services." From their various perspectives and lived experiences, they bring forth the notions of *legitimacy*, *fairness*, and *social justice* to implicate coercive psychiatric "care" in the implicit and explicit violence that might be enacted by people with psychosocial disabilities. Their analysis is demarcated by a focus on violence between staff and patients, and the use by staff of restraint and seclusion as a response to patient violence. The authors' position their analysis within a reformist frame underscoring the potential value of internal change strategies – an *"inside-out* strategy" – that promote staff reflection and re-conceptualizations of, and responses to, patient violence towards the revolutionary goals of external activist groups.

In line with emerging inquiries on the use of the graphic narrative (e.g., graphic novels, comics)[1] as a resource for health care professionals and service users, in chapter 17 Janet Lee-Evoy uses graphics to depict the implications of coercive psychiatric "care" examined in chapter 16. She offers an interpretation, from her perspective as a psychiatric resident-in-training, of Grace's interaction with psychiatry and the practices of the psychiatric institution to trouble the psychiatric narrative of "violence as benevolence." The reader is given a glimpse into the tension that she might have to negotiate as she is pulled into a psychiatric narrative of serving the "greater good" to justify the violence inherent in institutional responses to patient violence. Beyond these important insights, this graphic chapter speaks to the determination of risk and the fixed nature of risk (Grace's involuntary status is never revoked even though she never disputed her admission) and the use of chemical and physical restraints as institutionalize violence. Janet concludes by implying the impact of coercive psychiatric "care" through Grace's performance of docility.

Chapter 18 is the third examination of the ways in which psychiatric staff and institutions respond to patient "violence" through the lens of health care ethicist Kevin Reel. Drawing upon Simone Weil's discussion of the complimentary yet different forces of grace and gravity as important elements in human behaviour, and consultations with psychiatric staff about the practice of restraint and seclusion, Kevin argues that these practices should be taken as a form of institutional violence. In doing so, and in ways that are reminiscent of Janet Lee-Evoy's depiction of the "violence as benevolent" narrative in psychiatry, he troubles the institutional perspective that restraint and seclusion are legitimate responses to patient violence. The analysis counters individual and institutional dimensions of gravity that contribute to the use of restraint and seclusion, such as fear-based responses to patient violence and institutional policy undergirded by mistrust of clients/patients with complementary grace-supporting dimensions including service provider reflectivity on responses to fear and addressing the culture of mistrust that pervades the psychiatric institution.

In chapter 19 Jennifer Kilty and Sandra Lehalle explore the involvement of front-line staff in day-to-day practices of violence done to people within an institutional setting. However, they shift our gaze away from the psychiatric institution to examine the harmful physical and mental health consequences of carceral segregation practices. Using Teo's conceptualization of epistemological violence they explain how the interpretation of empirical data "pertaining to risks, needs and responsivity factor information" to produce knowledge of the Other as "risky" and "inferior" constitutes violence. Within the "correctional risk logic" model the conflation of risk and need transpires in people who experience more and greater needs being deemed to be greater risk, and subsequently, to be more vulnerable to institutional segregation policy and practices. The authors emphasize the uneven effect of "correctional risk logic" with Indigenous and Black people being "segregated at exceptional rates." Similar to Mick McKeown, Amy Scholes, Fiona Jones, and Will Aindow, and Kevin Reel, this chapter's authors theorize how front-line staff comes to the point of enacting violence on another, drawing upon the concepts of dehumanization and moral distancing.

In the book's final chapter, Ben Losman takes us from the geographical landscapes of the institution to the South Parkdale (Toronto) community as he explores gentrification as a form of "direct and indirect violence," particularly for its poor or racialized or Mad community members. Ben outlines the ways in which the interests of the state (urban development), the psychiatric institution (social integration), and the private sector (profit) violently converge to displace socially and economically marginalized community members from "their homes, communities, and historical sense of belonging," and re-populate the community with a "white, affluent, young, and sane" profit source. Importantly, he troubles the characterization of the simultaneous occurrence of South Parkdale's gentrification and the institution's strategy of social integration as coincidental by embedding his analysis in the historical relationship between the community and the institution. Ben's analysis points to the erasure of violence inherent in the psychiatric institution that happens through the emergence of an apparent socially progressive urban village, while also outlining how the urban village is contingent upon tamed madness achieved through social integration.

NOTE

1 See for example Williams, "Graphic Medicine"; Al-Jawad, "Comics Are Research."

BIBLIOGRAPHY

Al-Jawad, Muna. "Comics Are Research: Graphic Narratives as a New Way of Seeing Clinical Practice." *Journal of Medical Humanities* 36, no. 4 (2015): 369–74.
Williams, Ian. "Graphic Medicine: Comics as Medical Narrative." *Journal of Medical Humanities* 38, no. 1 (2012): 21–27.

16 Coercive Practices in Mental Health Services: Stories of Recalcitrance, Resistance, and Legitimation

MICK MCKEOWN, AMY SCHOLES, FIONA JONES, AND
WILL AINDOW

Introduction

This chapter is written by people with quite different experiences of violence in relation to the practice and organization of psychiatric services. It is our intention to draw upon our own collective experiences, including some relevant research studies to explore the notion of legitimacy with regard to violence and psychiatry. The social relations of care and associated power distribution demand more nuanced understandings than are often applied in practice, and critical reflection on the ways in which legitimacy is established, or appealed to, is similarly required.

Our intention is not to condone violence; rather we argue that complexities associated with coercive psychiatric practices are often unacknowledged in the justification for implicit and explicit violence. Furthermore, the idea that violence enacted by people subject to psychiatric care and treatment may have its own legitimacy is a neglected aspect of scrutiny and may be conceived of as a form of resistance, or recalcitrance, towards psychiatric power.[1] We highlight research and commentary beyond psychiatry that reinforce notions of legitimacy grounded in fairness and social justice, and refer to some illustrative accounts drawn from research of our own.

Locating Ourselves

First, let us clarify our positioning and personal journeys and how these situate us in terms of this subject matter. Mick is a sociologically inclined academic at a university who has an extensive background working in mental health nursing, including at the so-called hard end of psychiatry in secure care units. Despite a critical disposition towards psychiatry and a personal aversion to the use of coercive measures, never having used physical restraint or forcibly administered medication, he has undoubtedly shared complicity in psychiatric services as we know them. Amy is a research assistant, with a background in psychology, currently working on a large-scale study, with Mick, Fiona, and others, aimed at developing and evaluating practices in inpatient units designed to minimize or obviate the use of physical restraint. Fiona is a researcher and a survivor of mental health services with substantial experience of coercion, including time spent in secure facilities. Will has had numerous compelled admissions to acute psychiatric wards and is studying for a PhD focused upon contradictions in mental health policy. Both Will and Fiona have been subject to significant psychiatric violence, have also been violently recalcitrant, and are retrospectively troubled by both.

The policy and practice context is, arguably, replete with contradictions and we are aware that our contribution is also open to critique. Not least of these concerns relate to tensions between reformist as opposed to transformative objectives. To a greater or lesser degree, we are all involved in activist-inspired debates for revolutionizing mental health thinking and practice, such as those propounded in the insurgent Mad Studies field.[2] Yet we recognize that this movement is largely external to the concentrated psychiatric power that continues to dominate services. Large numbers of individuals remain legally compelled into coercive psychiatric services. Hence, we are committed to pragmatic efforts to minimize the violence that patients are, right now, subject to. Furthermore, we contend there is value in attempting to persuade the psychiatric workforce to consider the violence of their own actions together with alternative ways of understanding and responding to violence or its threat.

Violence Begets Violence: An Unfortunately Commonplace Experience

We set the scene for our focus on legitimacy with a first-person recollection from Will deriving from his most recent compulsory hospital admission:

I was on a PICU [psychiatric intensive care unit] ward and got put on depot medication by the psychiatrist. I argued against this during the consultation and refused to have it. The following day a nurse asked me at breakfast when I wanted to have the depot. I continued to say I did not want it. Then, about two days later, six or maybe seven men came into my room, led by a male nurse I quite liked, charged with administering the depot. I backed into the corner of my room. I told them that I disagreed with the legislation that empowered them. I also told them that I understood the consequences of resistance to me, both criminal and psychiatric. I removed my watch and threw it on the bed. I told them that I would drop the first person that came near me with a needle and probably get a punch in on someone else. There was a momentary stand off and then the attempt was called off. I didn't sleep at all that night, partly because I thought they would try again and partly because I had so much adrenaline sloshing about my system. That night I explained to the lead nurse the reasons for my refusal and self-defence.

Over a week and a half passed. I was asked every day to have the depot and politely declined. I learned from my medical notes that their next step had been to request the assistance of the police, who had refused to get involved. I was informed that my transfer to the acute ward had been postponed by my "recalcitrance." During that month on the ward I was physically assaulted twice by another patient. On both occasions I did not fight back but reported both incidents. Both assaults were violent, injurious, unprovoked, witnessed, and accurately documented by staff, including the absence of retaliation. My point is, I had sufficient insight to know when violence is permissible or warranted and to exercise restraint.

I was eventually administered the injection by guile. I was tricked out of my room by a nurse on the pretence of providing me with a nicotine replacement cartridge for my inhaler. On leaving my room there was a team in wait. My hands were grabbed from behind and I was marched along in a well-executed sting. I was sensible not to resist, like being thrown out of a club by an overzealous bouncer. I also had the composure to request that they march me into the medical room as their intention had been to administer the depot in the communal corridor. They then took me into the seclusion suite because I guess they assumed there may be some reaction. I remained calm and polite for a minute and requested to return to my room, which was allowed. I sulked for about three days, quit nicotine capsules, didn't eat, and read a book. I was able to think about the level of premeditation and the involvement of all the staff on the ward in cooperating and conspiring to do something most disagreeable to me.

I got out about a month later at a managers' hearing and avoided a CTO, refusing to engage with secondary services ever since because it has made me more recalcitrant and fucking angry.

Will's account evokes various responses for us. On one level, it is most apparent that the staff's and patients' interpretations on the course of such events can differ tremendously, and are not necessarily contemplated by all parties while circumstances unfold. Both staff and patients will, from different perspectives, claim legitimacy for their actions and in the staff's case may feel that the application of coercive measures are in a person's best interests, even as they forcibly resist. For us, however, the most profound impact of this narrative is the moment where purposeful deception by the staff is a precursor to physical restraint, and how this act is built upon a presentation of *kindness*. For us, this represents a microcosmic metaphor, for all that is wrong with that ultimate oxymoron – *coercive care*.

The actual and potential impact for patients appear obvious, leading to a breach of trust and diminution, if not complete negation, of any sense of therapeutic alliance. In addition, as Will describes, these staff tactics inculcate grievance at perceived unfairness and become the seed for legitimating a recalcitrant or violently pre-emptive response. The corruption of kindness speaks volumes of wider crises of legitimacy facing the so-called caring professions and raises deeper questions of morality and ethics, beyond instrumental considerations of effectiveness. If the consequence of efficiently applied coercion is fundamentally undermined therapeutic relations and provocation of recalcitrance on the part of patients, then even efficiency is called into question.

Coercive Mental Health Services

Unlike other health care contexts, mental health services are unique in legally mandating compulsion and coercion. The most obvious coercive measure used in the United Kingdom is physical restraint, and less extensively, seclusion, though in North America and other parts of the world mechanical restraints are also used. All forms of restraint and coercion predate psychiatry as a medical discipline and, indeed, modernity.[3] Restraint is most commonly used in response to violence on the part of patients but is a legitimated staff response to such diverse circumstances as absconding, refusing medication, self-harming, committing property damage, and being verbal aggressive; it is also reported in relation to staff refusing requests from patients.[4]

Physical restraint can have significant impacts for patients, including physical and psychological injury (on occasion associated with re-traumatization) or death. From an organizational perspective it can be distressing for other patient witnesses and staff, precipitate further aggression or violence, add to service costs, and damage therapeutic relations.[5] Moreover, the more coercive aspects of services and most restrictive environments are typically disproportionately visited upon ethnic minority group members, especially young Black men in the United Kingdom and Aboriginal populations in North America and the antipodes.[6] Hence, these groups are more likely to be subject to compulsion, be detained in secure services, receive physical treatments as opposed to talking therapies, and be secluded. A pernicious mix of racialized stereotyping and staff fears has been implicated in serious failings of care, including deaths while subject to restraint in psychiatric and other contexts.[7] There is some mixed evidence of disproportional use of physical restraint, but recording processes are often insufficiently systematic or thoroughly completed.[8]

Violence between patients and care staff can proceed in avoidably escalating, vicious cycles of conflict or avoidance.[9] Holmes and colleagues dispute the commonplace assumption that violence in health care settings is always perpetrated by patients, highlighting the violence implicit in the system and enacted by staff upon patients, distributed horizontally among staff or initiated by employers.[10] Similarly, Choiniere and colleagues emphasize the influence of clinical settings where biotechnologies are privileged to the detriment of relational care. Indeed, the systemic nature of violence within mental health care services has been conceptualized as inextricably bound up with the power of psychiatric knowledge to order and constrain human relations.[11] In this sense, the violence as a form of epistemic injustice makes the case for survivor research into coercion to resist professional and institutional framings of the topic and variables.[12] For Holmes and colleagues[13] the analysis of violence in health care settings needs turning on its head: *to look to health care and its organization for how violence is bred in its practices.*

The England and Wales Mental Health Act (MHA) was reformed most recently in 2007, and despite ambitions that new community treatment orders (CTOs) would reduce compelled hospital admissions the opposite has occurred. Levels of compulsion and coercion in hospital and community have risen annually since the Act came onto the statute book.[14] The quality of inpatient care has also been questioned, with concerns regarding over-occupancy, low staffing levels, overuse of agency staff, and limited alternatives to medication. For critics such as Bauman, much of the problem stems from unfettered neo-liberalism, condemning public sector services to benighted conditions of liquid uncertainty; a state of affairs implicated in notable systems failures and scandals.[15] To compound this, the Care Quality Commission (CQC) has warned that many positive aspirations of national mental health policy are relatively meaningless in the face of services characterized so much by compulsion, coercion, containment and control.[16] Arguably, these policies aspire to promote participation in decision making, other involvement practices and, essentially, forms of cooperation between staff and patients, ambitions that are thwarted by the tendency to control. We contend that tensions between coercion and cooperation expose more fundamental questions of legitimacy, and it is to these that we now turn.

Legitimacy: Rightful Violence

Numerous studies of wider society seem to show that people perceive violence on the part of the state, as exercised by the police, for example, to be legitimate if procedural justice and fairness principles are adhered to, and this underpins cooperation with authorities and deference to their power.[17] In this sense, societies expect that the police and the legal system hold a monopoly on the use of physical force, usually obviating the need for citizens to behave violently.[18] For Young, Hannah Arendt provides a critical perspective that "official violence is always questionable, and thus requires justification."[19] Where belief in the just exercise of power becomes diminished, trust breaks down between individuals or communities and the authorities. In such circumstances, citizens can understand a range of violent acts, such as those committed in the pursuance of protest or even riot, as fundamentally legitimate.

E.P. Thompson makes similar observations through a historical lens about the implicit morality of riotous behaviour in reaction to social injustice.[20] Jackson and colleagues hypothesized that public assumptions about the nature and quality of democracy may also be influential in their disposition towards violence on the part of themselves or fellow citizens.[21] From this general perspective, the legitimacy or otherwise of violence perpetrated by patients detained on mental health wards is open to understanding with regard to perceived unfairness at the hands of the psychiatric system, and this may extend to whether the public at large condones violence perpetrated by the system or in response to it. Furthermore, democratization of the social relations of care may prove to be important in the minimization of violence in either direction.

Legitimating Psychiatric Violence

Appreciation for progressive measures aimed at reducing or ameliorating coercive practices positively highlights such notions as recovery journeys, the value of different types of communication, the importance of different settings and places, and the quality of relationships. This results for many service users in the establishment of apparently cooperative relations with care staff, who also then experience reward and fulfilment in their work. We do not want to be overly critical at this juncture, as such scenarios seem preferable to the more austere, autocratic, and institutionalizing regimes that exist in contrast or combination. We do, however, suggest that a number of philosophical and practical problems exist with an uncritical affinity for these policy notions and practices. Psychiatry's adoption of seemingly progressive measures, some inspired by psychiatric survivor movements, indicates a wider colonization project, offering a legitimating smokescreen for more unpalatable coercive practices. Positive experiences of advocacy, recovery, and cooperation may mask the imperviousness and immutability of prevailing power dynamics: individuals may better enjoy the experience of care interventions or hospitalization, compelled or otherwise, but still have their core demands, wants, and needs denied.[22]

The extent to which patients are inclined to cooperate with mental health care is compounded by the entrenched dominance of biomedicine. One interesting aspect of legitimation is recourse to research evidence within a scientific paradigm. Psychiatry, on its own terms, faces a significant epistemological legitimacy crisis as the evidence underpinning medicalization of mental distress appears frayed at the edges or, indeed, coming apart at the seams.[23] Specifically, violent treatments, such as electroconvulsive therapy (ECT), are difficult to scientifically justify.[24] Similarly, the ways in which elderly patients are also subject to restraint, seclusion, ECT, and over-medication is more often than not contrary to established evidence and provokes unease and outrage.[25] Thus, evidence critiques supplement moral and ethical objections in framing campaigns of resistance.[26] That said, psychiatric orthodoxy is a long way from being transformed or de-legitimated, despite increasing appeals of alternative, more benign, democratic, relational options that minimize or eschew medication, such as Soteria, Open Dialogue, or the growing panoply of survivor-led or inspired alternatives.[27]

Practitioner staff embroiled in a risk management paradigm promote cooperation but doubt the sincerity of cooperating patients, while patients equally doubt the sincerity of staff claims to care.[28] Paradoxically, advocacy, cooperation, involvement, and recovery practices may actually constitute means for the *pacification of dissent* rather than living up to rhetorical transformational or even emancipatory claims.[29] As such, the apparently progressive becomes subsumed into more long-standing systems of governance and tyranny.

Numerous studies of psychiatric staff attitudes towards coercion and physical restraint in particular show that there is at the very least ambivalence over its use, and indeed a degree of consensus that there are counter-therapeutic consequences.[30] Closer reading of this body of work reveals that nurses and other staff when questioned about their views on violent interventions initiated by staff, such as physical or mechanical restraint or forced medication, offer a range of justifications. In one recent review, Riahi and colleagues describe various appeals for legitimacy that include necessity, maintaining safety for all, maintaining control over challenging situations, and the well-worn contention that such interventions are only used as a *last resort*.[31] Interestingly, this review also reveals circumstances where staff are conscious of the adverse psychological impact of physical interventions, for both patients and themselves, and critical of colleagues who are indiscriminate in their use of violence. All this applies in the context of legitimated coercive practices, but there is also a lengthy history of illegitimate and abusive use of coercion so much so that nursing in the United Kingdom is currently facing its own crisis of legitimacy, characterized by an alleged lack of compassion.[32]

The fact that health care staff and service users might see matters of violence differently is demonstrated in Rose and colleagues' research on UK wards.[33] In this study, nurses felt impotent to carry out care in the face of administrative burden, and patients in turn viewed the nurses as uncaring and inaccessible. These nurses saw coercion as a legitimate response to violence, caused by internal patient factors, whereas patients felt "driven to extreme behaviour" and viewed coercive measures as "unnecessary and heavy handed."[34] In our own study, ethnographic observations and interviews revealed a mixed picture, with legitimacy of nurse- or patient-initiated violence understood differently depending upon context and circumstances.[35] Some service users might object to coercive measures applied to themselves but see them as reasonably warranted for others or, indeed, on occasion resign themselves to proportional application of coercion.[36]

Debating notions of legitimacy concerning violence in mental health settings, on the part of patients or staff and services, is not new; though much of the available literature focuses upon understandings gleaned from the field of ethics rather than necessarily sociological theory.[37] A focus on ethics can result in a degree of pragmatism, upholding last resort rationalizations, ultimately validating physical restraint as a necessary evil.[38]

Chris Chapman in a searing, honest, and insightful reflection on working in a children's unit that routinely used physical restraint and seclusion observes that staff become enmeshed in their own narrative accounts of such events. These operate to legitimate, explain and exculpate actions that clearly are distressing for the children and provoke discomfort in staff sensibilities. Chapman draws insights from Arendt's thinking on violence, power, and legitimacy, as do Roberts and Ion in attempting to make sense of the abuse of patients in a series of recent UK scandals.[39] The essential feature of these staff narratives is to cast the person subject to coercion as the perpetrator of violent acts, such that violent staff responses, albeit controlled and formalized restraint techniques, are justified, and their own violence is reinterpreted in more palatable terms of necessity, protection, and safety. Chapman draws attention to the processes by which potential staff moral, ethical, or political objections are systematically dampened and contained by means, such as collective debriefings, which serve to consolidate legitimation narratives and, effectively, also individualize and psychologize patients *and* any staff who experience revulsion or upset:

> When we restrained children, we "debriefed" newer staff afterwards, knowing it was difficult to witness or participate in a restraint, and approaching it as something to address through something like a "talking cure" with a predetermined destination: to accept perpetrating violence as necessary.[40]

However, Prilleltensky and Nelson propose a *psychopolitical* framing that concentrates on unequal power dynamics and social causation, and argue for interventions to address these matters rather than simply respond to their effects.[41]

What other options are open to resistive psychiatric patients who might assert their will, reject diagnosis or treatment, and fight with care staff? In the wider context of civil disobedience, McWilliams discusses non-violent tactics as holding potential, but only if the oppressor is ultimately bound by sufficient moral conviction to be (eventually) moved by such protest. He wryly acknowledges that such tactics would not have prevailed in the context of Nazi oppression, where the final solution was locally legitimated, and the victims were effectively de-humanized.[42] We might consider that the formal legitimation of psychiatric violence would also substantially discount the value of non-violent patient protests, faced for example with the circumstances of forced medication. As an aside, the UK psychologist and survivor activist Rufus May offers training courses in non-violent communication for negotiating challenges in services.[43]

The Inevitability of Coercion and Restraint

We now present some illustrative snapshots of data from some of our research studies that support our arguments concerning legitimacy. These include the *ResTrain Yourself* project (RTY), designed to evaluate an initiative aimed at reducing the use of physical restraint and a study of views on the recovery concept in a high-secure hospital (HSR).[44] These excerpts are of necessity selective, but similar accounts have emerged in many of our studies and are apparent in the wider literature. The RTY study involved a substantial amount of ethnographic observation and interviews on 14 acute inpatient wards across the North West of England.

RTY Observation 1: The prior planning of a restraint to administer an intra-muscular injection, before the patient has even protested the treatment or before any violent incident has occurred.

Staff discussed the fact that handover will have to be brief because of a planned restraint at 2 pm, to administer a depot. Staff anxiety was clear from tone and body language. In the past few weeks there have been various incidents involving administering medication to this woman patient, some leading to seclusion. Handover was interrupted by an older male nurse, who stated that "2 big men have come over from X ward for the depot, and they want to leave, so can we do it now?" There was some awkwardness in the room as the staff seemed conscious of the presence of the research team, and the stark contradiction of the trauma-informed practice posters displayed above their heads. The NIC [nurse in charge] said they would have to wait until handover was finished, at which point the other nurse said he would draw up the injection. The incident concluded with the patient taking their medication without the need of a restraint team.

This decision to form a team with intention to administer medication against a person's will exposes the inadequacies of typical rationalizations of coercion, not least as last resort. Such claims are surely not sustainable in a context where physical restraint is preplanned. Whether it was the implicit threat or proximity of a team (including large men) that influenced compliance at this time is open to conjecture. Clearly, in this case prior violent incidents were understood as patient behaviour, without thinking about interaction with staff violence in terms of use of restraint and seclusion, and pragmatic concerns over staff safety overrode any inclination to do without restraint tactics. The case for legitimacy is also supplemented by belief that taking medication is ultimately beneficial:

> There has been a lot of planned restraints with the patients that have been
> non-compliant with medication. And they're informed and, obviously, in their
> treatment plan, we've got the power to give them this medication for their best
> interests. [nurse, RTY interview]

Violence as Legitimate Response?

Even when not looking for them, time and again we have elicited accounts of experiences illustrating how service responses precipitated violence, contemplation of violence, or other acts of resistance, which might in turn fuel further application of coercion. In the following excerpt a patient describes such a cycle:

> I can't remember what, I wasn't happy with something, so I ran for the push bar
> to get out. It was not like me. I ran for it and I was like, argh, get out. And then I
> think two members of staff got me in there, I think someone sat on me. And they
> said it was either take lorazepam or have this injection in the bum. So, I opted for
> the lorazepam … Yes, probably, I laugh at things that I should be crying about. But
> I don't find it funny being in here at all, so that's probably why I was trying to get
> out in the beginning. [patient, RTY interview]

UK public health policy has promoted prohibition of smoking in NHS units and their grounds. For detained persons this *best interest* initiative is yet another reminder that while a mental health patient, basic autonomous decisions regarding your lifestyle are controlled; adding to the plethora of mortifications to which you are subject. Predictable violence and aggression is often reported as a consequence of patient's resistance to these policies:

> We're saying to somebody, you're coming into hospital against your will, bringing you into this distressing environment, and saying you can't smoke. Even I think, oh my God, I'd go mad. And you know when you say you can't have one, you want one more, don't you? ... The doors were kicked in every single day trying to get out for fags [cigarettes]. Like the staff, we were attacked and all sorts for fags. [nurse, RTY interview]

Medication and specifically compliance with medication are pivotal issues relating to perceived cooperation, or its flipside, non-cooperation, typically referred to by services as noncompliance. As such, matters of compliance are at the centre of much violence and aggression. Medication and coercion often go hand in hand: the administration of medication can be replete with violence, is a trigger for patient violence, and is a front-line response to violence – in repeated cycles of anti-therapeutic practice and resistance, or submission, to it:

> ... first and foremost, I think they have to be in control of you. It's part of the psychiatric system, to be brought down a peg or two, shatter their confidence and then build it back up just enough for them to be able to leave hospital ... Because while a person is under the chemical cosh, or that type of medication, they do become aggressive ... I think if you harm somebody on the ward, you would be [put] on the harder medication. [patient, RTY interview]

In our framing of the notion of recalcitrance, people effectively position themselves in opposition to the psychiatric episteme when they link choices and behaviour to rejection of labelling, diagnosis, and medication:

> That was one of the things I questioned and because I've been labelled with "this" and because I was challenging something I didn't agree with, I was rebelling against how the system viewed me. [patient, HSR interview]

Mortification of the self can be seen to persist within modern psychiatric units given that most of them continue to exhibit characteristics of total institutions.[45] The interplay between staff and patient violence and the rhetorical valuation of cooperation amid the reality of coercion are indicative of the symbolic and actual interactions between individuals subject to institutionalizing mortification and their various coping strategies. Goffman pinpointed the means by which cooperation becomes singularly defined in terms of compliance with the institutional perspective:

> The difficulties caused by a patient are closely tied to his version of what has been happening to him, and if cooperation is to be secured, it helps if this version is discredited. The patient must "insightfully" come to take, or affect to take, the hospital's view of himself.[46]

Faced with psychiatry as *the only show in town*, persons who resist diagnostic labelling and medication, especially more coercive forms, can be compelled to take on the identity of *recalcitrant*. Individuals who defy the system and practitioners within it have previously been referred to as *difficult patients* or exhibiting *challenging behaviour* as they confront layers of psychiatric control and struggle to assert their own agency.[47] Will's opening story demonstrates that the descriptor *recalcitrance* can be both a pejorative applied by staff or a positive claim by patients themselves. The term has been deployed similarly in the context of movement activism and resistance to the vicissitudes of neoliberalism.[48] For some individuals subject to psychiatric coercion, the struggle erupts in violence and quite literally fighting against institutional regimes and the staff who service them. We have attempted to theorize recalcitrance in terms of resisting the psychiatric episteme and, in these terms, as a legitimate and rational response to illegitimate coercion.[49]

Alliances for Change: Possibilities and Perils

If the problem of violence within psychiatric services is one of interaction between an oppressive system, staff working within it, and detained patients, then arguably solutions have to involve all interested parties. Revolutionary solutions demand total transformations. More pragmatic approaches seek to reform the most egregious aspects of the system. Peter Sedgwick in his arguments for a left-leaning *psychopolitics* made the case for cross-sectional coalitions between survivor and labour movements.[50] At least one possibility is to frame efforts to reduce workplace violence as an employment relations matter, holding out potential for politicized alliances between the health care workforce and survivor activists.[51] Of course, to some extent practitioner workers' unions have always been visible on this territory. Unfortunately, however, their contribution has been, more often than not, implicitly conservative. Hence, in the UK, employers in conjunction with unions have designed *zero tolerance* campaigns that appear to locate the entire responsibility for hospital violence with patients and the public, neglecting to consider wider contributory factors and care staffs' own role in precipitating or perpetrating violence.

One set of possibilities is that survivor movements and unions seek mutual interest in challenging both psychiatry *and* the neo-liberal forces that weaken worker interests and stigmatize and impoverish disabled and Mad citizens.[52] Models of community mobilization offer a helpful starting point, and survivor activists are already formulating their demands.[53] For trade unions to make credible efforts towards forging alliances on this and other territory, issues of asymmetrical power need to be faced up to.[54]

Without holding to any great optimism for a revolution in psychiatry, we prefer to posit an *inside-out* strategy – reforming from inside while simultaneously working towards a transformative ideal, and opening up the system to be receptive to alternative organizational forms articulated externally. The obvious counter argument to such tactics is this may do little to dismantle psychiatric hegemony. Yet, not to directly engage beyond critique and protest appears to cede all ground *within* services to the current orthodoxy. Alternative models of care emphasize the appeal of deliberative, democratized dialogue and relationships that also might inspire or sustain political activism and alliances on the same territory. There is so much room for improvement in rendering psychiatric services as we know them more humane, respectful of rights, less coercive, and free of violence. This much is in our scope right now, without anything like a revolution, however desirable that might be.

The implicit violence and injustices that flow from epistemic and hegemonic power are something else. These require much more substantial remediation or transformation, and the forms of equality and democratization that are necessary may need to be realized as much in wider society as in the micro-territory of psychiatric services. That said, to paraphrase Sedgwick, if the social relations of psychiatry can be thus transformed we have a blueprint for a desirable transformation of society as a whole. For Arendt, absolute power is deferred to, not requiring violence to exert control; places replete with violence indicate "where power is in jeopardy."[55] For psychiatry this may be the case, reflecting profound crises of legitimacy. The struggle is ongoing, and perhaps the recalcitrants will win.

NOTES

1　McKeown et al., "Looking Back."
2　Lefrançois, Menzies, and Reaume, *Mad Matters*; Reville and Church, "Mad Activism"; Russo and Beresford, "Between Exclusion and Colonisation"; Russo and Wallcraft, "Resisting Variables."
3　Paterson and Duxbury, "Restraint."
4　Bowers et al., "Manual Restraint"; Gudjonsson, Rabe-Hesketh, and Szmukler, "Management of Psychiatric"; Ryan and Bowers, "An Analysis"; Southcott and Howard, "Effectiveness and Safety."
5　Ashcraft and Anthony "Eliminating Seclusion"; Fisher, "Curtailing the Use"; Foster, Bowers, and Nijman, "Aggressive Behaviour"; Moran et al., "Restraint and Seclusion"; Sequeira and Halstead, "The Psychological Effects."
6　Gone, "'We Never Was Happy'"; Stowell-Smith and McKeown, "Race, Stigma and Stereotyping"; Zubrick et al., "Social Determinants."
7　Aiken, Duxbury, and Dale, "Deaths in Custody"; Anthony, "Deaths in Custody"; Keating and Robertson, "Fear, Black People and Mental Illness"; Prins, *Big, Black and Dangerous*; Razack, *Dying from Improvement*; Ambalavaner, *Deadly Silence*.
8　Stewart et al., "Manual Restraint."
9　Duxbury, "The Eileen Skellern Lecture"; Whittington and Wykes, "An Observational Study."
10　Holmes et al., "Introduction."
11　Choiniere et al., "Conceptualizing Structural."
12　Carel and Kidd, "Epistemic Injustice"; Fricker, *Epistemic Injustice*; Liegghio, "A Denial of Being"; Russo and Beresford, "Between Exclusion"; Russo and Wallcraft, "Resisting Variables."
13　Holmes et al., "Introduction," 9.
14　Care Quality Commission, *Monitoring*.
15　Bauman, *Liquid Modernity*. See also Randall and McKeown, "Editorial."
16　Care Quality Commission, *Mental Health Act*.
17　See Jackson et al., "Monopolizing Force?"; Tyler, *Why People Obey*; Tyler, "Psychological Perspectives."
18　Weber, *Politics as a Vocation*.
19　Young, "Power, Violence, and Legitimacy," 277.

20 Thompson, "The Moral Economy."
21 Jackson et al., "Monopolizing."
22 McKeown et al., "Independent Mental Health Advocacy."
23 Bentall, *Madness Explained*; Whitaker, *Anatomy of an Epidemic*.
24 Breggin, "ECT Damages the Brain," 83; Weitz, "Struggling."
25 Andrews, "Managing Challenging Behaviour," 741; Banerjee, *The Use of Antipsychotic Medication*; Thompson Coon et al., "Interventions to Reduce"; Foebel et al., "Physical Restraint," 184e9; Muir-Cochrane, Baird, and McCann, "Nurses' Experiences."
26 Burstow, "Legitimating Damage and Control."
27 For Soteria see Mosher, "Soteria and Other Alternatives"; for Open Dialogue see Seikkula, Alakare, and Aaltonen, "The Comprehensive Open-Dialogue Approach"; for survivor-led or inspired alternatives, see Russo and Sweeney, *Searching for a Rose Garden*.
28 McKeown et al., "Looking Back."
29 McKeown et al., "Independent Mental Health Advocacy."
30 Bonner et al., "Trauma for All."
31 Riahi, Thompson, and Duxbury, "An Integrative Review."
32 Department of Health, *Transforming Care*; Hopton, "Towards a Critical Theory"; McKeown and White, "The Future of Mental Health Nursing"; Flynn and Mercer, "Is Compassion Possible"; Spandler and Stickley, "No Hope without Compassion"; Stenhouse et al., "Exploring the Compassion Deficit Debate."
33 Rose et al. "Life in Acute Mental Health Settings."
34 Ibid., 1.
35 Duxbury et al., "Implementing the Six Core Strategies."
36 See also Dickens, Piccirillo, and Alderman, "Causes and Management"; Duxbury and Whittington, "Causes and Management."
37 See Paterson and Duxbury, "Restraint."
38 Perkins et al., "Physical Restraint in a Therapeutic Setting."
39 Chapman, "Becoming Perpetrator"; Roberts and Ion, "Thinking Critically."
40 Chapman, "Becoming Perpetrator," 25.
41 Prilleltensky and Nelson, *Doing Psychology Critically*.
42 McWilliams, "On Violence and Legitimacy."
43 May, "How I've Found."
44 Duxbury et al., "Implementing," 2015; McKeown et al., "Looking Back," 2016.
45 Goffman, *Asylums*.
46 Ibid., 143.
47 See Breeze and Repper, "Struggling for Control."

48 Clarke, "Citizen-Consumers"; Law and Mooney, "The Maladies."
49 It is not our intention here to essentialize the notion of recalcitrance or in any way support a meaning that overly internalizes the opposition of the person or, indeed, infers pathology. We do, however, make links to matters of personal agency, as likely to connect with wider forms of collective resistance and considerations of power.
50 Sedgwick, *Psycho Politics.*
51 McKeown and Foley, "Reducing Physical Restraint"; McKeown, Cresswell, and Spandler, "Deeply Engaged Relationships."
52 McKeown, "Stand Up." In this regard it is possible for members of the psy-workforce and other external commentators to adopt the identity of recalcitrant, adopting movement aims and activist strategies commensurate with resistance to the dominance of bio-medicine and its entanglement with neo-liberalism.
53 See Psychiatric Disabilities Anti-violence Coalition, *Clearing a Path.*
54 McKeown et al., "Deeply Engaged Relationships."
55 Arendt, *On Violence,* 76.

BIBLIOGRAPHY

Aiken, Frances, Joy Duxbury, and Colin Dale. "Deaths in Custody: The Role of Restraint." *Journal of Learning Disabilities and Offending Behaviour* 2 (2011): 178–90.
Andrews, Gavin J. "Managing Challenging Behaviour in Dementia." *British Medical Journal* 332, no. 7544 (2006): 741.
Anthony, Thalia. "Deaths in Custody: 25 Years after the Royal Commission, We've Gone Backwards." *Green Left Weekly* 1092 (2016). https://www.greenleft.org.au/content/deaths-custody-25-years-after-royal-commission.
Arendt, Hannah. *On Violence.* Orlando, FL: Harvest Books/Harcourt, 1970.
Ashcraft, Lori, and William Anthony. "Eliminating Seclusion and Restraint in Recovery-Oriented Crisis Services." *Psychiatric Services* 59, no. 10 (2008): 1198–202.
Banerjee, Sube. *The Use of Antipsychotic Medication for People with Dementia: Time for Action.* London, UK: Department of Health, 2009.
Bauman, Zygmunt. *Liquid Modernity.* Cambridge, UK: Polity Press, 2000.
Bentall, Richard. P. *Madness Explained: Psychosis and Human Nature.* London, UK: Penguin, 2004.
Bonner, G., T. Lowe, D. Rawcliffe, and N. Wellman. "Trauma for All: A Pilot Study of the Subjective Experience of Physical Restraint for Mental Health

Inpatients and Staff in the UK." *Journal of Psychiatric and Mental Health Nursing* 9 (2002): 465–73.

Bowers, Len, Marie Van Der Merwe, Brodie Paterson, and Duncan Stewart. "Manual Restraint and Shows of Force: The City-128 Study." *International Journal of Mental Health Nursing* 21, no. 1 (2012): 30–40.

Breeze, Jayne Ann, and Julie Repper. "Struggling for Control: The Care Experiences of "Difficult' Patients in Mental Health Services." *Journal of Advanced Nursing* 28, no. 6 (1998): 1301–11.

Breggin, Peter. "ECT Damages the Brain: Disturbing News for Patients and Shock Doctors Alike." *Ethical Human Psychology and Psychiatry* 9, no. 2 (2007): 83–6.

Burstow, Bonnie. "Legitimating Damage and Control: The Ethicality of Electroshock Research." *Intersectionalities: A Global Journal of Social Work Analysis, Research, Polity, and Practice, Special Issue: The Ethics and Politics of Knowledge Production* 5, no. 1 (2016): 94–109.

Carel, Havi, and Ian James Kidd. "Epistemic Injustice in Healthcare: A Philosophical Analysis." *Medicine, Health Care and Philosophy* 17 (2014): 529–40.

Care Quality Commission. *Mental Health Act Annual Report 2011/12.* Newcastle, UK: CQC, 2012.

Care Quality Commission. *Monitoring the Mental Health Act in 2013/14.* Newcastle, UK: CQC, 2015.

Chapman, Chris. "Becoming Perpetrator: How I Came to Accept Restraining and Confining Disabled Aboriginal Children." In *Psychiatry Disrupted: Theorizing Resistance and Crafting the (R)evolution,* edited by Bonnie Burstow, Brenda A. Lefrançois, and Shaindl Diamond, 16–33. Montreal, QC: McGill-Queen's University Press, 2014.

Choiniere, Jacqueline A., Judith, A. MacDonnell, Andrea L. Campbell, and Sandra Smele. "Conceptualizing Structural Violence in the Context of Mental Health Nursing." *Nursing Inquiry* 21 (2014): 39–50.

Clarke, John. "Citizen-Consumers and Public Service Reform: At the Limits of Neo-liberalism?" *Policy Futures in Education* 5 (2007): 239–48.

Coon, Jo Thompson, Rebecca Abbott, Morwenna Rogers, Rebecca Whear, Stephen Pearson, Ian Lang, Nick Cartmell, and Ken Stein. "Interventions to Reduce Inappropriate Prescribing of Antipsychotic Medications in People with Dementia Resident in Care Homes: A Systematic Review." *Journal of the American Medical Directors Association* 15, no. 10 (2014): 706–18.

Department of Health. *Transforming Care: A National Response to Winterbourne View Hospital – Final Review Report.* London, UK: Department of Health, 2012.

Dickens, Geoffrey, Maria Piccirillo, and Nick Alderman. "Causes and Management of Aggression and Violence in a Forensic Mental Health Service: Perspectives of Nurses and Patients." *International Journal of Mental Health Nursing* 22, no. 6 (2013): 532–44.

Duxbury, Joy. "The Eileen Skellern Lecture 2014. Physical Restraint: In Defence of the Indefensible?" *Journal of Psychiatric and Mental Health Nursing* 22, no. 2 (2015): 92–101.

Duxbury, Joy, John Baker, Soo Downe, Fiona Edgar, Paul Greenwood, Mick McKeown, Owen Price, Amy Scholes, Gillian Thomson, and Richard Whittington. "Implementing the Six Core Strategies (6CS) to Reduce Physical Restraint in the UK: The "REsTRAIN YOURSELF' project" [Abstract]. In *Violence in Clinical Psychiatry: Proceedings of the 9th European Congress*, edited by P. Callaghan, N. Oud, J. H. Bjørngaard, H. Nijman, T. Palmstierna, and Joy Duxbury, 195–6. Amsterdam: Kavanah, 2015.

Duxbury, Joy, and Richard Whittington. "Causes and Management of Patient Aggression and Violence: Staff and Patient Perspectives." *Journal of Advanced Nursing* 50, no. 5 (2005): 469–78.

Fisher, Jennifer Atieno. "Curtailing the Use of Restraint in Psychiatric Settings." *Journal of Humanistic Psychology* 43, no. 2 (2003): 69–95.

Flynn, Maria, and Dave Mercer. "Is Compassion Possible in a Market-Led NHS?" *Nursing Times* 109, no. 7 (2012): 12–14.

Foebel, Andrea D, Graziano Onder, Harriet Finne-Soveri, Albert Lukas, Michael Denkinger, Angela Carfi, Davide L. Vetrano, Vicenzo Brandi, Roberto Bernabei, and Rosa Liperoti. "Physical Restraint and Antipsychotic Medication Use among Nursing Home Residents with Dementia." *Journal of the American Medical Directors Association* 17, no. 2 (2016): 184e9–184e14.

Foster, Chloe, Len Bowers, and Henk Nijman. "Aggressive Behaviour on Acute Psychiatric Wards: Prevalence, Severity and Management." *Journal of Advanced Nursing* 58, no. 2 (2007): 140–9.

Fricker, Miranda. *Epistemic Injustice: Power and the Ethics of Knowing*. Oxford, UK: Oxford University Press, 2007.

Goffman, Erving. *Asylums: Essays on the Social Situation of Mental Patients and Other Inmates*. New York: Anchor Books, 1961.

Gone, Joseph P. "'We Never Was Happy Living Like a Whiteman': Mental Health Disparities and the Postcolonial Predicament in American Indian Communities." *American Journal of Community Psychology* 40, nos. 3–4 (2007): 290–300.

Gudjonsson, Gisli H., Sophia Rabe-Hesketh, and George Szmukler. "Management of Psychiatric In-Patient Violence: Patient Ethnicity and Use of Medication, Restraint and Seclusion." *British Journal of Psychiatry* 184, no. 3 (2004): 258–62.

Holmes, Dave, Trudy Rudge, Amelie Perron, and Isabelle St-Pierre. "Introduction: (Re)thinking Violence in Health Care Settings." In *(Re) Thinking Violence in Health Care Settings: A Critical Approach*, edited by Dave Holmes, Trudy Rudge, and Amelie Perron. Surrey, UK: Ashgate Publishing, 2012.

Hopton, John. "Towards a Critical Theory of Mental Health Nursing." *Journal of Advanced Nursing* 25, no. 3 (1997): 492–500.

Jackson, Jonathon, Aziz Z. Huq, Ben Bradford, and Tom R. Tyler. "Monopolizing Force? Police Legitimacy and Public Attitudes toward the Acceptability of Violence." *Psychology, Public Policy, and Law* 19, no. 4 (2013): 479–97.

Keating, Frank, and David Robertson. "Fear, Black People and Mental Illness: A Vicious Circle?" *Health and Social Care in the Community* 12, no. 5 (2004): 439–47.

Law, Alex, and Gerry Mooney. "The Maladies of Social Capital II: Resisting Neo-liberal Conformism." *Critique* 34, no. 3 (2006): 253–68.

Lefrançois, Brenda A., Robert Menzies, and Geoffrey Reaume. *Mad Matters: A Critical Reader in Canadian Mad Studies*. Toronto, ON: Canadian Scholars' Press, 2013.

Liegghio, Maria. "A Denial of Being: Psychiatrization as Epistemic Violence." In *Mad Matters: A Critical Reader in Canadian Mad Studies*, edited by Brenda A. Lefrançois, Robert Menzies, and Geoffrey Reaume, 122–9. Toronto, ON: Canadian Scholars' Press, 2013.

May, Rufus. "How I've Found Nonviolent Communication Helpful." 2017. http://rufusmay.com/index.php/news-and-views/136-how-i-ve-found -nonviolent-communication-helpful.

McKeown, Mick. "Stand Up for Recalcitrance!" *International Journal of Mental Health Nursing* 25 (2016): 481–3.

McKeown, Mick, M. Cresswell, and H. Spandler. "Deeply Engaged Relationships: Alliances between Mental Health Workers and Psychiatric Survivors in the UK." In *Psychiatry Disrupted: Theorizing Resistance and Crafting the (R)evolution*, edited by Bonnie Burstow, Brenda. A. Lefrançois, and Shiandl Diamond, 145–62. Montreal, QC: McGill-Queen's University Press, 2014.

McKeown, Mick, and Paul Foley. "Reducing Physical Restraint: An Employment Relations Perspective." *Journal of Mental Health Nursing* 35, no. 1 (2015): 12–15.

McKeown, Mick, Fiona Jones, Paul Foy, Karen Wright, Tracey Paxton, and Michael Oakes Blackmon. "Looking Back, Looking Forward: Recovery

Journeys in a High Secure Hospital." *International Journal of Mental Health Nursing* 25 no. 3 (2016): 234–42. https://doi.org/10.1111/inm.12204.

McKeown, Mick, D. Poursanidou, L. Able, K. Newbigging, J. Ridley, and M. Kiansumba. "Independent Mental Health Advocacy: Still Cooling Out the Mark?" *Mental Health Today*, November/December (2013): 20–1.

McKeown, Mick, and Jacquie White. "The Future of Mental Health Nursing: Are We Barking up the Wrong Tree?" *Journal of Psychiatric and Mental Health Nursing* 22, no. 9 (2015): 724–30.

McWilliams, Wilson Carey. "On Violence and Legitimacy." *Yale Law Journal* 79, no. 4 (1970): 623–46.

Moran, A., A. Cocoman, P. A Scott, A. Matthews, V. Staniuliene, and M. Valimaki. "Restraint and Seclusion: A Distressing Treatment Option?" *Journal of Psychiatric and Mental Health Nursing* 16, no. 7 (2009): 599–605.

Mosher, Loren. "Soteria and Other Alternatives to Acute Psychiatric Hospitalization: A Personal and Professional Review." *Journal of Nervous and Mental Disease* 187 (1999): 142–9.

Muir-Cochrane, C. Eimear, John Baird, and Terance V. McCann. "Nurses' Experiences of Restraint and Seclusion Use in Short-Stay Acute Old Age Psychiatry Inpatient Units: A Qualitative Study." *Journal of Psychiatric and Mental Health Nursing* 22, no. 2 (2015): 109–15.

Paterson, Brodie, and Joy Duxbury. "Restraint and the Question of Validity." *Nursing Ethics* 14, no. 4 (2007): 535–45.

Perkins, Elizabeth, Helen Prosser, David Riley, and Richard Whittington. "Physical Restraint in a Therapeutic Setting: A Necessary Evil?" *International Journal of Law and Psychiatry* 35, no. 1 (2012): 43–9.

Prilleltensky, Isaac, and Geoffrey Nelson. *Doing Psychology Critically: Making a Difference in Diverse Settings.* Basingstoke, UK: Palgrave Macmillan, 2002.

Prins, H. *"Big, Black and Dangerous." Report of the Committee of Inquiry into the Death in Broadmoor Hospital of Orville Blackwood and a Review of the Deaths of Two Other Afro-Caribbean Patients.* London, UK: SHSA, 1993.

Psychiatric Disabilities Anti-violence Coalition. *Clearing a Path: A Psychiatric Survivor Anti-Violence Framework.* Toronto, ON: PDAC, 2015.

Randall, Duncan, and Mick McKeown. "Editorial: Failure to Care: Nursing in a State of Liquid Modernity?" *Journal of Clinical Nursing* 23, nos. 5–6 (2014): 766–7.

Razack, Sherene. *Dying from Improvement: Inquests and Inquiries into Indigenous Deaths in Custody.* Toronto, ON: University of Toronto Press, 2015.

Reville, David, and Kathryn Church. "Mad Activism Enters its Fifth Decade: Psychiatric Survivor Organizing in Toronto." In *Organize! Building from* the Local for Social Justice, edited by Aziz Choudry, Jill Hanley, and Eric Shragge, 189–201. Oakland, CA: PM Press, 2012.

Riahi, Sanaz, Gill Thompson, and Joy Duxbury. "An Integrative Review Exploring Decision-Making Factors Influencing Mental Health Nurses in the Use of Restraint." *Journal of Psychiatric and Mental Health Nursing* 23 (2016): 116–28.

Roberts, Marc, and Robin Ion. "Thinking Critically about the Occurrence of Widespread Participation in Poor Nursing Care." *Journal of Advanced Nursing* 71, no. 4 (2014): 768–76.

Rose, D., J. Evans, C. Laker, and T. Wykes. "Life in Acute Mental Health Settings: Experiences and Perceptions of Service Users and Nurses." *Epidemiology and Psychiatric Sciences* 24, no. 1 (2013): 90–6.

Russo, Jasna, and Peter Beresford. "Between Exclusion and Colonisation: Seeking a Place for Mad People's Knowledge in Academia." *Disability and Society* 30, no. 1 (2015): 153–7.

Russo, Jasna, and Angela Sweeney, eds. *Searching for a Rose Garden: Challenging Psychiatry, Fostering Mad Studies.* Wyastone Leys, UK: PCCS Books, 2016.

Russo, Jasna, and Jan Wallcraft. "Resisting Variables: Service User/Survivor Perspectives on Researching Coercion." In *Coercive Treatment in Psychiatry: Clinical, Legal and Ethical Aspects,* edited by Thomas Kallert, Juan Mezzich, and John Monahan, 213–34. Oxford, UK: Wiley-Blackwell, 2011.

Ryan, Carl J., and Len Bowers. "An Analysis of Nurses' Post-incident Manual Restraint Reports." *Journal of Psychiatric and Mental Health Nursing* 13, no. 5 (2006): 527–32.

Sedgwick, Peter. *Psycho Politics.* 1982. London, UK: Unkant, 2015.

Seikkula, Jaakko, Birgitta Alakare, and Jukka Aaltonen. "The Comprehensive Open-Dialogue Approach in Western Lapland: II. Long-term Stability of Acute Psychosis Outcomes in Advanced Community Care." *Psychosis* 3, no. 3 (2011): 192–204.

Sequeira, Heather, and Simon Halstead. "The Psychological Effects on Nursing Staff of Administering Physical Restraint in a Secure Psychiatric Hospital: 'When I Go Home, It's Then That I Think about It.'" *British Journal of Forensic Practice* 6, no. 1 (2004): 3–15.

Sivanandan, Ambalavaner. *Deadly Silence: Black Deaths in Custody.* London, UK: Institute of Race Relations, 1991.

Southcott, John, and Allison Howard. "Effectiveness and Safety of Restraint and Breakaway Techniques in a Psychiatric Intensive Care Unit." *Nursing Standard* 21, no. 36 (2007): 35–41.

Spandler, Helen, and Theodore Stickley. "No Hope without Compassion: The Importance of Compassion in Recovery-Focused Mental Health Services." *Journal of Mental Health* 20 (2011): 555–66.

Stenhouse, Rosie, Robin Ion, Michelle Roxburgh, Patric Devitt, and Stephen D. M. Smith. "Exploring the Compassion Deficit Debate." *Nurse Education Today* 39 (2016): 12–15.

Stewart, Duncan, Len Bowers, Alan Simpson, Carl Ryan, and Maria Tziggili. "Manual Restraint of Adult Psychiatric Inpatients: A Literature Review." *Journal of Psychiatric and Mental Health Nursing* 16 (2009): 749–57.

Stowell-Smith, Mark, and Mick McKeown. "Race, Stigma and Stereotyping: The Construction of Difference in Forensic Care." In *Stigma and Social Exclusion in Healthcare*, edited by Caroline Carlisle, Tom Mason, Caroline Watkins, and Elizabeth Whitehead, 158–69 London, UK: Routledge, 2001.

Thompson, E. P. "The Moral Economy of the English Crowd in the Eighteenth Century." *Past and Present* 50 (1971): 76–136.

Tyler, Tom R. "Psychological Perspectives on Legitimacy and Legitimation." *Annual Review of Psychology* 57 (2006): 375–400.

Tyler, Tom R. *Why People Obey the Law*. Princeton, NJ: Princeton University Press, 2006.

Weber, Max. *Politics as a Vocation*. Philadelphia, PA: Fortress Press, 1968.

Weitz, Don. "Struggling against Psychiatry's Human Rights Violations: An Antipsychiatry Perspective." *Radical Psychology* 7 (2008): 7–8.

Whitaker, Robert. *Anatomy of an Epidemic: Magic Bullets, Psychiatric Drugs and the Astonishing Rise of Mental Illness in America*. New York: Broadway Books, 2010.

Whittington, R., and T. Wykes. "An Observational Study of Associations between Nurse Behaviour and Violence in Psychiatric Hospitals." *Journal of Psychiatric and Mental Health Nursing* 1, no. 2 (1994): 85–92.

Young, Iris Marion. "Power, Violence, and Legitimacy: A Reading of Hannah Arendt in an Age of Police Brutality and Humanitarian Intervention." In *Breaking the Cycles of Hatred: Memory, Law, and Repair*, edited by Nancy L. Rosenblum and Martha Minow, 260–87. Princeton, NJ: Princeton University Press, 2002.

Zubrick, Stephen R., Pat Dudgeon, Graham Gee, Belle Glaskin, Kerrie Kelly, Yin Paradies, Clair Scrine, and Roz Walker. "Social Determinants of Aboriginal and Torres Strait Islander Social and Emotional Wellbeing." In *Working Together: Aboriginal and Torres Strait Islander Mental Health and Wellbeing Principles and Practice,* edited by Nola Purdie, Pat Dudgeon and Roz Walker, 75–90. Canberra, Australia: Office of the Prime Minister and Cabinet, 2010.

17 Institutional Oppression and Violence as Self-Defence

JANET LEE-EVOY

Through the practice of psychiatry, I've learned ways of seeing the world that can invalidate other ways of seeing. One learned narrative that is both seductive and dangerous is that of violence as benevolence: that psychiatry's violent actions are justified because they serve the greater good. This is an understanding that allows for, and in fact celebrates, the institutionalization of violence. This is the narrative that, through this work, I hope to explore and challenge.

FAR FROM A CRY FOR HELP

I MET GRACE ONE MORNING IN LATE SEPTEMBER.

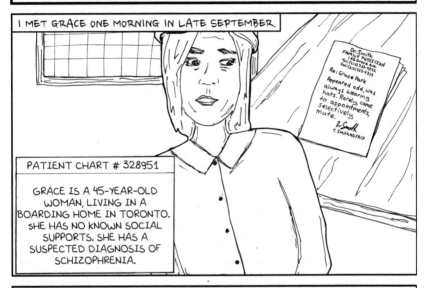

PATIENT CHART # 328951

GRACE IS A 45-YEAR-OLD WOMAN, LIVING IN A BOARDING HOME IN TORONTO. SHE HAS NO KNOWN SOCIAL SUPPORTS. SHE HAS A SUSPECTED DIAGNOSIS OF SCHIZOPHRENIA.

SHE HAD BEEN ADMITTED TO THE PSYCHIATRY FLOOR OF A HOSPITAL WHERE I WAS WORKING, COMPLETING MY RESIDENCY TRAINING IN PSYCHIATRY. WE DIDN'T KNOW MUCH ABOUT HER, BUT I READ ABOUT HOW SHE HAD COME TO BE WITH US.

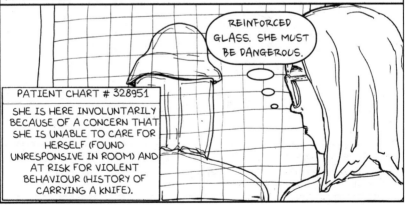

REINFORCED GLASS. SHE MUST BE DANGEROUS.

PATIENT CHART # 328951

SHE IS HERE INVOLUNTARILY BECAUSE OF A CONCERN THAT SHE IS UNABLE TO CARE FOR HERSELF (FOUND UNRESPONSIVE IN ROOM) AND AT RISK FOR VIOLENT BEHAVIOUR (HISTORY OF CARRYING A KNIFE).

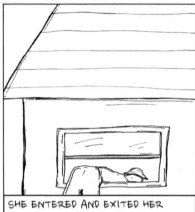
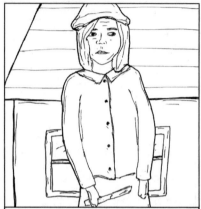
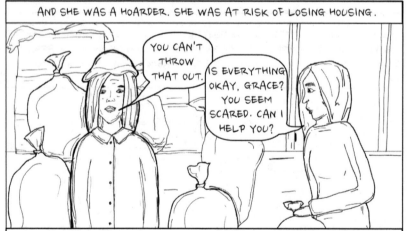

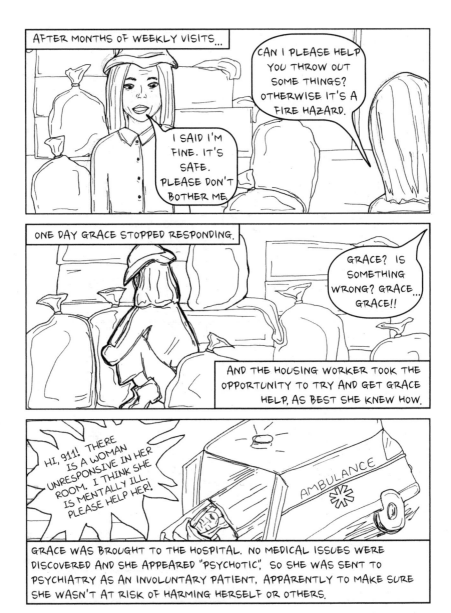

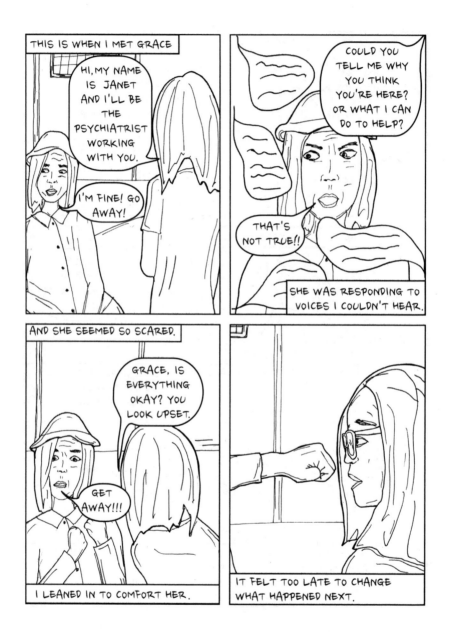

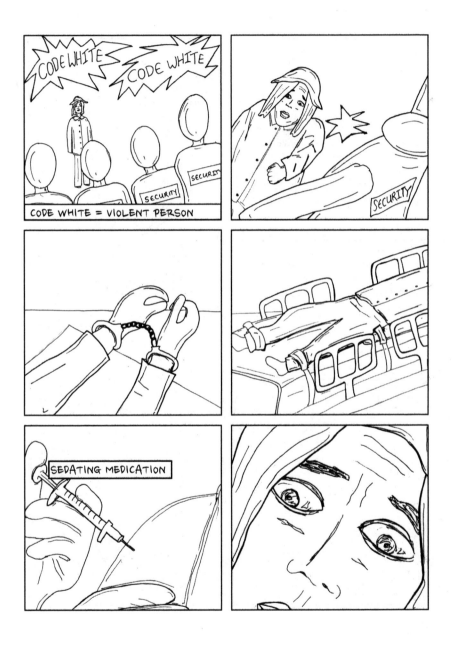

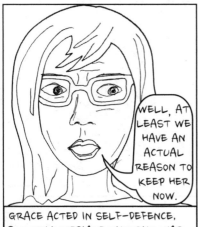

WELL, AT LEAST WE HAVE AN ACTUAL REASON TO KEEP HER NOW.

GRACE ACTED IN SELF-DEFENCE, BUT MY IMMEDIATE THOUGHT WAS TO JUSTIFY OUR VIOLENT IMPRISONMENT, OUR ONGOING VIOLENT ACTIONS.

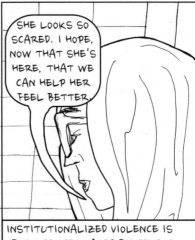

SHE LOOKS SO SCARED. I HOPE, NOW THAT SHE'S HERE, THAT WE CAN HELP HER FEEL BETTER.

INSTITUTIONALIZED VIOLENCE IS OFTEN PERPETRATED BY PEOPLE WHO THINK THEY ARE DOING THE "RIGHT THING."

AFTER THAT DAY GRACE WAS ALWAYS COOPERATIVE, OR AT LEAST SCARED INTO COOPERATION.

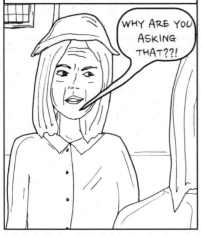
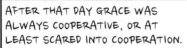

WHY ARE YOU ASKING THAT??!

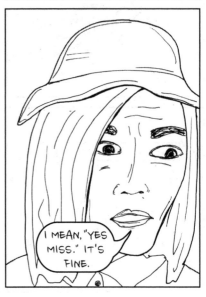

I MEAN, "YES MISS." IT'S FINE.

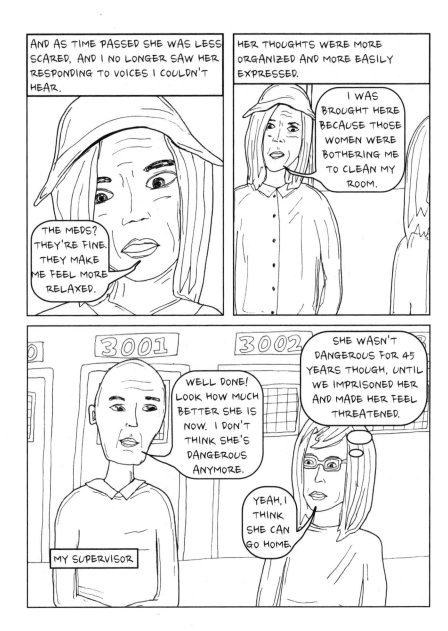

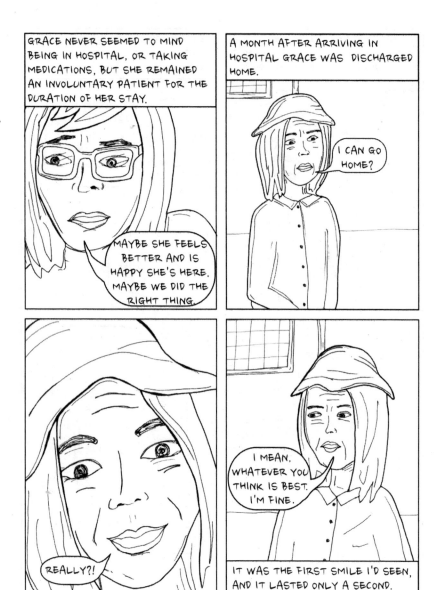

18 "Gravity and Grace": Acknowledging Restraint and Seclusion as a Violence

KEVIN REEL

Introduction

As a practising health care ethicist, I often consult with individual staff members and teams about their moral unease with the practice of restraint and seclusion. I hear about feeling like a perpetrator, victim, and guilty bystander in turn. The directives of the institution can require restraint and seclusion in response to certain behaviours by clients, regardless of questions about the true necessity and usefulness of these actions. This chapter will present some pondering about these charged and complex human interactions, and a proposition that service providers and institutions consider the idea that restraint and seclusion is itself a violence, even described as "one of the most brutal interventions within the nursing domain" facilitated by the "psychiatric apparatus of capture."[1]

The ideas that lie ahead are based on a deceptively profound three-word phrase: *gravity and grace*. This phrase is a translation from the writings of French philosopher Simone Weil.[2] I will first explore the concepts of slow violence and atmospheric violence in the hope of making it possible, if unpleasant, to conceive of restraint and seclusion as violence, or at least part of an atmosphere of violence. I will then describe Weil's idea of gravity and grace, two complementary but differentially dominant elements of human behaviour. Factors that emphasize gravity and enable grace are discussed. I will conclude with some thoughts offered about the challenge of repairing moral wrongs.

In what follows, I will use the terms *staff* and *clients* to refer to all service providers and those who are using their services, respectively. The word *good* (in italics) will be used in the ethical sense (as in a good person) to differentiate it from the notion of quality (as in a good pizza). This presupposes some clear values-based deliberation about what is *good*. This is not meant to include a simplistic sense of "obedient" or "well-behaved," especially where these notions are drawn from normative frames that are based in repressive ideas of madness, gender, race, or other identities.

I want also to say that I support the goals of "zero restraint" or "restraint-free" environments, and I also accept that this may not be universally achievable. It is probably an uneasy fact that there will be instances of "treatment failure" (where non-violent health care support fails to achieve the effect desired) just as in other realms of health care.[3] Using restraint and seclusion may, at times, be ethically defensible for some people.[4] But even if one accepts this line of argument, effective safeguards against its abuse are less likely to be given the necessary attention. More often than any defensible restraint and seclusion event, there will be indefensible and unnecessary acts of restraint and seclusion because of institutional climates and cultures – often influenced by poor policies, inadequate institutional processes, and incompetent, poorly supported practice.[5] However, even if one argues it may be genuinely defensible, I would propose it remains a type of wrongdoing.

For many, though, the idea of restraint and seclusion being a "brutal intervention" within the "psychiatric apparatus of capture" may be too extreme a characterization.[6] At a minimum, however, I propose we need to have some notion of these acts being a form of violence. However, conventional definitions of violence as constructed by institutions must necessarily leave the impression that the prescribed response is altogether different in nature; restraint and seclusion are not violence themselves but legitimate responses to violence or the threat of it. Two broader conceptions of violence offer the possibility of seeing what some would argue as "defensible" restraint and seclusion as forms of violence nonetheless. These are the ideas of *slow violence* and *atmospheric violence*.

Nixon's notion of "slow violence" might be a more palatable lens through which to see these interventions. He describes this in the context of environmental destruction as violence that is unseen, "attritional violence that is typically not viewed as violence at all."[7] It might be described as the result of generally accepted ways of being that carry deleterious effects borne disproportionately. For Nixon, environmental damage is a largely unseen outcome of our daily lifestyle in the developed world that disproportionately burdens the poor. Restraint and seclusion might similarly be characterized as largely out of sight and presenting disproportionate burdens to an already disadvantaged few, with some persons and their bodies (racialized, poor people) more likely to be restrained or secluded.

A second concept is that of "atmospheric violence," as described by Aciksoz who applies the idea to more extreme contexts of state violence to control citizen protests.[8] One of the elements contributing to his idea is the notion of *atmosphere* described by Stewart as "not an inert context but a force field in which people find themselves ... It is an attunement of the senses, of labours, and imaginaries to potential ways of living in or living through things."[9] In contexts of significant power differentials, combining the ideas of Stewart and Aciksoz offers a way to begin to examine how the practices of restraint and seclusion might significantly contribute to an atmosphere of violence, if not constitute a form of violence. The impressions conveyed by these ideas capture what many report when asked about their experience of restraint and seclusion. The fact remains, however, that many who are involved in the practice will resist this characterization of seclusion and restraint; many neither understand nor appreciate the experience of the client when they themselves or those acting under their aegis are the perpetrators of violence.

While I focus here on staff and institutional responsibility and argue restraint and seclusion is a form of violence, I appreciate that many clients would likely have the moral responsibility to do what is within their capacities to help prevent and minimize aggressive behaviours. Given the general inclination is towards a focus on the latter, I will unapologetically attend to the former. While we all have our part in understanding, recognizing, and countering it, I would maintain that more power-invested individuals have higher duties to do so than those over whom they wield power. I believe that obligations to cultivate *grace* follow power, given its *gravity*.

Simone Weil and "Gravity and Grace"

Simone Weil was an early-twentieth-century philosopher, mystic and political and military activist. Since her death at the age of 34, she has been a subject for many fascinated authors. Many have commented on the complexity of her mental health, wrapped up as it was in her mystically inclined mind. Reflecting on the nature of human behaviour and interactions, she developed the idea of "gravity and grace" in her notebook entries, a collection of which were posthumously published under the same title.[10] Partial to science metaphors, she compares her "gravity" to conventional gravity: weightiness, heaviness, or seriousness but with a decidedly negative, destructive character. Like conventional gravity, its effects are evident around us. Weil's gravity is manifest in its pull on behaviour towards survival and protection.[11]

Grace is something entirely different, opposing the pull of gravity. For Weil, grace is definitely something divine and comes from outside, from God, in fact. For others, like myself, whose world view does not involve a god, I propose that the notion of grace can be captured by the idea of *good*. Most of us regularly think through choices and actions, both great and small – asking, what is the *right* thing to do? This often involves resisting automatic, expedient, or self-serving responses. In this generally shared aim of promoting *good*, I believe we align with Weil's notion of grace – with a vision of something larger than ourselves, often directing our actions away from gravity's pull.

Weil saw gravity woven within us, and typically dominating our thinking and behaviour, leading to self-protective outcomes. She describes an example in her own experience:

> I must not forget that at certain times when my headaches were raging I had an intense longing to make another human being suffer by hitting him in exactly the same part of the forehead ... When in this state, I have several times succumbed to the temptation at least to say words which cause pain. Obedience to the force of gravity ... Thus we corrupt the function of language, which is to express the relationship between things.[12]

Weil's intense headaches created an inclination to be a perpetrator. What prevented such harm was grace, a sort of influencing perspective from outside herself, moderating the gravity within. In the context of restraint and seclusion, gravity might be evident in the default policy positions through which institutions wield the power to restrain or seclude in lieu of more complex, nuanced responses. Individual accountability and responsibility can be the victims of gravity here – the policy is the rule, regardless of any individual sense of a *better* response (in the sense of *ethically* better). The question for me is how to enable the influence of grace (either God or *good*, as you prefer) to prevent gravity from obscuring any possibility of better responses at both individual and institutional levels.

Weil constructs this pairing of gravity and grace with the idea that when grace is enabled to enter the frame, it does not replace gravity. The two dimensions coexist as complementary parts of a larger whole, albeit far from equals.[13] Where this complementarity is emphasized, our understanding of our actions might become fuller. Recognizing how and when our own thinking and behaviour tends to be drawn by gravity offers the chance to work on bringing grace to them. It can also help us see others as whole persons. Rather than slipping into reductionist stereotyping or stigmatizing, we might be more likely to see the many dimensions of any person, even when we perceive them to present a threat. In the context of restraints and seclusion, is there a way to appreciate the gravity of the behaviour while letting grace maintain that the whole perpetrator is worthy of even more and varied efforts directed towards their care? I believe many staff members do hold both perspectives at the same time, but many do not. This is lamentable but also understandable because gravity has amplifiers.

What Gives Gravity the Upper Hand?

If you accept that humans normally aim to do what is *good* during daily interactions, then it is perplexing to know how often that aim is foiled. If we aim for grace, why are we drawn so readily by gravity? A number of factors contribute to this pull of gravity. Perhaps first among them is the powerful reaction Goleman described as "emotional hijack" which leads to the fight or flight response.[14] Put simply, our brain has developed to have a reflex reaction to any perception of threat to keep us from harm. This automatic physiological response is, however, a real problem in some circumstances. It doesn't give us time to properly assess the actual versus perceived risk – that happens after the response. This pre-reflective response is a brilliant survival mechanism in the face of many real dangers in the world, but it often causes us grief in daily human social interaction. Once triggered, self-protection is the preconscious goal as "hijack" closes the mind to grace.

Another enabler of gravity is how the mind simplifies and categorizes the world, to make complexity and incompleteness tidier, but ends up overgeneralizing, stereotyping, and often stigmatizing. Banaji and Greenwald explore the subconscious assumptions we hold about people around us – biases of which we may not be aware.[15] While we do not imagine that we are inclined to think in sexist, racist/racialized, and other discriminatory ways, their work suggests we hold implicit biases and associations between groups of people and other positive or negative things. These biases may fall short of overt prejudice and concrete acts of discrimination; however, they manifest in our judgments, choices, and behaviours, which reflect our implicit cognitive inclinations. These implicit biases may ultimately prevent us from upholding our own ethical principles as we do not recognize when our own behaviours run contrary to the values we wish to promote.[16]

Another enabler of gravity, and barrier to grace, is power. Implicit power, like implicit assumptions, is particularly problematic as those who possess it may not reflect on and work to be conscious of its impact. By implicit power I mean the structural and relational power that is inherent in the health care system and the relationships between leaders and staff, clients and staff, and individual staff members and various staff groupings. These differentials are particularly pervasive in mental health care as staff members have duties to exercise powers arising from the statutory and regulatory frameworks that govern mental health care practice. The circumspect deployment of these powers and duties can be critical to preventing harm and promoting "recovery" or attaining of other desired goals. The institutional policy framework to support this deployment of power can vary dramatically in the way it promotes or prevents slow and atmospheric violence. The need for circumspect institutional perspectives is heightened when we consider the vagaries of clinical assessment and judgment – risk assessment tools are still debated in the literature and the "epidemic of overdiagnosis" has been much discussed.[17] So, too, has the legitimacy of diagnostic categories used in psychiatric practice.[18]

To prevent abuse of power, mental health services are often placed in the context of a human rights framework beginning with those same laws. In addition to these, most organizations have staff codes of conduct. Some organizations have gone further and state more clearly the rights of clients using mental health services specifically, often termed a bill of client rights.[19] These rights may be eroded in the grey zones of health care practice where laws, policies, and procedures must be interpreted and implemented by numerous individuals who are themselves subject to the pull of *gravity*.

Perhaps counterintuitively, a core factor in human relationships may be another potential driver towards gravity – empathy. It is important to acknowledge here that empathy is an increasingly complex entity – subject to various implicit biases in its conception and thus how it is measured. These biases can follow our assumptions about gender,[20] culture,[21] and even the neuroscience[22] we use to understand them and empathy itself. These dimensions of empathy are beyond the scope of this chapter. Here, the intent is to consider how one notion of empathy and its relationship to compassion and stress might have an impact on the work of those who impose seclusion and restraint upon others.

This idea of the relationship between empathy and compassion is premised upon the work of Singer and Bolz.[23] They have demonstrated that empathizing with another person in distress is itself an experience of stress. Their studies using functional magnetic resonance imaging reveal that the act of empathizing activates stress response areas of the brain. Where empathy alone is the experience, there is a risk that empathy fatigue (or "empathic distress fatigue"[24]) may manifest. When empathy fatigue sets in, gravity can overpower grace as we may default to a position of avoiding empathy, and perhaps caring about others, for our own self-protection.

What Might Give Grace Support to Counter Gravity?

First, each of the factors above can be seen as having a complementary grace-supporting dimension. Feeling empathy remains stressful until it can be translated into an act of compassion, which is more of a satisfaction experience.[25] By acting on empathy and communicating compassion, we will typically see the distressed individual benefit from empathy. In turn, we may benefit from this because grace pays dividends. But a significant problem arises if we are unable to communicate compassion. Empathy remains a stress and it soon becomes something we may seek to avoid. Thus, efforts to create a compassionate exchange can counter the effects of empathetic distress fatigue.

In the case of emotional hijack, our innate tendency towards physiologically triggered reflex reactions is not insurmountable. Rather than hoping to deprogram a reflex that has physiological roots, the key lies in recognizing it and its power when activated. This creates the possibility of managing it. Similarly, implicit assumptions require first that we recognize them. From there, we might be able to counter them, if not unlearn them. Here, the onus falls on individuals and institutions alike to enable staff to understand and manage these gravity-leaning phenomena. Grace is most likely to be found in continuing and expanding efforts that promote awareness and appreciation of our reflex fear reactions that are grounded in implicit bias about who is a threat to us, when, and why.

A More Involved Approach to Fostering Grace – Moral Repair

Many initiatives aim to reduce restraint and seclusion, drawing from both philosophies of care and evidence-based best practices, including trauma-informed care plans, client-identified comfort measures, and more meaningful therapeutic engagement throughout a hospital stay.[26] In addition to these, I am proposing to bring grace into our responses – to encourage a reflective rather than reflex response and restore relationships between both the perpetrators of "conventional" violence (such as harm to others by assault) and those who perpetrate institutional violence (conceived perhaps as slow or atmospheric violence).

To consider what is involved in restoring these relationships, I turn to an exploration of more extreme circumstances. Walker examines wrongdoings of a particularly large degree and/or scale (the horrific litany of political violence and oppression in the last century) as well as isolated individual acts.[27] For Walker, moral repair is the work of "restoring or creating trust and hope in a shared sense of value and responsibility."[28] I propose applying this to the damage done to therapeutic relationships and milieu in hospital settings where atmospheric and slow violence may be characteristics of incidents involving restraint and seclusion.

Walker outlines a series of tasks to promote moral repair. I adapt the list here and outline some recommendations for ways in which grace might be allowed to enter situations where fear, reflex responses and implicit assumptions might otherwise see gravity overwhelm its chances.

Place Responsibility Where It Belongs

I acknowledged that some incidents of restraint and seclusion might be defensible and others not, falling short of the ultimate in quality care, perhaps achieving a defensible second best. The challenge is to acknowledge that restraint and seclusion itself might still be, or lie within the territory of, a moral wrong. It may arise from one or more other wrongs such as noncompliance of staff with previously determined individual treatment plans and misapplication of policy and procedure. Gravity's allies pull us away from pondering this prospect. It is threatening to our self-image and self-esteem to think our own failure might have been the cause of a restraint or seclusion incident.

Address the Wrong(s) Done

Only when we acknowledge the prospect that restraint and seclusion are experienced as moral wrongs can we begin to address them as such. Typical debrief procedures focus on the staff, and this support is essential. Debriefing with clients has become more commonplace; however, it occurs within the context of power differentials when conducted by staff according to institutionally defined procedures. Peer debriefing is likely more productive, more so if the process is co-created with clients.

Reinstate or Establish Moral Terms and Standards and Foster Trust

These terms and standards are understood and supported by all those who have been involved in the restraint/seclusion (those restrained/ secluded and those who perpetrated the restraint/seclusion event), and the people involved in this moral repair endeavour (those who have been retrained/secluded and those who perpetrated the restraint/seclusion event) are themselves trustworthy. Bok asserted that "whatever matters to human beings, trust is the atmosphere in which it thrives."[29] If this is true, and if reduction of restraint and seclusion (even to minimal levels, if not zero) is embraced as something that matters, then trust will be essential to establishing the necessary moral terms and standards for moral repair. This involves accepting the possibility that using restraint and seclusion might have breached moral terms and standards. If we accept this, how might we reinstate terms and standards in a manner that all affected will see the breach and then understand, support, and trust such a process of reinstatement? Baier observed, "Trust is much easier to maintain than it is to get started and is never hard to destroy."[30] If trust is to characterize the regular interactions between staff and clients in mental health care service contexts (throughout the day, evening, and overnight), then it likely also needs to be developed among and between the staff group itself.[31] From there, consistency in the interpretation of policy and procedure will further the trustworthiness of the team and their practice – both trust of the team among those to whom they provide care, and trust within and among the care team members themselves.

Other organizational practices need reviewing. Some organizations have begun "flagging" individuals with colour coded wristbands as a public identifier of an assessment of risk of violence.[32] While possibly sensible at first glance, the evidence base to support flagging is far from conclusive.[33] At a more fundamental level, some colleagues have called into question the very paradigm of assessments that purport to predict risk of violence.[34] A better set point might be one in which they seek to make earlier detections of possible risk and complementary prevention opportunities. The former feels like gravity; the latter, more like grace.

Another subtle manifestation of distrust of clients beyond the use of wristbands as flags is the commonplace practice of omitting full names on staff identification badges in many mental health settings. These practices reinforce our invalid implicit assumptions about the inherent violence of patients, create further grey zones of individual judgment, and increase the imbalances of power   probably contributing to an atmosphere that is ultimately permeated by something like a Nixon's "slow violence," and thus a subtle version of what Aciksoz's termed "atmospheric violence."

Finally, the investigation and public reporting of restraint and seclusion incidents must be far more transparent. Available statistics are rarely straightforward, and the legal frameworks protecting the information relating to adverse events involving restraint and seclusion typically mean that only very limited findings and recommendations are made available to the victim or family.

It must also be asserted that trust among staff requires that organizational responses to violence in the workplace are seen to be genuine, acknowledging the wrong done and supporting the staff who have been harmed. But the same approaches must avoid strengthening the pull of gravity (by reinforcing emotionally hijacked reactions and implicit assumptions) and actively create space for grace (by enabling compassionate communication between those involved).

Reconnect or Connect the People Involved When Possible

This is where compassion serves us well towards a very challenging goal. Immense stresses are inherent in situations where violence and power manifest themselves. These stresses are real in many ways but may also be prone to the exaggerating effects of gravity. As mentioned above, empathy on its own is a stress experience, whereas communicating compassion is often something different with a potentially very different effect. Creating ways to enable the communication of compassion will require focused effort. Reimagined debriefings may be one possibility, along with "unit council meetings" or other forums enabling safe, semi-structured exchange between clients and staff. Ideally, strategies for enabling communication will be identified and developed collaboratively between various groups typically seen as stakeholders in the restraint/seclusion experience: mental health care staff, the recipients of care and the administrators responsible for ensuring that policies, procedures, and practice combine to ensure safety for all clients and staff. There may be greater or lesser need to involve external facilitators in this process; this will be a reflection of the current state of readiness for change within staff-client relationships.

I have placed the onus here on both the provider organization and its staff to consider that their own actions might constitute a type of violence or at the very least lean into the realm of a moral wrong. I suggest this in the service of enabling a greater appreciation of the experience of restraint and seclusion from the client perspective. I propose that there are significant challenges in mechanisms that create a confluence of forces that lead to some of these behaviours – the pull of gravity. These mechanisms include those at play within us as individuals: emotional hijack, implicit assumptions, and empathy fatigue. They also include the contexts in which we function, which can be seen to be inclined towards Aciksoz's idea of "atmospheric violence," because of the institutional climate. The idea of complementary "gravity and grace" could be a helpful lens with which to hold much of this in mind, despite the discomfort it might induce, to realize the benefits of more just and compassionate relationships. It costs nothing, other than taking a small conceptual risk and thinking differently.

NOTES

1 Jacob et al., "Sovereign Power," 80.
2 Weil, *Gravity and Grace*.
3 Knox and Holloman Jr., "Use and Avoidance"; Mildred, *Seclusion and Restraints*.
4 Herrera, "Justifying Restraint-Use."
5 Office of the Chief Coroner, "Inquest"; "Use of Physical Restraint."
6 Jacob et al., "Sovereign Power," 80, 82.
7 Nixon, *Slow Violence*.
8 Aciksoz, "Medical Humanitarianism."
9 Stewart, "Atmospheric Attunements," 452.
10 Weil, *Gravity and Grace*.

11 Plant, *Simone Weil.*
12 Weil, *Gravity and Grace*, 2–3.
13 Ibid.
14 McKeever, "The Brain."
15 Banaji and Greenwald, *Blindspot.*
16 FitzGerald, "A Neglected Aspect."
17 Wand, "Investigating the Evidence"; Moynihan et al., "Public Opinions."
18 McKenzie, "Mind Games."
19 Citizens Commission on Human Rights, "Mental Health Declaration"; Empowerment Council, "The Centre for Addiction"; Canadian Mental Health Association, "Our Client Bill of Rights."
20 Bluhm, "Gender and Empathy."
21 Hollan, "Empathy across Cultures."
22 Cong Guo, "The Neuroscience of Empathy."
23 Singer and Bolz, *Compassion.*
24 Klimecki and Singer, "Empathic Distress Fatigue."
25 Solon, "Compassion over Empathy."
26 Safewards, "Resources for Safewards Implements"; Restraint Free World, "Welcome to Restraint Free World."
27 Urban Walker, *Moral Repair.*
28 Ibid., 28.
29 Bok, *Lying*, 32.
30 Baier, "Trust and Antitrust," 242.
31 Glauser, Bournes, and Tepper, "Should Hospital Staff."
32 Toronto East General Hospital, *Workplace Violence Prevention.*
33 Public Services Health and Safety Association, *Flagging Toolkit.*
34 Wand, "Investigating the Evidence," 2–7.

BIBLIOGRAPHY

Aciksoz, Salih Can. "Medical Humanitarianism under Atmospheric Violence: Health Professionals in the 2013 Gezi Protests in Turkey." *Culture, Medicine and Psychiatry* 40 (2015): 198–222.
Baier, Annette. "Trust and Antitrust." *Ethics* 96, no. 2 (1986): 231–60.
Banaji, Mahzarin R., and Anthony G. Greenwald. *Blindspot: Hidden Biases of Good People.* New York: Delacorte Press, 2013.
Bluhm, Robyn. "Gender and Empathy." In *The Routledge Handbook of Philosophy of Empathy*, edited by Heidi L. Maibom, 377–87. London, UK: Routledge, 2017.

Bok, Sissela. *Lying*. New York: Pantheon Books, 1978.

Boysen, Philip G. "Just Culture: A Foundation for Balanced Accountability and Patient Safety." *Ochsner Journal* 13, no. 3 (2013): 400–6.

Canadian Mental Health Association. "Our Client Bill of Rights." Accessed February 16, 2017. https://toronto.cmha.ca/about-us/our-client -bill-of-rights/.

Citizens Commission on Human Rights. "Mental Health Declaration of Human Rights." Accessed February 16, 2017. https://www.cchr.org/ about-us/mental-health-declaration-of-human-rights.html.

Cong Guo, Christine. "The Neuroscience of Empathy." In *The Routledge Handbook of Philosophy of Empathy*, edited by Heidi L. Maibom, 44–53. London, UK: Routledge, 2017.

Empowerment Council. "The Centre for Addiction and Mental Health Bill of Client Rights." Accessed February 16, 2017. http://www .empowermentcouncil.ca/PDF/client_bill_rights.pdf.

FitzGerald, Chloë. "A Neglected Aspect of Conscience: Awareness of Implicit Attitudes." *Bioethics* 28, no. 1 (2014): 24–32.

Glauser, Wendy, Debra Bournes, and Joshua Tepper. "Should Hospital Staff Satisfaction Survey Results Be Public?" *Healthy Debate*, January 29, 2015. http://healthydebate.ca/2015/01/topic/staff-satisfaction.

Herrera, Christopher D. "Justifying Restraint-Use in Psychiatric Care." *Journal of Ethics in Mental Health* 6 (2011). http://www.jemh.ca/issues/v6/ documents/JEMH_Vol6_Article_Justifying_Restraint_Use_In_Psychiatric_ Care.pdf.

Hollan, Douglas. "Empathy across Cultures." In *The Routledge Handbook of Philosophy of Empathy*, edited by Heidi L. Maibom, 341–52. London, UK: Routledge, 2017.

Jacob, Jean Daniel, Marilou Gagnon, Amelie Perron, and Dave Holmes. "Sovereign Power, Spectacle and Punishment: A Critical Analysis of the Use of the Seclusion Room." *International Journal of Culture and Mental Health* 2, no. 2 (2009): 75–85.

Klimecki, Olga, and Tania Singer. "Empathic Distress Fatigue Rather than Compassion Fatigue? Integrating Findings from Empathy Research in Psychology and Social Neuroscience." In *Pathological Altruism*, edited by Barbara Oakley, 368–83. New York: Oxford University Press, 2012.

Knox, Daryl, K., and Garland H. Holloman Jr. "Use and Avoidance of Seclusion and Restraint: Consensus Statement of the American Association for Emergency Psychiatry Project BETA Seclusion and Restraint Workgroup." *Western Journal of Emergency Medicine* 13, no. 1 (2012): 35–40.

McKeever, Monty. "The Brain and Emotional Intelligence: An Interview with Daniel Goleman." *Tricycle*, May 18, 2011. http://tricycle.com/blog/brain-and-emotional-intelligence-interview-daniel-goleman.

McKenzie, Kwame. "Mind Games." *Walrus*, May 2013. https://thewalrus.ca/mind-games/.

Mildred, Laurel. *Seclusion and Restraints: A Failure, Not a Treatment*. Sacramento: California Senate Office of Research, 2002. https://sor.senate.ca.gov/sites/sor.senate.ca.gov/files/Seclusion%20and%20Restraints.pdf.

Moynihan, Ray, B. Nickel, J. Hersch, E. Beller, J. Doust, and S. Compton. "Public Opinions about Overdiagnosis: A National Community Survey." *PLoS ONE* 10, no. 5 (2015). https://doi.org/10.1371/journal. pone.0125165.

Nixon, Rob. *Slow Violence and the Environmentalism of the Poor*. Cambridge, MA: Harvard University Press, 2011.

Office of the Chief Coroner. "Inquest into the Death of Jeffrey James: Jury Recommendations." 2008. http://www.empowermentcouncil.ca/PDF/Jeffery%20James%20Inquest.pdf.

Plant, Stephen. *Simone Weil: A Brief introduction*. Maryknoll, NY: Orbis Books, 1997.

Public Services Health and Safety Association. *Communicating the Risk of Violence: A Flagging Program Handbook for Maximizing Preventative Care*. Toronto, Ontario: Public Services Health and Safety Association, 2016. https://www.pshsa.ca/wp-content/uploads/2017/04/VWVMNAEN0616-Communicating-Risk-of-Violence-Flagging-Prevention-Program-V1.1-2017.04.21.pdf.

Restraint Free World."Welcome to Restraint Free World." Accessed February 17, 2017. http://www.restraintfreeworld.org/.

Safewards. "Resources for Safewards Implements." Accessed February 17, 2017. http://www.safewards.net/.

Singer, Tania, and Matthias Bolz. *Compassion. Bridging Practice and Science*. Munich: Max Planck Society, 2013. http://www.compassion-training.org/.

Solon, Olivia. "Compassion over Empathy Could Help Prevent Emotional Burnout." *Wired*, July 12, 2012. https://www.wired.co.uk/article/tania-singer-compassion-burnout.

Stewart, Kathleen. Atmospheric Attunements. *Environment and Planning D: Society and Space* 29, no. 3 (2011): 445–53.

Toronto East General Hospital. *Workplace Violence Prevention: Flagging Process for Patients Exhibiting Acting Out Behaviour*. https://www.ona.org/wp-content/uploads/tegh_flagging_201310.pdf?x72008.

Urban Walker, Margaret. *Moral Repair: Reconstructing Moral Relations after Wrongdoing*. New York: Cambridge University Press, 2006.

"Use of Physical Restraint on Mental Health Patients at 'Disturbing Levels.'"
   Guardian, June 19, 2013. https://www.theguardian.com/society/2013
   /jun/19/physical-restraint-mental-health-patients.
Wand, T. "Investigating the Evidence for the Effectiveness of Risk Assessment
   in Mental Health Care." *Issues in Mental Health Nursing* 33, no. 1 (2012): 2–7.
Weil, Simone. *Gravity and Grace*. London, UK: Routledge, 2002.

19 Mad, Bad, and Stuck in the Hole: Carceral Segregation as Slow Violence

JENNIFER M. KILTY AND SANDRA LEHALLE

Introduction

Before the election of Conservative federal political leadership in 2006, scholars dismissed the notion that Canada was experiencing the kind of a "punitive turn" witnessed in either the United States or Britain.[1] However, under the direction of then prime minister Stephen Harper, the federal government demarcated a dramatic ideological shift in crime control and punishment strategies that when taken together indicate a transformation of Canada's historically moderate approach to penality.[2] The Conservative party's aggressive law-and-order style of governing crime, exemplified by the introduction of 90 new pieces of criminal justice legislation, including two massive omnibus style bills,[3] suggests we are experiencing a kind of "penal intensification" that is characterized by longer custodial sentences, the creation of new imprisonable offences, and the erosion of legal protections.[4] These routes to penal expansion not only amplify the use of "hard power" in prison settings[5] but also disproportionately affect the poor, racialized minorities,[6] and individuals experiencing mental illness or distress.[7] Notably, all of these groups are already considered to be especially vulnerable to processes of criminalization.

While many studies examine the harmful physical and mental health consequences of carceral segregation practices, this chapter considers how it is that institutional staff can use these practices without serious moral quandaries. We conceptualize the correctional risk logic used to govern carceral institutions and individual prisoners as a form of epistemological violence that leads to a kind of dehumanization of the penal subject, which allows us to theorize carceral segregation practices as enacting a form of *slow violence* – violence that occurs incrementally and oftentimes systematically over time – to which correctional actors are socially and morally indifferent. We begin by showcasing how segregation is a key feature of penal intensification.

Segregation and Penal Intensification

One significant consequence of penal intensification is the increasing and prolonged usage of segregation, also known as solitary confinement, as a population management strategy and as a punishment for institutional infractions or misconduct. Carceral systems around the world continue to isolate political prisoners, prisoners who are mentally distressed, and any incarcerated person deemed dangerous or threatening to the security of the institution. Shalev found that in Europe, solitary confinement occurs on a "much smaller scale" than in the United States, but it is still "a common prison practice."[8] That isolation would occur on a smaller scale in Europe is not surprising given that the United States incarcerates more people than any other country in the world, and forty-four states and the federal system have supermax units comprising only isolation cells. Leading human rights organizations like Amnesty International and the United Nations identify prolonged isolation and the segregation of mentally distressed prisoners as cruel and unusual punishment, torture, and a violation of human rights. Notably, Human Rights Watch released in 2016 a report on France's "inadequate conditions for prisoners with psychosocial disabilities," emphasizing that female prisoners with psychosocial disabilities face especially harsh prison conditions.

In Canada, the number of admissions to segregation increased significantly from 7572 in 2005–2006 to 8309 in 2014–2015.[9] There are approximately 850 federal prisoners housed in segregation units at any given time, 44% of whom are segregated for 30 days or less while 16.5% are segregated for more than 120 days.[10] These numbers show the growing frequency of the use of segregation as an everyday (rather than a last resort) carceral management strategy and the increasingly lengthy time some prisoners are sentenced to spend segregated.[11] Admission to segregation is notably racialized; the Office of the Correctional Investigator (OCI) reports that between 2005 and 2015 the rate of admission to segregation for Aboriginal prisoners increased 52.4% (from 2296 to 3500) and 77.5% for Black prisoners (from 792 to 1406).[12] In fact, admissions to segregation for Black prisoners have grown at a faster rate than the incarcerated population of Black offenders, while Aboriginal prisoners consistently experience the longest lengths of stay in segregation.

The Correctional Service of Canada (CSC) uses two security classifications to describe the legal practice of isolating individual prisoners.[13] *Disciplinary segregation* is the status designated to those who breach an institutional rule or act violently towards staff or other prisoners.[14] It is a form of punishment legally sanctioned by the Corrections and Conditional Release Act (CCRA) and set out in Commissioner's Directive (CD) 580. In contrast to disciplinary segregation, prisoners may go into *administrative segregation* voluntarily or involuntarily.[15] In accordance with Section 31 of the CCRA (1992), an individual may be segregated for one of three administrative reasons: they are thought to pose a danger to staff, other prisoners, or to the security of the institution; they have the potential to interfere with an ongoing investigation; or for their own safety. Because administrative segregation is not *meant* to be punitive, prisoners with this classification status are legally required to receive the same rights, privileges, and conditions of confinement as the general prisoner population, barring those that institutional authorities believe to be a security concern and the limitations of the segregation area. However, given the failure to institute definitive limits regarding the length of time correctional authorities may isolate a prisoner in segregation, it is unsurprising that segregation is one of the most frequently cited grievance issues prisoners report.[16] According to the OCI, 2.2% of all admissions to segregation during 2011–2012 were for disciplinary reasons and the remaining 97.8% of cases involved administrative segregation.[17] It is important to point out that prisoners segregated for administrative and disciplinary reasons occupy the same cells and experience similar restrictions – for example, with respect to barred access to programs, no communication with other prisoners, and the inability to experience more than one hour outside their cell a day.

Segregation, Psychological Harm, and Ashley Smith

The extant literature consistently demonstrates that there are negative emotional and psychological harms derived from experiencing institutional isolation and the types of restrictive punishments commonly employed in this form of holding. These include, but are not limited to, violent cell extractions, physical and chemical restraints, extreme levels of material deprivation and removal of personal items, lack of meaningful activity, sensory deprivation (e.g., by leaving the lights on in the cell 24 hours a day, delivering food through a mail slot in the cell door, denial of utensils), strip-searching, lack of access to programming, and limited access to yard time.[18] The most common concerns centre on the deleterious mental health effects of time spent isolated. The longer the time the individual spends segregated the greater the likelihood that they will experience difficulties related to social interaction (including social isolation, greater association with criminal acquaintances, being more easily influenced by others, and difficulty communicating with others); personal and emotional orientation (including cognition problems, hostility, poor conflict resolution skills, low frustration tolerance, and thrill seeking); and attitude (including negative attitudes towards the criminal justice system, pro-criminal attitudes, being disrespectful and lacking direction, and non-conformance).[19]

Isolating an individual who is clearly in emotional distress is widely panned for aggravating personal suffering and damaging the possibility for a positive therapeutic relationship between the individual prisoner and front-line staff members.[20] In December 2014 the *Canadian Medical Association Journal* published an editorial stating that the isolation and lack of stimulation experienced while in segregation can lead to mental health distress and anger, which increase the risk of self-harm and suicide.[21] The 2014 and 2015 OCI annual report indicate that when prisoners commit suicide they do so more often in segregation cells and other maximum-security units than while housed among the general population.[22] The carceral deaths of 19-year-old Ashley Smith in 2007 and 24-year-old Edward Snowshoe in 2010 while housed in prolonged segregation demonstrate this fact.[23] Throughout this chapter we refer to the Smith case to exemplify the manifest ways that prolonged carceral segregation gradually creates and amplifies psychiatric distress and thus acts as a form of slow violence. To humanize Ashley we introduce her as a central character by highlighting her personhood – notably, the intersection of her gender, youth, and experiences of mental distress.

At the age of 15, Ashley Smith was sentenced as a juvenile to a one-month custodial term in the New Brunswick Youth Centre (NBYC) for the minor transgression of throwing crab apples at a postal worker. Because of numerous institutional infractions, the majority for self-injurious behaviour, Ashley's sentence was repeatedly extended culminating in a three-year period of incarceration in NBYC before her transfer to the adult federal correctional system at the age of 18. Ashley's psychological distress and self-injurious behaviour intensified in federal custody, where she was kept in permanent seclusion for nearly a year before strangling herself to death in Grand Valley Institution in 2007. In violation of correctional policy, institutional staff members were instructed not to intervene until Smith passed out from ligature use. As a result of this order, on the day of her death a group of correctional officers watched from the hallway for nearly ten minutes before entering her segregation cell to cut the ligature off.[24] Ashley Smith's horrific carceral treatment was facilitated by the guiding correctional philosophy of governing through risk, a logic we conceptualize as a form of epistemological violence.

Governing through Risk as Epistemological Violence

Feeley and Simon famously argued that in the "new penology" of contemporary risk societies, correctional administrators have sacrificed rehabilitation efforts in favour of strategies aimed at "managing costs and controlling dangerous populations."[25] The CSC has long-governed its institutions through risk management logic, embracing the risk-need-responsivity model and a variety of actuarial risk assessment tools. While the CSC attempts to assess both the risks and needs of each offender to determine their security level and the details of their correctional plan, critics problematize the conflation of risk and need, especially for criminalized women, the mentally distressed, and Indigenous prisoners, such that the greater the number and salience of a person's needs the greater the risk they are seen to pose – potentially to themselves, other prisoners, prison staff, and the public upon their release.[26] We suggest that governing through risk contributes to the creation of what Haney describes as "a culture of harm" shored up by "ideological toxicity" that sees exceptional danger lurking in every prisoner, especially in Indigenous and Black prisoners who are segregated at exceptional rates, and manifests extreme forms of deprivation and violence in this form of holding that are sustained by the "dynamics of cruelty" at play in maximum-security environments.[27]

Haney suggests that this culture of harm encourages guards to be hyper-sensitive to even the slightest provocation or rule infraction, as well as an empathic indifference to the suffering isolated prisoners endure. In turn, this leads to an acceptance of punitive and violent expressions of power between prisoners and staff, so much so that "the interactions between guards and prisoners in these units are always at risk of devolving into increasingly tight spirals of negative expectation, conflict, and recrimination."[28] This was clearly exemplified in the Ashley Smith case; Ashley was placed in administrative segregation for repeatedly self-injuring, tying ligatures around her neck, and being belligerent, defiant, and sometimes violent with staff members. Correctional authorities responded with tasers and pepper spray, and by increasing her material and interpersonal deprivations (e.g., she was denied all clothing but a security gown, writing utensils, cutlery, and sufficient amounts of items like toilet paper, sanitary napkins or tampons, and deodorant).[29] As her conditions of confinement grew more and more austere, she became increasingly defiant and despondent, while guards gradually became exasperated by and then indifferent to the suffering of a teen girl.

Given the ongoing placement of self-injuring and suicidal prisoners into administrative segregation under the ideological guise that it is an institutional safety and security measure, we must consider how correctional authorities understand these behaviours and thus what interpretive framework they draw from to explain them. Following traditional biomedical frameworks that locate the origin of mental distress in the individual's inherently flawed psychology, correctional authorities tend to characterize prisoners who self-harm or who attempt suicide as "mentally ill," irrational, potentially manipulative, and attention seeking but also as rebellious, insubordinate, and manipulative and thus as risks to the security of the institution.[30]

We take up Teo's concept of epistemological violence (EV) to problematize the reductionist and individualizing effects of risk analyses and biomedical frameworks that constitute self-injurious and suicidal behaviours as evidence of a mentally ill subjectivity and the individual as a risky and dangerous Other.

The epistemological part of this concept suggests that these theoretical interpretations are framed as knowledge about the Other when in reality they are interpretations regarding data. The term *violence* denotes that this "knowledge" has a negative impact on the Other or that the theoretical interpretations are produced to the detriment of the Other. The negative impact can range from misrepresentations and distortions to a neglect of the voices of the Other, to propositions of inferiority, and to the recommendations of adverse practices or infringements concerning the Other. The term *epistemological violence* as it is used in the argument does not refer to the misuse of research in general but is specific to theoretical interpretations of empirical results that have negative connotations for the Other in a given community.[31]

Teo's formulation is useful because it does not necessarily problematize the empirical data set, but rather the hermeneutics of its interpretation given that plural meanings can be attributed depending on the researcher's theoretical framework. Teo contends that at least two forms of EV occur when data are interpreted: "the interpretation itself is a form of violence and the interpretation is violent because specific policy recommendations are made or accepted."[32] In this theoretical orientation, empirical social researchers and front-line correctional staff (the subject) work to interpret data pertaining to the risks, needs, and responsivity factor information (which is presented as knowledge) that is collected with respect to the Other (the gendered and racialized individual prisoner as the object). They do this by reviewing the individual's case file to see if they have a history of self-harming behaviours (a static and thus unchanging factor), observing the individual, and conducting an interview with them (if they agree). Akin to a caged zoo animal, if placed in a high suicide watch segregation cell (as Ashley Smith was) the prisoner is under constant direct observation by a correctional officer or primary worker while experiencing extreme material and interpersonal deprivations.

The logic underpinning this policy response is embedded in the historic practice of secluding agitated psychiatric patients with as little mental and physical stimulation as possible to try to calm them.[33] This interpretive framework focuses exclusively on using increasingly austere deprivations to try to eliminate the possibility of self-injury in the present moment and fails to consider the long-lasting harms that this inflicts upon the individual. An alternative interpretation might instead emphasize that,

> When combined with the sheer starkness and deprivation of the environment, the technologies and implements of forceful custodial restraint and control, a special ecology is created. This ecology is fairly described as "cruel" for the simple reason that it inures people to the suffering of others and because it is designed and operated in ways that give staff members little choice but – by merely following procedure – to likely add to that suffering.[34]

This interpretive frame supports the erroneous belief that these particular offenders are

> somehow impervious to the pains of imprisonment, [which] allows the compassion and empathy that would otherwise be extended to persons who are held in desperate and degraded conditions, who are in crisis or

in need, anguished or disconsolate, to be suspended, so that their pain not only does not register but becomes something that they have earned, asked for, or otherwise simply deserve.[35]

The epistemological violence done by routinely framing penal subjects as risky and inferior Others paves the way for their dehumanization, which throws the moral performance of the prison into disrepute.[36] In the next section we conceptualize the moral distancing and dehumanization process and outline how this occurs within the context of carceral segregation.

Moral Distancing and Dehumanization

The institutionalization of penal segregation practices illustrates a dehumanization process, which relies on bureaucracy to create distance between institutional actors and penal subjects and to normalize institutional activities (i.e., segregation), the justifications provided for those activities (i.e., risk), and the vocabulary used (i.e., mentally ill; administrative versus disciplinary segregation). Beyond procedures and technical terms, normalization ensures that it is easy to forget that penal subjects are human beings. We draw from Kelman and Hamilton who outline three conditions that facilitate moral distancing.[37] The first condition is the authorization of violence. Segregation is a legal practice that is outlined in official government documents and validated by different levels of authority (legislative, executive, and judicial). Therefore, while segregation might be explicitly ordered in some cases and tacitly encouraged in others, it is always used with the seal of approval of someone in a position of authority (i.e., the courts, correctional officers, mental health workers, nurses, wardens, and bureaucrats).

The second condition involves the routinization of segregation practices. Repeatedly performing violent cell extractions, strip searches, and using punitive technologies to physically and chemically restrain prisoners can, over time, habituate correctional staff to inflicting pain and degradation as a customary component of their work. With no alternative strategies to manage secluded prisoners, front-line correctional staff can become desensitized to the suffering that their uses of force inflict upon segregated prisoners. The daily routine of performing these activities over and over again enables correctional staff to act without thinking and without facing the moral dilemmas and consequences of their actions.[38] Authorization and routinization encourage front-line staff to prioritize obedience to authority and acquiescence to institutional rationale over conventional moral values. When employees' main concern is being accountable to their superiors, despite being aware of the negative consequences, they are more likely to use punitive institutional techniques. This occurred with Ashley Smith after correctional officers were reprimanded on at least one occasion for removing a ligature from her neck before allowing her to fall unconscious – which was their (illegal) bureaucratic instruction.[39]

While correctional actors might adopt a technical responsibility for their actions (that were approved by the bureaucratic hierarchy), they are likely to refuse moral responsibility for the harms that might flow from their actions. In this context, normalization can lead correctional staff to become desensitized to the point where "behavioural drift" – the blurring of the line between ethical and unethical treatment– becomes possible.[40] As a result, the moral evaluation of the practice falls outside of and becomes foreign to the practice itself so that the actor becomes a "non subject."[41] Although correctional employees act violently when performing segregation practices, these actions do not involve their subjectivity; rather, by following orders and institutional procedures the violence they inflict upon prisoners loses moral meaning and comes to reflect an instance of submission to a lawful authority by the "non subject."

The final condition is dehumanization, which is a process through which an individual is excluded from the actor's "moral universe." The universe of moral obligation refers to the circle of individuals and groups "toward whom obligations are owed, to whom rules apply, and whose injuries call for amends."[42] In other words, if a person is reframed in such a way that they are excluded from the moral universe, then we are no longer faced with a moral dilemma regarding how they are treated. The individual may then be perceived as deserving of the treatment they are forced to endure. This process takes place through the use of segregation, which is designed to house "the worst of the worst" – an idea that has created a kind of mythology around those so imprisoned as "fundamentally 'other' and dehumanizes, degrades, and demonizes them as essentially different, even from other prisoners."[43]

The epistemological violence done by designating a self-injuring prisoner as risky, mentally ill, attention seeking, and manipulative facilitates this Othering process. As segregation practices are normalized and routinized, correctional actors have been found to act as though carceral institutions are places where ordinary rules, norms, and standards of decency do not apply.[44] When this occurs, segregated prisoners become "morally excluded," placed in a kind of alternative moral universe that is free of conventional ethical constraints and moral accountability with respect to their institutional treatment, which leads to their dehumanization.[45] The social and moral indifference and dehumanizing treatment that correctional actors express towards prisoners constituted as dangerous "Others" exemplifies how segregation enacts a kind of "slow violence," an invisible violence that creates "displacement in place."[46]

Segregation as Slow Violence Lacking Visibility

Prison is a desolate and uninviting habitation space, and segregation units are even more so; they are often described as a *prison within a prison*, playing host to the most austere forms of material and interpersonal deprivation in the penal sphere. We take up Nixon's notion of slow violence to conceptualize the long-term harms of carceral segregation.

By slow violence we mean a violence that occurs gradually and out of sight, a violence of delayed destruction that is dispersed across time and space, an attritional violence that is typically not viewed as violence at all. Violence is customarily conceived as an event or action that is immediate in time, explosive and spectacular in space, and as erupting into instant sensational visibility. We need, we believe, to engage a different kind of violence, a violence that is neither spectacular nor instantaneous, but rather incremental and accretive, its calamitous repercussions playing out across a range of temporal scales.[47]

What is especially unique and important about Nixon's conceptualization is his consideration of the notion of time and temporality, such that the harms that flow from acts of slow violence may take months or years to appreciate. This can present a "major representational challenge" given that violence, as it is typically conceived, is hyper-visible, sensational, and visually spectacular. The slow violence of segregation exists in a strangely liminal space that is hyper-visible, as per the constant direct or closed circuit television surveillance monitoring, yet simultaneously invisible, given that prisons are largely "insulated places [that] allow the staff to establish a social reality that is largely immune from critical evaluation, challenge, and debate and [that is] exempted from normal forms accountability."[48] It is also invisible because it operates by slowly and systematically destroying connection to others through both physical and psychological isolation. This displacement adds to the emotional and psychological torture of isolation and can lead to long-lasting emotional suffering and even psychological and physical death.

Segregation practices rarely generate negative moral reactions from the people using them (staff) or the people in the name of whom they are used (society) precisely because correctional actors constitute them as adiaphoric.[49] Originally a medical term, *adiaphoria* refers to insensitivity and even nonresponse to pain stimuli, which is crucial for the body's ability to defend itself, as a result of previous exposure. More recently, it has been used to refer to a society's loss of sensitivity to perceive and react to the first signs of dysfunction.[50] The routine harms of carceral segregation practices typically go unnoticed by the media and thus the public. Nixon suggests that the passage of time allows "the memory of catastrophe [to] readily fade from view as the casualties incurred typically pass untallied and unremembered. Such discounting in turn makes it far more difficult to secure effective legal measures for prevention, restitution, and redress."[51] The federal government has been known to try to prevent the public from viewing images of prisoners enduring forms of violent victimization and extreme deprivation – as it did in the Ashley Smith case.[52] Despite the state's best efforts, when the image of a teenage girl, her hands and feet already manacled, duct-taped to her airplane seat with a mesh hood over her head during an institutional transfer was made available to the public, Ashley became the instant star of a public, political, and eventually legal debate surrounding the harms of carceral segregation practices and the lack of institutional oversight and transparency in federal corrections.

Given that many of the harms of segregation are intensely psychological and thus typically unseen, Ashley Smith's experiences gave "figurative shape to formless threats whose fatal repercussions are dispersed across space and time," making her an "iconic symbol" of the harms of carceral isolation for a population that is dangerously out of sight, out of mind.[53] The tragedy of her death "draws together the domains of perception, emotion, and action"[54] to demonstrate that the harms flowing from the repeated violent interactions Ashley had with correctional staff and the material and interpersonal deprivations to which she was steadfastly subject built slowly, layer upon layer, over the four years she was incarcerated. Spending over a quarter of her young life in prison segregation cells, Ashley provided critics with both visible and written documentary evidence to make the invisible world of segregation known to the public.

In the end, the ground-breaking coroner's inquest into Ashley's death concluded by making 104 recommendations, including the abolition of indefinite segregation and the elimination of segregation for self-injuring and mentally or emotionally distressed prisoners.[55] The United Nations Special Rapporteur on Torture[56] and Amnesty International made similar recommendations, yet the federal government refuses to implement them. As a result, on January 19, 2015, the British Columbia Civil Liberties Association and the John Howard Society of Canada filed a joint lawsuit against the Attorney General of Canada to challenge the use of administrative segregation in Canadian prisons. One week later, the Canadian Civil Liberties Association filed a similar petition in Ontario Superior Court.

In December 2017 Associate Chief Justice Frank Marrocco of the Ontario Superior Court struck down Canada's laws on segregation as unconstitutional, citing the lack of independent review and the harms caused by isolation. While the Canadian Civil Liberties Association applauded the decision, they are now launching an appeal to prohibit segregation beyond 15 days and for certain vulnerable groups (e.g., the mentally distressed, young people, and those seeking safety). In January 2018 just one month after the Ontario decision, the British Columbia Supreme Court went even further by declaring that segregation laws violate Sections 7 and 15 of the Charter of Rights and Freedoms because they permit prolonged indefinite isolation, fail to provide an independent review of segregation placements, deprive prisoners of the right to counsel at segregation review hearings, and authorize administrative segregation for the mentally distressed, and because the regime discriminates against Indigenous prisoners.[57]

Conclusion

While only time will tell whether the Ontario Supreme courts will rule in favour of the appeal seeking to abolish the use of segregation for mentally distressed prisoners, we maintain that the CSC's refusal to stop segregating prisoners who are experiencing emotional distress exemplifies that the correctional obsession with risk management and security continues to supersede the moral and ethical treatment of incarcerated people. We disagree with the correctional discourse that frames segregated prisoners like Ashley Smith as ticking time bombs, as this type of characterization generates fear of and hostility towards the dangerous Other of our cultural imaginary, which then contributes to the erosion of moral impulses towards them. Once they are excluded from the obligations of the moral universe, isolated prisoners become the objects of different segregation practices that inflict slow violence upon them. It is our position that the extreme forms of deprivation that prisoners experience while isolated in segregation aggravates mental and emotional distress, which can lead to both self-harming and externally-directed aggressive behaviour, and offers nothing by way of therapeutic care or safe and humane conditions of confinement.

In this chapter we argued that as an interpretive frame, risk logic and assessment perpetrates epistemological violence that facilitates the use of certain correctional practices that come to inflict slow violence upon segregated prisoners. The normalization and routinization of these practices can lead to the dehumanization of isolated prisoners and to a "culture of harm" inside maximum-security units similar to what Ashley Smith experienced while housed in permanent segregation.[58] The slow violence that everyday correctional practices like violent cell extractions, strip and body cavity searches, and physical and chemical restraint procedures enact is often invisible or misrecognized, where only the passage of time will reveal the lasting harms.

The legal right to deprive criminals of their liberty and the unruly prisoner of even the most basic material and interpersonal conditions that might make their confinement bearable problematically justifies the use of carceral segregation. Therefore, these everyday acts of violence consist of conduct that is socially permitted, encouraged, and enjoined as components of the correctional actor's requisite duty. Segregation, then, can be conceived as a form of institutionalized slow violence that dehumanizes specific populations in a way that is almost invisible to others. As such, it may be considered an example of the "small wars and invisible genocides" as conceived by Scheper-Hugues,[59] where segregated prisoners, and Indigenous, Black, and mentally distressed prisoners in particular, who are the targets of institutionalized violence disproportionately encounter the social and moral indifference of their captors.

NOTES

1 Doob and Webster, "Countering Punitiveness"; Meyer and O'Malley, "Missing the Punitive Turn?"; Webster and Doob, "Punitive Trends."

2 Doob, "Principled Sentencing"; Doob and Webster, "The Harper Revolution."

3 Doob and Webster, "The Harper Revolution"; Webster and Doob, "Punitive Trends."

4 Sim, *Punishment and Prisons*.

5 Ben Crewe, "Soft Power in Prison," 456, describes hard power as "the use of direct command or coercion" whereas soft power "comprises those aspects of treatment and regulation that are accomplished directly through staff–prisoner relationships and indirectly through the policies that officers assist or put into effect."

6 Razack, "Racial Terror."

7 Haney, "Mental Health Issues"; Haney, "A Culture of Harm."

8 Shalev, "Solitary Confinement," 145. The Arthur Liman Public Interest Program at Yale Law School and the Association of State Correctional Administrators ("Time-in-Cell") estimated that between 80,000 and 100,000 people in state prisons were held in isolation in 2014. They based this estimate on data obtained from 34 states, housing 73 percent of all prisoners, which found over 66,000 people in restrictive housing. This figure does not include local jails, juvenile, military, and immigration facilities.

9 Office of the Correctional Investigator, *Administrative Segregation*.

10 Zinger, *Ending the Isolation*.

11 For the use of segregation as an everyday management strategy, see Guenther, *Solitary Confinement*; Haney, "A Culture of Harm"; Kerr, "The Chronic Failure"; Martel, "Women in the Hole." For discussions on the length of segregation see Haney, "A Culture of Harm"; Kerr, "The Chronic Failure"; Kilty, "Examining the 'Psy-Carceral Complex'"; Martel, "Women in the Hole"; Martel, "To Be, One Has to Be Somewhere"; Martel, "Les Femmes"; McGill, "An Institutional Suicide Machine"; Razack, "Racial Terror."

12 Office of the Correctional Investigator, "Administrative Segregation."

13 CSC oversees the imprisonment, correctional rehabilitation, and carceral release of federally sentenced men and women – those who are sentenced to a period of incarceration of two years or more. While segregation is also problematically overused in provincial corrections, we focus on the

federal level because prisoners spend lengthier periods of time segregated in federal prisons and there is no publicly accessible data for the provincial sector.

14 An individual may be sentenced to up to 30 days in disciplinary segregation, unless she is already serving a period of segregation for another serious offence, in which case the adjudication committee will determine whether the two periods are to be served concurrently or consecutively. If the sanctions are to be served consecutively, the total period of segregation imposed may not exceed 45 days.

15 The CCRA does not specify the maximum length of time an individual may be kept in administrative segregation; prisoners are expected to return to the general population at the earliest possible moment, with institutional and regional reviews conducted after five, thirty, and then after each sixty days that pass. This review practice has allowed the CSC to house prisoners in segregation for over one, two, and in Ashley Smith's case more than three hundred consecutive days.

16 Zinger, *Ending the Isolation.*

17 Ibid.

18 Guenther, *Solitary Confinement*; Haney, "Mental Health Issues"; Haney, "A Culture of Harm"; Liebling, "Moral Performance"; Martel, "Women in the Hole"; Martel, "To Be"; Martel, "Les Femmes"; Sapers, *A Preventable Death.*

19 Kane, *Commitment to Legal Compliance*, 11.

20 Bonner, "Stressful Segregation Housing"; Haney, "Mental Health Issues"; Haney, "A Culture of Harm"; Lanes, "The Association"; Liebling, "Moral Performance"; Alison Liebling et al., "Revisiting Prison Suicide."

21 Kelsall, "Cruel and Usual Punishment," 1345.

22 Office of the Correctional Investigator, *A Three Year Review*; Office of the Correctional Investigator, "Administrative Segregation."

23 Edward Snowshoe was a First Nations man who hung himself after serving 162 consecutive days in segregation in the federal Edmonton Institution for men. The fatality report suggests that he "fell through the cracks of a system and no one was aware of how long he had been in segregation even though that information was readily available" (4). Province of Alberta, *Report to the Minister of Justice.*

24 Although the jury for the 2013 provincial coroner's inquest stopped short of a finding of criminal or civil liability, in a ground-breaking decision they ruled that because the actions and inactions of other people contributed to Ashley Smith's death, it was a homicide.

25 Feeley and Simon, "The New Penology," 465.

26 Hannah-Moffat, "Criminogenic Needs"; Kilty, "Under the Barred Umbrella"; McGill, "An Institutional Suicide Machine"; Razack, "Racial Terror."

27 Haney, "A Culture of Harm."

28 Ibid., 974.

29 Sapers, *A Preventable Death*.

30 Kilty, "Under the Barred Umbrella"; Kilty, "Examining."

31 Teo, "What Is Epistemological Violence?", 298.

32 Ibid., 296.

33 Sim, *Punishment and Prisons*.

34 Haney, "A Culture of Harm," 973–4.

35 Ibid., 963.

36 Liebling, "Moral Performance"; Liebling et al., "Revisiting Prison Suicide."

37 Kelman and Hamilton, *Crimes of Obedience*.

38 Liebling, "Moral Performance"; Liebling et al., "Revisiting Prison Suicide."

39 Sapers, *A Preventable Death*.

40 Haney, "A Culture of Harm," 972.

41 Wievorka, *Evil*.

42 Fein, *Accounting for Genocide*, 33.

43 Haney, "A Culture of Harm," 963.

44 Ibid.; Kilty, "Examining"; Liebling, "Moral Performance"; Liebling et al., "Revisiting Prison Suicide"; Sapers, *A Preventable Death*.

45 Fein, *Accounting for Genocide*.

46 Nixon, *Slow Violence*.

47 Ibid., 2.

48 Haney, "A Culture of Harm," 967.

49 Jensen, "Beyond Good and Evil."

50 Bauman and Donskis, *Moral Blindness*.

51 Nixon, *Slow Violence*, 8.

52 The CSC filed a motion to seal the video footage and documents related to Smith's forced restraint and sedation while imprisoned in Quebec, arguing that the Coroner's inquiry should only consider the immediate events preceding her death; when the motion was denied, the CSC requested a temporary injunction to stay the inquest proceedings through Ontario Divisional Court, which was also denied.

53 Nixon, *Slow Violence*, 10.

54 Ibid., 14.

55 These recommendations can be retrieved from Correctional Service Canada, "Coroner's Inquest."

56 Méndez, *Interim Report of the Special Rapporteur of the Human Rights Council on Torture and Other Cruel, Inhuman or Degrading Treatment or Punishment*, United Nations General Assembly, 66th Session, UN Doc A/66/268, 2011.
57 In December 2018, the Canadian federal government received a four-month extension to make its segregation oversight process compliant with the Charter of Rights and Freedoms. The government has proposed Bill C-83, which would create "Structured Intervention Units" in each prison where prisoners could access better health care and programming than exists in segregation, as well as four hours a day outside their cells (up from two hours) and two hours a day of "meaningful human contact" (up from one hour). With no hard cap on the number of days someone can spend in an SIU and no provision for the meaningful independent review prescribed by Justice Marrocco, critics suggest that this is simply segregation by a different name that fails to substantively alter the experience of isolation and would thus remain in violation of the Charter.
58 Haney, "A Culture of Harm."
59 Scheper-Hugues, "The Gray Zone."

BIBLIOGRAPHY

Bauman, Zygmunt, and Leonides Donskis. *Moral Blindness: The Loss of Sensitivity in Liquid Modernity*. Cambridge, UK: Polity Books, 2013.
Bonner, Ronald L. "Stressful Segregation Housing and Psychosocial Vulnerability in Prison Suicide Ideators." *Suicide and Life-Threatening Behavior* 36, no. 2 (2006): 250–4.
British Columbia Civil Liberties Association. "BCCLA and JHSC v. AG of Canada: Challenging Solitary Confinement in Canadian Prisons." January 19, 2015. https://bccla.org/our_work/bccla-and-jhsc-v-ag-of-canada-challenging-solitary-confinement/.
Correctional Service Canada. "Coroner's Inquest Touching the Death of Ashley Smith." May 2014. http://www.csc-scc.gc.ca/publications/005007-9009-eng.shtml.
Crewe, Ben. "Soft Power in Prison: Implications for Staff-Prisoner Relationships, Liberty and Legitimacy." *European Journal of Criminology* 8, no. 6 (2011): 455–68.
Doob, Anthony N. "Principled Sentencing, Politics, and Restraint in the Use of Imprisonment: Canada's Break with its History." *Champ Penal/Penal Field* 9 (2012). http://journals.openedition.org/champpenal/8335.
Doob, Anthony N., and Cheryl M. Webster. "Countering Punitiveness: Understanding Stability in Canada's Imprisonment Rate." *Law and Society Review* 40, no. 2 (2006): 325–67.

Doob, Anthony N., and Cheryl M. Webster. "The Harper Revolution in Criminal Justice Policy … and What Comes Next." *Policy Options* (May–June 2015): 24–31.

Feeley, Malcolm, and Jonathan Simon. "The New Penology: Notes on the Emerging Strategy of Corrections and its Implications." *Criminology* 30 (1992): 449–74.

Fein, Helen. *Accounting for Genocide*. New York: Free Press, 1979.

Guenther, Lisa. *Solitary Confinement: Social Death and its Afterlives*. Minneapolis: University of Minnesota Press, 2013.

Haney, Craig. "A Culture of Harm: Taming the Dynamics of Cruelty in Supermax Prisons." *Criminal Justice and Behavior* 35, no. 8 (2008): 956–84.

Haney, Craig. "Mental Health Issues in Long-Term Solitary and 'Supermax' Confinement." *Crime and Delinquency* 49, no. 1 (2003): 124–56.

Hannah-Moffat, Kelly. "Criminogenic Needs and the Transformative Risk Subject: Hybridizations of Risk/Need in Penality." *Punishment and Society* 7, no. 1 (2005): 29–51.

Jackson, Michael. "The Psychological Effects of Administrative Segregation." *Canadian Journal of Criminology and Criminal Justice* 43 (2001): 109–16.

Jensen, Tommy. "Beyond Good and Evil: The Adiaphoric Company." *Journal of Business Ethics* 96 (2010): 425–34.

Kane, D. *Commitment to Legal Compliance, Fair Decisions and Effective Results*. Task Force Reviewing Administrative Segregation. Ottawa, ON: Correctional Service of Canada, 1997.

Kelsall, D. "Cruel and Usual Punishment: Solitary Confinement in Canadian Prisons." *Canadian Medical Association Journal* 186 (2014): 1345.

Kelman, Herbert C., and V. Lee Hamilton. *Crimes of Obedience: Toward a Social Psychology of Authority and Responsibility*. New Haven, CT: Yale University Press, 1989.

Kerr, Lisa Coleen. "The Chronic Failure to Control Prisoner Isolation in US and Canadian Law." *Queen's Law Journal* 40, no. 2 (2015): 483–529.

Kilty, Jennifer M. "Examining the "Psy-Carceral Complex' in the Death of Ashley Smith." In *Criminalizing Women: Gender and (In)Justice in Neo-Liberal Times*, edited by Gillian Balfour and Elizabeth Comack, 236–354. Halifax, NS: Fernwood Press, 2014.

Kilty, Jennifer M. "Under the Barred Umbrella: Is There Room for a Women Centred Self-Injury Policy in Canadian Corrections?" *Criminology and Public Policy* 5, no. 1 (2006): 161–82.

Lanes, Eric. "The Association of Administrative Segregation Placement and Other Risk Factors with the Self-injury-free Time of Male Prisoners." *Journal of Offender Rehabilitation* 48 (2009): 539–46.

Liebling, Alison. "Moral Performance, Inhuman and Degrading Treatment and Prison Pain." *Punishment and Society* 13, no. 5 (2011): 530–50.

Liebling, Alison., L. Durie, A. Stiles, and S. Tait. "Revisiting Prison Suicide: The Role of Fairness and Distress." In *The Effects of Imprisonment*, edited by Alison Liebling and Shad Maruna, 209–31. Cullompton, UK: Willan Publishing, 2005.

Martel, Joane. "Les Femmes et L'Isolement Cellulaire au Canada: Un Défit de L'Esprit sur la Matière." *Revue Canadienne de Criminologie et de Justice Pénale* 48, no. 5 (2006) 781–801.

Martel, Joane. "To Be, One Has to Be Somewhere: Spatio-Temporality in Prison Segregation." *British Journal of Criminology* 46, no. 4 (2006): 587–612.

Martel, Joane. "Women in the Hole: The Unquestioned Practice of Segregation." In *An Ideal Prison: Critical Essays on Women's Imprisonment in Canada*, edited by Kelly Hannah-Moffat and Margaret Shaw, 128–35. Halifax, NS: Fernwood Press, 2000.

McGill, Jena. "An Institutional Suicide Machine: Discrimination against Federally Sentenced Aboriginal Women in Canada." *Race/Ethnicity: Multidisciplinary Global Contexts* 2, no. 1 (2008): 89–119.

Méndez, Juan. *Interim Report of the Special Rapporteur of the Human Rights Council on Torture and Other Cruel, Inhuman or Degrading Treatment or Punishment*. United Nations General Assembly, 66th Session, UN Doc A/66/268, 2011. Geneva: UN.

Meyer, Diana, and O'Malley, Pat. "Missing the Punitive Turn? Canadian Criminal Justice, 'Balance,' and Penal Modernism." In *The New Punitiveness: Trends, Theories, Perspectives*, edited by John Pratt, David Brown, Mark Brown, Simon Hallsworth, and Wayne Morrison, 201–17. Portland, OR: Willan Publishing, 2005.

Nixon, Rob. *Slow Violence and the Environmentalism of the Poor*. Cambridge MA: Harvard University Press, 2011.

Office of the Correctional Investigator. *Administrative Segregation in Federal Corrections: Ten Year Trends*. Ottawa, ON: Office of the Correctional Investigator, 2015. http://www.oci-bec.gc.ca/cnt/rpt/pdf/oth-aut/oth-aut20150528-eng.pdf.

Office of the Correctional Investigator. *A Three Year Review of Federal Inmate Suicides (2011–2014)*. Ottawa, ON: Office of the Correctional Investigator, 2014. http://www.oci-bec.gc.ca/cnt/rpt/pdf/oth-aut/oth-aut20140910-eng.pdf?texthighlight=inmate+suicide+segregation.

Province of Alberta. *Report to the Minister of Justice and Attorney General Public Fatality Inquiry*. Calgary: Province of Alberta, 2005. https://open.alberta.ca/dataset/d8bedb35-398a-4e24-befa-bef1d49531de/resource/2736fe62-60e2-4179-b919-eb4febbb93ed/download/2014-fatality-report-Snowshoe.pdf.

Razack, Sherene. "Racial Terror: Torture and Three Teenagers in Prison." *Borderlands* 13, no. 1 (2014): 1–27.

Sapers, Howard. *A Preventable Death*. Ottawa, ON: Office of the Correctional Investigator, 2008. http://www.oci-bec.gc.ca/cnt/rpt/pdf/oth-aut/oth-aut20080620-eng.pdf.

Scheper-Hugues, Nancy. *The Gray Zone: Small Wars, Peacetime Crimes, and Invisible Genocides*. In *The Shadow Side of Fieldwork*, edited by Athena McLean and Annette Leibing, 159–84. Oxford, UK: Blackwell Publishing, 2007.

Shalev, Sharon. "Solitary Confinement: The View from Europe." *Canadian Journal of Human Rights* 4, no. 1 (2015): 143–65.

Sim, Joe. *Punishment and Prisons: Power and the Carceral State*. London: Sage Publications, 2009.

Teo, Thomas. "What Is Epistemological Violence in the Empirical Social Sciences?" *Social and Personality Psychology Compass* 4, no. 5 (2010): 295–303.

"Time-In-Cell: The ASCA-Liman 2014 National Survey of Administrative Segregation in Prison." Lineman Program. 2015. http://www.law.yale.edu/system/files/documents/pdf/asca-liman_administrative_segregation_report_sep_2_2015.pdf.

Webster, Cheryl M., and Anthony N. Doob. "Punitive Trends and Stable Imprisonment Rates in Canada." *Crime and Justice* 36 (2007): 297–369.

Wieviorka, Michel. *Evil*. Cambridge, UK: Polity Press, 2012.

Zinger, Ivan. "Segregation in Canadian Federal Corrections A Prison Ombudsman's Perspective." Paper presented at Ending the Isolation: An International Conference on Human Rights and Solitary Confinement, Winnioeg, Manitoba, March 22–23, 2013. http://www.oci-bec.gc.ca/cnt/comm/presentations/presentations20130322-23-eng.aspx.

20 Madness and Gentrification on Queen West: Violence and the Transformations of Parkdale and the Queen Street Site

BEN LOSMAN

Introduction

In June 2015, corporate real estate developer BSäR Group took possession of 1521 Queen Street, a mixed-use building in the West Toronto neighbourhood of South Parkdale.[1] At the time, there were 27 people living on the second floor in a rooming house known as the Queen's Hotel.[2] As in other rooming houses throughout the city, many of the tenants were receiving disability pensions for issues with physical or mental health that interfered with their ability to work; many had also previously experienced homelessness.[3] In mid-July, BSäR demanded that tenants pay rent on a weekly (rather than monthly) basis – a technicality the corporation would soon use to circumvent tenant protection laws (by claiming that the Queen's was actually operating as a hotel rather than as a rooming house, and its occupants were therefore temporary guests rather than long-term tenants).[4] By that point, BSäR had already been taking deliberate action towards making the building unliveable. Not only did the firm refuse to exterminate a severe property-wide bedbug and rodent infestation, but tenants also allege that BSäR went so far as to remove the privacy walls between toilets in the common washrooms.[5]

On July 29, tenants received notice that they had seven days to vacate the premises, despite the fact that the Landlord and Tenant Protection Act requires such notices to be delivered with 90 days of warning.[6] As tenants and housing advocates scrambled to mount a legal challenge contesting BSäR's contravention of the law, BSäR ratcheted up its intimidation campaign, allegedly hiring someone to pound on unit doors at nights and scream threats at tenants throughout the night.[7] On

August 7, the corporation officially evicted all 27 tenants. According to Victor Willis, executive director of Parkdale Activity-Recreation Centre (PARC), tenants had the "legal right" to continue living in their rooms, but between the unliveable conditions, alleged intimidation, and overwhelming uncertainty of the situation, none did.[8] On the day of the eviction, PARC and the Red Cross were able to help seven tenants find temporary emergency housing; the other 20 simply fled. "We have no idea where they are," Willis said.[9] Willis and other advocates fear that many of those who fled became homeless.[10]

Within six months, the rooms once occupied by impoverished Mad people had been renovated and converted into the Roncey Hotel & Artist Studios, a combined hotel and gallery dedicated to providing space for "local emerging artists that are exquisitely talented."[11] The reinvention of a low-income rooming house as hip hotel/gallery reflects the wave of intense gentrification that is currently transforming South Parkdale; the pushing out of tenants on disability into the streets puts the trauma of this phenomenon in stark relief.

Indeed, Paula Johnson argues that we must understand gentrification to be a very real form of "direct and structural violence"; perpetrated in "collusion among state, private, and institutional actors," gentrification severs poor or racialized long-term residents from their homes, communities, and historic sense of belonging so that "affluent White populations" can take their place.[12] In studying the "forced removal" of Black residents from Harlem and New Orleans, Johnson observed a complex set of "physical, psychological, cultural, and political traumas" among the dispossessed, all of which culminate in a condition similar to post-traumatic stress disorder that psychiatrist Dr Mandy Fulillove terms "root shock."[13]

I begin with the violence of gentrification because it is a major theme within this chapter, and it is a violence that is constantly transpiring in cities around the world.[14] My specific focus is on how this violence is uniquely brought to bear on the residents of South Parkdale, because, as Johnson says, "gentrification must be understood in the specific societal context in which it occurs."[15] Like Harlem and New Orleans, South Parkdale is a racialized space – since the 1930s, it has served as a geographic container for a number of non-white populations, including West Indians, Hispanics, Filipinos, Sikhs, Tamils, Roma, and Tibetans.[16] It is also a space of madness.[17] The neighbourhood is adjacent to the Centre for Addictions and Mental Health (CAMH), Canada's largest mental health facility, which has existed on the same grounds on Queen

Street West since 1850 (because of multiple name changes through-out its history, I'll refer to the CAMH campus as the *Queen Street site* throughout this chapter).[18] Thanks to its proximity to the Queen Street site, Parkdale has long been home to a significant population of Mad residents, many of whom are impoverished and precariously housed.[19] As gentrification in Parkdale intensifies, with corporate landlords buy-ing up low-income rental properties and forcing poor residents into homelessness, the neighbourhood's Mad population becomes ever more vulnerable to direct and structural violence.

While the forces of gentrification – private developers, city planners, and affluent white residents – transform the space of South Parkdale, there is a parallel project of spatial change unfolding within the Queen Street site itself. Transforming Lives Here is a multi-decade, multi-billion dollar redevelopment initiative aimed at dissolving the architectural and metaphorical boundaries between the Queen Street site and surround-ing neighbourhoods of Queen West and South Parkdale.[20] According to CAMH, the goal of the project is to turn its "once-stigmatized institution into an urban village."[21] By demolishing many of the old hospital build-ings, extending city roads to cut through campus, and inviting corpo-rate developers to build mixed-use retail and residential buildings on the site, CAMH seeks to create an "inclusive, healing neighbourhood" where the Mad and sane share space in parks, residences, and cafes.[22] According to the project's website, "This integration with the commu-nity is very important to address the stigma long associated with the property and will improve and normalize the care environment for CAMH's clients."[23]

CAMH's goal of dismantling the stigma of mental illness is certainly laudable, as is the fact that, upon its completion, the redevelopment initiative will have added 179 units of desperately needed affordable housing to the area.[24] But what impact does the reinvention of the Queen Street site as a borderless "urban village" within a rapidly gentrifying Parkdale have on the neighbourhood's Mad population? What protec-tion does Transforming Lives Here offer the Mad from the direct and structural violence of gentrification? How does the utopian discourse around the area as a socially inclusive urban village mask the fact that the poor, the Mad, and the racialized are being forcibly removed from the places they call home?

At this point, these are questions without concrete answers – Trans-forming Lives Here is still years away from completion, and Park-dale's gentrification has not yet peaked. However, such a complex transformation is not without precedent, and historical attempts to convert slums into utopian spaces have often yielded catastrophic results for marginalized residents. In her book *The Blackest Streets: The Life and Death of a Victorian Slum*, Sarah Wise explores the combined efforts of city planners, philanthropists, clergy, and industrialists to "save" the Nichol, one of Victorian London's most notorious slums.[25] While their concern about disease and overcrowding may well have been sincere, many of the Nichol's self-styled saviours were profiteering social Darwinists who used charity as a veil to grab power and land. For many of the Nichol's residents, "salvation" came in the form of forced labour, incarceration, housing demolitions, evictions, dispossession, and utter disempowerment. Ultimately, the "solution" enacted upon the Nichol was a slum clearance and rehousing scheme – one marketed as the creation of a "utopian workers' village" – that Wise describes as a "disaster" for the local poor.[26]

I bring up Wise's analysis to illuminate the necessity for a sceptical approach towards urban utopian projects, particularly when spearheaded by institutional powers with vested financial interests in redeveloping poor communities. In this chapter, I propose that such scepticism is a necessary response to the discourse around transforming Parkdale into an inclusive urban village. To understand the combined impact of Parkdale's gentrification and Transforming Lives Here on marginalized populations, however, scepticism is not enough – we must also consider the historical spatial relationship between Parkdale and the Queen Street site. This is a relationship that goes deeper than physical proximity. According to Sherene Razack, although we tend to think of spaces such as Parkdale and the Queen Street site as being "neutral" geographic containers for buildings, streets, and parks, space is actually the product of interlocking social forces that afford privileges to certain people by oppressing others.[27] In Toronto, this hierarchy emerges from the fact that the city was founded – and continues to exist – as a settler colonial city, a place in which the *respectable, civilized public* (the sane, white, and affluent) maintain dominance over *uncivilized, degenerate* "Others" (the Mad, the racialized, the Indigenous, and the poor).[28]

The constant struggle to evict degeneracy from the settler colonial city is upheld by the economic ideology of neo-liberal urbanism. According to Neil Smith, neo-liberal urbanism transforms the relationship between the power of the state and the power of globalized capitalism: instead of regulating the market, the state serves as an agent of market forces, collaborating with them in an alliance that extends "the reach of global capital down to the local neighbourhood scale."[29] In other words, neo-liberal powers consider the local neighbourhood to be less of a human tapestry comprising a community and more of a source of potential corporate profit. To maximize this profit, the neighbourhood must be populated with those who will buy the most expensive private properties, pay the most in taxes, and spend the most disposable income. In the case of Parkdale, neo-liberalism's model citizen is the respectable settler – white, affluent, young, and sane. Those who don't fit this ideal are forcibly ejected from the space.

All this creates a profoundly unjust social order, one that requires tremendous amounts of violence to uphold.[30] Sometimes, the violence is as brazen as the 1997 police killing of Edmond Yu, a Mad Parkdale resident from Hong Kong shot to death on an emptied city bus while brandishing a small hammer.[31] More often than not, however, the violence is hidden. The transformation of the Queen's Hotel into the Roncey Hotel, for example, serves to obscure the public memory of BSäR's forced removal of nearly 30 vulnerable people from their homes and into the streets. Jihan Abbas and Jijian Voronka argue that the transformation of the Queen Street site into an urban village functions as a similar erasure:[32] "opening up" the site so that the respectable public (read: the sane, white, middle class) can shop, dine, and live upon the grounds of a former asylum makes it seem as if the violence visited upon Mad people – whether by police, the psychiatric establishment, or corporate landlords – is a thing of the past. And yet changes to the built environment coupled with the project's "language of inclusivity" belie the fact that "many people within the site are still being held and undergoing [psychiatric] treatments against their will."[33]

Because I am a sane, white, middle-class Toronto resident, I do not have to bear the brunt of any of this violence. In fact, I stand to benefit from it – the gentrification of Parkdale affords me the opportunity to eat at trendy restaurants, drink at hip bars, and even purchase affordable property. And according to CAMH, by simply moving through its new urban village, I am helping Mad people by making them feel less socially isolated; this in turn makes me feel like a compassionate, empathetic person. In unpacking these benefits, we encounter a hidden truth: the success of Transforming Lives Here depends on the gentrification of Parkdale, and vice versa. CAMH cannot build a "safe, comfortable, and welcoming" urban village on Parkdale's border if Parkdale remains a slum, just as Parkdale cannot become a rich, white neighbourhood if the Queen Street site remains a place of concentrated madness. It would be misguided and unfair to blame the violence of Parkdale's gentrification upon the redevelopment of the Queen Street site – these two phenomena are interrelated, but one does not cause the other. Instead, I'm interested in interrogating the social forces that are driving these simultaneous transformations. By looking at the historical and contemporary spatial relationship between Parkdale and the Queen Street site, it becomes clear that the struggle between respectability and degeneracy has shaped both spaces for more than a century and a half.

Examining the interplay between these social forces, a fundamental question emerges: in the utopian urban village, who benefits and at what cost?

A Shared History of Violence

According to CAMH CEO Catherine Zahn, the parallel timing of Transforming Lives Here and Parkdale's gentrification is simply a happy accident. "We have a big piece of land that *just happens to be* in a very up-and-coming area that's a very lively, socially conscious area of the neighbourhood," Zahn says.[34] But to conceive of these two transformations as coincidental is to ignore a spatial relationship that has existed for more than 165 years. The Queen Street site has played a major role in shaping Parkdale's social, economic, and physical landscape since 1850, when the Provincial Lunatic Asylum first opened its gates on the grounds that would eventually become CAMH.[35] The inverse is also true, as for more than a century and a half, Parkdale has been a primary stakeholder in the evolution of the Queen Street site, as it reinvented itself from a nineteenth-century asylum into a twentieth-century psychiatric hospital, and now to its current incarnation as a burgeoning urban village. Examining the history of each space reveals a cycle of violence, one in which the forces of settler colonial respectability are waging a constant struggle to evict, confine, and erase degeneracy.

Like all of Canada, South Parkdale and the Queen Street site are built on stolen land. The connection that Indigenous Peoples such as the Huron, Haudonesaunee, and Mississauga peoples have to the territory now called Toronto dates back thousands of years;[36] according to the Eurocentric logic of settler colonialism, this connection was (and still is) conceived of as a fundamental obstacle in building a respectable, civilized nation. Throughout the nineteenth century, the colonial Government of

Canada employed a variety of interlocking strategies to displace, contain, and eliminate Indigenous Peoples. Through manipulation tactics such as treaties, the implementation of dehumanizing legal policies (most notably the "extremely repressive body of colonial law" known as the Indian Act of 1876),[37] and the institution of a violent residential school system that ripped Native children from their families and cultures, the white settler regime embarked upon a structural genocide of Indigenous Peoples that it pursues to this day.[38]

During the early days of nation building, Indigenous bodies were not the only ones considered in need of social cleansing. As Mad Studies scholar Jijian Voronka notes, anyone "existing outside of the Victorian ideal (the poor, the mad, the criminal, the deviant)," as well as the racialized and the female, were considered "the antithesis of white middle class respectability."[39] According to critical race theorist David Goldberg, colonialism dictated that these Othered bodies be "prevented at all costs from polluting the body politic or sullying civil(ized) society."[40] And so colonial powers applied a similar set of violent tactics – containment, eviction, and elimination – on any population they deemed degenerate.

To examine the historical relationship between the Queen Street site and South Parkdale is to witness these tactics playing out in spectacular clarity. In 1850 the Provincial Lunatic Asylum (the original name of the Queen Street site) institutionalized its first cohort of 211 "patients" (all had been previously held in a former jail).[41] A self-contained fortress beyond Toronto's western city limits, the Provincial Lunatic Asylum allowed for the complete segregation and regulation of Mad bodies; Voronka describes the asylum as a prison-like "carceral space" designed to prevent plague-like outbreaks of madness among the civilized public.[42] Within this space, Mad people were subjected to "treatments" that included "arsenic, insulin and metrazol 'therapies,' electroconvulsive shock, and lobotomies," as well as unpaid hard labour – in fact, inmates built the 12-foot-tall brick walls surrounding the campus, a portion of which has been preserved as a heritage site and remains standing today.[43] In addition, the asylum was packed beyond capacity; at one point it held more than seven hundred inmates, although there was only room for four hundred.[44] Throughout the second half of the nineteenth century, hygiene was poor, outbreaks of cholera were common, and many inmates suffered abuse at the hands of the staff.[45]

Wealthy, "sane" Torontonians must have taken comfort in the asylum's capacity to seal in degeneracy, because in the 1870s they flocked to the adjacent neighbourhood of Parkdale.[46] Attracted by its proximity to Lake Ontario, the upper-middle class built Victorian mansions overlooking the water; by 1879, the neighbourhood's wide roads, leafy trees, and prestigious shopping district had earned Parkdale the title of the city's "floral suburb."[47] The City of Toronto annexed the neighbourhood in 1889, and for the next two decades it was one of the city's most affluent, desirable areas.[48]

However, by World War I, Parkdale's reputation began to slide. For one thing, the rich were moving away, and the Victorian mansions they left behind were being subdivided and converted into boarding houses and apartments. The availability of affordable rental housing attracted an influx of single working women (whose independence was considered inherently promiscuous by mainstream Canadian society) and Eastern European immigrant families ("whose ideas of sanitation are not our own," read one city report).[49] In the sexist, Anglo-centric metropolis of Toronto, the presence of unmarried women and non-British bodies was considered to be so degenerate that, by World War II, the area had been designated a slum.[50] As a slum space, Parkdale was considered "unhealthy, unsafe, and immoral," and was therefore a threat to Toronto's colonial respectability.[51]

In much the same way that they would lobby for gentrification under the banner of *urban revitalization* decades later, politicians and city planners in the 1930s were obsessive in their proposals to "clear" slums such as Parkdale. Historian Carol Whitzman's analysis of city reports shows how urban planners continuously depicted poor and racialized communities as a serious threat to public health. The city then utilized this "threat" to advance an infrastructure development agenda that required massive displacement of poor and racialized people. According to critical geographer Tom Slater, by the 1950s, Toronto had become a "prime site of experimental modernist planning, with expressways leading to suburban expansion seen as signs of progress."[52] Plans for the Gardiner Expressway, a road meant to restore western Toronto's nineteenth-century prestige, ran straight through Parkdale. Slater notes that "South Parkdale was in the path of ... the Gardiner ... and, thus, in the way of 'progress.'" Fortunately for the city planners, Parkdale's designation as a slum meant that it could (in fact, must) be demolished "under the ideological banners of 'slum clearance' and 'urban renewal.'"[53]

And so in the early 1950s the city embarked upon construction of the Gardiner Expressway by demolishing 170 Parkdale houses and displacing eight hundred people. To entice dispossessed middle-class homeowners to remain in the neighbourhood and bolster property values, the city invited developers to build a series of modern high-rise apartment buildings.[54] However, the middle class fled and did not return. In their wake, two dramatic demographic shifts would cement Parkdale's degenerate slum status for the remainder of the twentieth century.

By the time the Gardiner was completed in 1966, the Queen Street site (then known as the Queen Street Mental Health Centre) had embraced deinstitutionalization and begun significantly reducing hospital beds. From the late 1960s throughout the early 1980s, thousands of former psychiatric residents (both from the Queen Street site and the Lakeshore Mental Hospital, which closed in 1979) were discharged into Parkdale, ostensibly to receive mental health care and social support at residential "group homes."[55] However, according to Mad activist and former group home resident Pat Capponi, conditions were "dehumanizing."[56] A lack of regulation and oversight meant that operators were not compelled to provide an adequate standard of living or care. Residents lived in overcrowded, filthy quarters, and were kept docile and obedient through the use of heavy medication.[57] What's more, by 1985, there were only thirty-nine group homes to serve a population of more than a thousand people. Many Mad people who could not secure housing in a group home became homeless; others rented "bachelorettes," or self-contained, single occupant mini-apartments within boarding homes.[58]

Deinstitutionalization coincided with a spike in non-white immigration that began in the 1970s and lasted until the turn of the century. Thanks in large part to the presence of Mad bodies, the average rent was cheaper in Parkdale than in the rest of the city; recent immigrants, many of whom were political refugees, were drawn to the affordable housing and social services in the area.[59] Parkdale became an important "gateway neighbourhood" (informally known as the "landing strip") where West Indians, Tamils, Tibetans, Hispanics, Sikhs, and Filipinos lived among the Mad.[60] As the home of the Mad, non-white, impoverished Other, Parkdale was once again an affront to Toronto's colonial respectability – a degenerate space that demanded intervention.

The twentieth century laid the groundwork for what Slater calls *municipally managed gentrification*, a process in which city planners, private developers, and middle-class business/resident associations collude to push out degenerate bodies in the name of revitalization. The phenomenon follows the same pattern as historical projects of social cleansing: dispossess, destroy, and rebuild. Between 1996 and 2006, Parkdale real estate development shot up by 123%, rent values increased by 45%, and at least forty-five rooming homes were shut down – staggering numbers for an area in which, in 2006, renters comprised 91% of the population, and 45% of the population fell below the low-income cut-off.[61] In the decade since then, gentrification has only intensified in pace and force. At the helm are corporate landlords such as BSäR, the company that orchestrated the eviction of 1521 Queen West, and Akelius, a Swedish firm that now owns fifty-six buildings in Toronto, five of which are in Parkdale.[62] Akelius has gained both notoriety and market share by exploiting loopholes in provincial guidelines for tenant protection: in 2014, although Ontario limited annual rent increase to 0.8%, Akelius successfully increased rents in one Parkdale property by 4.1%. In 2015 the firm applied to increase rent in that property again, this time by 4.6%. In addition to manipulating rents, Akelius also removed the building's superintendent and refused to fix cracking walls, mouldy bathrooms, and insect infestations in the units of low-income renters, many of whom are Tibetan refugees.[63]

The gentrification crisis has inspired some impressive acts of resistance. The Parkdale Neighbourhood Land Trust (PNLT), for example, seeks to "acquire land and use it to meet the needs of Parkdale by leasing it to non-profit partners who can provide affordable housing, furnish spaces for social enterprises and non-profit organizations, and offer urban agriculture and open space."[64] If successful in securing community ownership rights to a majority of Parkdale lands, PNLT could provide Mad, racialized, and impoverished residents a crucial measure of protection against the violence of gentrification. It's an ambitious vision, one that aims to fundamentally shift power away from corporate developers and towards community residents.

Can Transforming Lives Here be considered a similarly vital act of resistance? It certainly is proving to yield some tangible benefits to the community. By providing 179 units of affordable housing "for seniors living on low income, people with disabilities and other low-income households" – with 10% of those units reserved specifically for "CAMH clients" – CAMH is helping vulnerable people with critical housing needs.[65] And the benefits aren't limited to housing. In a neighbourhood where, social space for Mad people is shrinking,[66] the CAMH campus provides indoor and outdoor public spaces that are clean and well-maintained. The redevelopment has also created jobs: Out of this World Cafe is a social enterprise with two on-campus locations, and both employ Mad people. And the urban village concept will certainly be appealing to psychiatric consumers who would prefer to access

services in a place that feels more like a neighbourhood than an institution. Finally, it is entirely possible that, for many sane residents, living
among the Mad will indeed increase empathy and help dissolve the
stigma of madness.

However, is this enough to stem the tide of Parkdale's gentrification?
Not necessarily. As local columnist Marcus Gee points out, "Who would
want to live right next to a huge mental-health institution? Plenty of
people, it turns out. The converted factory just next to CAMH commands
top dollar for its loft residences. Some houses on nearby streets go for a
million dollars and more."[67] In other words, the conversion of the Queen
Street site into a thriving urban village – a conversion made possible
through billions of dollars' worth of investment from the private sector
and the municipal government – is a potential neighbourhood selling
point for gentrifiers. After all, CAMH states that "nothing quite like this
[the creation of a mixed Mad/sane urban village] has ever been done
before."[68] The novelty of this prospect might be enticing for socially
conscious people with money who wish to play a leading role in a
progressive social experiment. This could well be a contributing factor
towards rising property values, which shot up 65% in South Parkdale
between 2008 and 2013.[69] Ironically, this means that the creation of an
"inclusive, healing neighbourhood" in and around the Queen Street site
may ultimately fuel gentrification-driven displacement, making the area
unaffordable and inaccessible for South Parkdale's Mad population.

Mad in the Village

Recently, my wife and I strapped our six-month-old daughter into a
baby carrier and walked from 1521 Queen Street (former home of the
Queen's Hotel) to the Queen Street site. Although we don't live in Parkdale, as a young, white, sane family drinking lattes from to-go cups, we
looked the part of neighbourhood gentrifiers.

According to the Toronto real estate website, "Not everyone can find
the appeal in the remaining gritty pockets of Parkdale."[70] However,
few places felt off-limits to us on our walk down Queen Street. Clearly,
we are the target patron for the neighbourhood's bohemian cafes and
vegan restaurants, and we are far from being the only middle-class
white people who come to Parkdale for cheap Tibetan momos and
West Indian roti. According to critical geographers Katie Mazer and
Katherine Rankin, this feeling of universal access is an exclusive privilege. "In Parkdale, although rooming-house tenants have most of their

material needs (besides housing) met through public service providers, they nonetheless identify the recent arrival of trendy boutique hotels and shops as markers of a different kind of place: one geared towards the tastes and capacities of the rich."[71] In their interviews with the tenant population, Mazer and Rankin discovered that, "in relation to new commercial establishments, most rooming-house tenants experienced this subtle form of exclusion rooted in the dynamics of shaming."[72]

When my family and I arrived at the Queen Street site, I remembered a walking tour I had recently done across the CAMH campus. Gesturing at the pedestrian, bike, and vehicle traffic on Queen Street, the guide had explained that the *animation* – another word for human activity, as I understood it – on Queen Street played an important role in the recovery process for CAMH clients. (My interpretation of this is that seeing the bustle of the city is meant to make psychiatric consumers feel less isolated, which is assumed to benefit their emotional well-being.) The guide had gone on to explain that one of the primary goals of Transforming Lives Here is to invite the public to enter the site and make it our own; as sane people, CAMH wants us to feel completely comfortable playing with our children on the campus' green spaces, buying coffee at the cafes, and walking our dogs around the paths.

The social integration that CAMH seeks to foster within its urban village is ostensibly for the benefit of Mad people. This goal is made explicit in the Transforming Lives Master Vision document: "A model of care focused on clients' recovery requires a normalized treatment environment for a person with mental illness and/or addictions. On a large scale, the urban integration is key to this normalizing process ... A community that is inclusive and one that erases barriers reduces stigma."[73] But what exactly does the urban village normalize? Or as Abbas and Voronka ask: "Should a site that still continues to enact forced incarceration, forced medical treatment, seclusion and restraints, and conditional releases be considered a normal site within our everyday community?"[74]

As my family and I wandered deeper into the campus, we eventually encountered a caged off area, enclosed in prison-like fencing. Against the backdrop of the open, green campus, it was a shocking sight. I would later discover that this is a secure entrance to one of the forensic units, where people who have committed crimes and "have been legally found to be either Not Criminally Responsible (NCR) or Unfit" are held.[75] It was a strange feeling to stumble upon this area – if someone had been admitted into the forensic unit while we were standing there, we would have been able to watch this process take place, and the incarcerated person would have been able to watch us watching.

Encountering this acutely carceral space reveals a disparity in spatial access, much like the disparity present in gentrifying Parkdale. According to the rhetoric of social inclusion, life in the urban village is barrier free. And indeed, for a sane, white, middle-class person like me, this is true. I encounter few barriers as I move through the space – I can go almost anywhere without being stopped or feeling like I don't belong. Mad people, on the other hand, don't have this privilege. Their bodies are subject to intense regulation; they are evicted from rooming homes, shot by police, and incarcerated in plain sight. And yet the Mad body is essential to the urban village – it is what justifies the language of social inclusion and progress. Through contact with the Mad body, the gentrifying subject comes to understand himself as respectable, compassionate, politically progressive, and sane – the *good kind of gentrifier*, the kind who believes in his own presence as emancipatory force.

The urban village can only become the gentrified ideal if the Mad are powerless and thus pose no threat to neo-liberal progress. And so instead of brutalizing the Mad body, as the asylum did in the past, the urban village tames madness through the gentle manoeuvre of social integration. In conquering the Mad without resorting to visible violence, the urban village emerges as a utopia of respectability – much like Parkdale was in the 1850s, when it was completely white.

The Transforming Lives Here redevelopment is scheduled for completion later this decade. At that point, the CAMH campus will have been completely subsumed by the surrounding neighbourhood. What will happen to the Mad then? And what will happen to the racialized immigrant population? Will the "respectable public" claim Parkdale's public spaces as their own, pushing Mad bodies out of parks, lawns, and street corners until they become placeless? Will developers succeed in converting the last of the neighbourhood's affordable housing into high-end condos, displacing anyone who is not young, rich, and white?

Perhaps, having served its purpose, madness will no longer be considered essential and will be memorialized along with the institutional violence of the Queen Street site, considered a tragic part of history but non-existent in the present. And perhaps Parkdale's "ethnicity" will follow a similar course, invoked by trendy restaurants to generate authenticity in neighbourhood of whiteness. Until then, the degenerate body will remain both emplaced and out of place, "a thing that [seems] slightly human and a human being that [seems] slightly thing-like,"[76] but powerless, caught up in the endless dance between degeneracy and respectability.

NOTES

1 Khandaker, "Parkdale Residents."
2 Ibid. The City of Toronto defines a rooming house as a "house, apartment or building where four or more people that pay individual rent share a kitchen and/or washroom." Rent is typically much lower than in other forms of housing; tenants usually pay rent on weekly, bi-monthly, or monthly bases. In 2013, there were 80 rooming homes that were licensed or pending licensing in Parkdale, making it one of the highest concentrations of such housing in the city. See City of Toronto, "Bylaw Enforcement," and Advocacy Centre for Tenants Ontario, "Rooming Houses in Toronto."
3 See Parkdale Villager, "Parkdale Activity Recreation Centre Finds Homes for Seven Tenants of the Queen's Hotel," *Inside Toronto*, August 10, 2015, https://www.insidetoronto.com/news-story/5791603-parkdale-activity -recreation-centre-finds-homes-for-seven-tenants-of-the-queen-s-hotel/; Khandaker, "Parkdale Residents"; Bob Rose, Presentation at Here to Stay: A Community Forum on Gentrification Driven Displacement, hosted by Parkdale Activity-Recreation Center, Toronto, ON, September 21, 2015.
4 Parkdale Villager, "Parkdale Activity Recreation Centre."
5 See Khandaker, "Parkdale Residents" and Anonymous Tenants of 1521 Queen Street West, Presentation at Here to Stay: A Community Forum on Gentrification Driven Displacement, hosted by Parkdale Activity-Recreation Center, Toronto, ON, September 21, 2015.
6 See Khandaker, "Parkdale Residents" and Parkdale Villager, "Parkdale Activity Recreation Centre."
7 See Khandaker, "Parkdale Residents" and Anonymous Tenants, Presentations.
8 Parkdale Villager, "Parkdale Activity Recreation Centre."
9 Ibid.
10 Ibid.
11 Caton, "The Former Queen's Hotel."
12 Johnson, "Beyond Displacement," 80.
13 Ibid., 81.
14 Smith, "New Globalism," 427.
15 Johnson, "Beyond Displacement," 80.

16 Whitzman, *Suburb, Slum, Urban Village*, 103.
17 Menzies, Lefrançois, and Reaume, "Introducing Mad Studies," 10. I use
   the terms "mad" and "sane," privileging the language of Mad Theory
   over the biomedical vocabulary of "mental illness." Menzies, Lefrançois,
   and Reaume explain: "Following other social movements including queer,
   black, and fat activism, madness talk and text invert the language of
   oppression, reclaiming disparaged identities and restoring dignity and
   pride to difference."
18 Centre for Addiction and Mental Health, "History."
19 Slater, "Municipally Managed Gentrification," 303.
20 Centre for Addiction and Mental Health, "Innovative Site Design."
21 Centre for Addiction and Mental Health, "Transforming Lives."
22 Charity Village, "CAMH Launches."
23 Centre for Addiction and Mental Health, "Innovative Site Design."
24 Centre for Addiction and Mental Health, "New Neighbours."
25 Wise, *The Blackest Streets*.
26 Ibid., 262, 266.
27 Razack, "When Place Becomes Race," 7.
28 Voronka, "Re/moving Forward?", 46.
29 Smith, "New Globalism," 441.
30 Razack, "When Place Becomes Race," 5.
31 History in Practice, "Because of Edmond."
32 Abbas and Voronka, "Remembering Institutional Erasures," 129.
33 Ibid.
34 Barba, "Back to Old Roots" [emphasis added].
35 Centre for Addiction and Mental Health, "History."
36 Methot, "'Toronto' Is an Iroquois Word."
37 Lawrence, *"Real" Indians*, 31.
38 Wolfe, "Settler Colonialism," 387.
39 Voronka, "Re/moving Forward?", 46.
40 Goldberg, "Polluting the Body Politic," 187.
41 Centre for Addiction and Mental Health, "Historical Chronology."
42 Voronka, "Re/moving Forward?", 48.
43 Abbas and Voronka, "Remembering Institutional Erasures," 128.
44 Voronka, "Re/moving Forward?", 51.
45 Ibid.; Reaume, *Remembrance of Patients Past*, 247.
46 Whitzman, *Suburb*, 62.
47 Slater, "Municipally Managed Gentrification," 307; Whitzman, *Suburb*, 106.
48 Whitzman, *Suburb*.
49 Ibid., 112.

50 Ibid., 103; Reaume, *Remembrance*, 31. Female promiscuity was also grounds for institutionalization at the Queen Street site around the turn of the twentieth century; it was "highly associated with the lower classes," and therefore, with criminality.
51 Whitzman, *Suburb,* 104.
52 Slater, "Municipally Managed Gentrification," 307.
53 Ibid.
54 Ibid., 146, 309.
55 Slater, "Municipally Managed Gentrification," 309.
56 McPherson, "Pat Capponi," 6.
57 Ibid.
58 Slater, "Municipally Managed Gentrification," 309, 310.
59 Whitzman, *Suburb,* 159.
60 Slater, "Municipally Managed Gentrification," 309.
61 Goodmurphy and Kamizaki, "A Place for Everyone."
62 Akelius Properties, "Our Properties."
63 "Parkdale Residents Protest."
64 Parkdale Neighbourhood Land Trust, "About."
65 Ontario Ministry of Municipal Affairs and Housing, "Governments of Canada and Toronto."
66 Mazer and Rankin, "The Social Space of Gentrification," 822.
67 Gee, "Toronto's West Queen West."
68 Centre for Addiction and Mental Health, "The Queen Street Site."
69 Ireland, "Toronto's Once Scruffy Neighbourhoods."
70 BREL Team, "Parkdale."
71 Mazer and Rankin, "The Social Space," 829.
72 Ibid.
73 Liang, "Master Vision."
74 Abbas and Voronka, "Remembering," 132.
75 Centre for Addiction and Mental Health, "Forensic Secure."
76 Mbembe, "Aesthetics of Superfluity," 381.

BIBLIOGRAPHY

Abbas, Jihan, and Jijian Voronka. "Remembering Institutional Erasures: The Meaning of Histories of Disability Incarceration in Ontario." In *Disability Incarcerated: Imprisonment and Disability in the United States and Canada,* edited by Liat Ben-Moshe, Chris Chapman, and Allison C. Carey, 121–38. New York: Palgrave Macmillan, 2014.

Akelius Properties. "Our Properties." Accessed January 7, 2019. https://www
.akelius-properties.ca/searchlisting.aspx.

Advocacy Centre for Tenants Ontario. "Rooming Houses in Toronto." July
2017. https://www.acto.ca/production/wp-content/uploads/2017/07/
Overview_RoomingHousesinToronto_ENG.pdf.

Anonymous Tenants of 1521 Queen Street West. Presentations at Here to Stay:
A Community Forum on Gentrification Driven Displacement, hosted by
Parkdale Activity-Recreation Centre, Toronto, ON, September 21, 2015.

Barba, Lindsay. "Back to Old Roots with a New Facility." *Behavioral
Healthcare*, May 1, 2010. https://www.behavioral.net/article/back
-old-roots-new-facility.

BREL Team. "Parkdale." Accessed June 2, 2016. https://www.getwhatyou
want.ca/toronto-neighbourhood/parkdale.

Caton, Hillary. "The Former Queen's Hotel Is Rebranded the Roncey Hotel,
an Artist Studio and Event Space," *Inside Toronto*, May 10, 2016.

Centre for Addiction and Mental Health. "Forensic Secure Unit A (3-2) and
B (3-3)." Accessed May 29, 2016. https://www.camh.ca/en/your-care/
programs-and-services/forensic-secure-units.

Centre for Addiction and Mental Health. "Historical Chronology of CAMH's
Queen Street Site." Accessed October 10, 2015. https://www.camh.ca/en
/driving-change/building-the-mental-health-facility-of-the-future/
history-of-queen-street-site.

Centre for Addiction and Mental Health. "History of the Queen Street Site."
Accessed October 10, 2015. https://www.camh.ca/en/driving
-change/building-the-mental-health-facility-of-the-future/
history-of-queen-street-site.

Centre for Addiction and Mental Health. "Innovative Site Design."
Accessed October 10, 2015. https://www.camh.ca/en/driving-change/
building-the-mental-health-facility-of-the-future.

Centre for Addiction and Mental Health. "New Neighbours in the
Urban Village." Accessed October 10, 2015. https://www.camh.ca/en
/driving-change/building-the-mental-health-facility-of-the-future/
vision-and-guiding-principles.

Centre for Addiction and Mental Health. "The Queen Street Site: The Vision—
Transforming Lives Here." Accessed October 10, 2015. https://www.camh
.ca/en/driving-change/building-the-mental-health-facility-of-the-future.

Centre for Addiction and Mental Health. "Transforming Lives." Accessed
June 2, 2016. https://www.camh.ca/en/driving-change/about-camh/
camh-leadership-team-directory.

Charity Village. "CAMH Launches Art Competition to Enhance Therapeutic Spaces." June 22, 2016. https://www.camh.ca/en/camh-news-and-stories/camh-launches-art-competition-to-enhance-therapeutic-spaces.

City of Toronto. "Bylaw Enforcement – Illegal Rooming Houses." Accessed June 1, 2016. https://www.toronto.ca/311/knowledgebase/07/101000038007.html.

Gee, Marcus. "Toronto's West Queen West Shows Acceptance for the Mentally Ill." *Globe and Mail*, May 20, 2016. https://www.theglobeandmail.com/news/toronto/torontos-west-queen-west-shows-acceptance-for-the-mentally-ill/article30112048/?cmpid=rss1&click=sf_globe%E2%80%8E.

Goldberg, David Theo. "Polluting the Body Politic: Race and Urban Location." In *Racist Culture*, 185–205. Malden, MA: Blackwell, 1993.

Goodmurphy, Brendon, and Kuni Kamizaki. "A Place for Everyone: How a Community Land Trust Could Protect Affordability and Community Assets in Parkdale." *Parkdale Activity-Recreation Centre*. November 2011. https://parkdalecommunityeconomies.files.wordpress.com/2011/11/a-place-for-everyone-parkdale-community-land-trust-november-20111.pdf.

History in Practice. "Because of Edmond: A Place of Safety and Hope." Accessed June 2, 2016. http://historyinpractice.ca/en/node/85.

Ireland, Carolyn. "Toronto's Once Scruffy Neighbourhoods Are Newly Cool." *Globe and Mail*, February 13, 2014. https://www.theglobeandmail.com/real-estate/torontos-once-scruffy-neighbourhoods-are-newly-cool/article16860102/.

Johnson, Paula. "Beyond Displacement: Gentrification of Racialized Spaces as Violence – Harlem, New York and New Orleans, Louisiana." In *Accumulating Insecurity: Violence and Dispossession in the Making of Everyday Life*, edited by Shelley Feldman, Charles Geisler, and Gayatri A. Menon, 79–102. Athens, GA: University of Georgia Press, 2011.

Khandaker, Tamara. "Parkdale Residents Left without a Home: Infested Building Was Abode for Low-Income Downtowners, Who Now Face Uncertain Future." *Toronto Star*, August 22, 2015.

Lawrence, Bonita. *"Real" Indians and Others: Mixed-blood Urban Native Peoples and Indigenous Nationhood*. Lincoln: University of Nebraska Press, 2004.

Liang, Alice. "Master Vision: Transforming Lives." Centre for Addiction and Mental Health. January 2008. https://www.camh.ca/-/media/files/redevelopment-project/012008-master-vision-pdf.pdf?la=en&hash=A75793936B6DF62C4AE47FDA01DA2805C040A076.

Mazer, Katie, and Katherine Rankin. "The Social Space of Gentrification: The Politics of Neighbourhood Accessibility in Toronto's Downtown West." *Environment and Planning D: Society and Space* 29, no. 5 (2011): 822–39.

Mbembe, Achille. "Aesthetics of Superfluity." *Public Culture* 16, no. 3 (2004): 373–405.

McPherson, Cathy. "Pat Capponi: Parkdale's No. 1 Shit Disturber." *Phoenix Rising* (1980): 5–9.

Menzies, Robert, Brenda Lefrançois, and Geoffrey Reaume. "Introducing Mad Studies." In *Mad Matters: A Critical Reader in Canadian Mad Studies*, edited by Brenda Lefrançois, Robert Menzies, and Geoffrey Reaume, 1–22. Toronto, ON: Canadian Scholars' Press, 2013.

Methot, Susan. ""Toronto' Is an Iroquois Word." August 20, 2012. http://dragonflycanada.ca/toronto-is-an-iroquois-word/.

Ontario Ministry of Municipal Affairs and Housing. "Governments of Canada and Toronto Celebrate New Affordable Housing in Toronto." November 9, 2012. https://news.ontario.ca/mma/en/2012/11/governments-of-canada-and-ontario-celebrate-new-affordable-housing-in-toronto-7.html.

Parkdale Neighbourhood Land Trust. "About." Accessed May 27, 2016. http://www.pnlt.ca/about/.

"Parkdale Residents Protest Back-to-back Rent Increases by Akelius." *CBC News*, March 23, 2015. http://www.cbc.ca/news/canada/toronto/parkdale-residents-protest-back-to-back-rent-increases-by-akelius-1.3005265.

Parkdale Villager. "Parkdale Activity Recreation Centre Finds Homes for Seven Tenants of the Queen's Hotel." *Inside Toronto*, August 10, 2015. https://www.insidetoronto.com/news-story/5791603-parkdale-activity-recreation-centre-finds-homes-for-seven-tenants-of-the-queen-s-hotel/.

Razack, Sherene. "When Place Becomes Race." In *Race, Space, and the Law: Unmapping a White Settler Society*, edited by Sherene Razack, 1–20. Toronto, ON: Between the Lines, 2002.

Reaume, Geoffrey. *Remembrance of Patients Past: Patient Life at the Toronto Hospital for the Insane, 1870–1940*. Toronto, ON: University of Toronto Press, 2009.

Rose, Bob. Presentation at Here to Stay: A Community Forum on Gentrification Driven Displacement, hosted by Parkdale Activity-Recreation Center, Toronto, ON, September 21, 2015.

Slater, Tom. "Municipally Managed Gentrification in South Parkdale, Toronto." *Canadian Geographer/Le Géographe Canadien* 48 (2004): 303–25. https://doi.org/10.1111/j.0008-3658.2004.00062.x.

Smith, Neil. "New Globalism, New Urbanism: Gentrification as Global Urban Strategy." *Antipode* 34, no. 3 (2002): 427–50. https://doi.org/10.1111/1467-8330.00249.

Spurr, Ben. "New Rent Monster." *NOW Toronto,* July 31, 2014. https://nowtoronto.com/news/new-rent-monster/.

Voronka, Jijian. "Re/Moving Forward? Spacing Mad Degeneracy at the Queen Street Site." *Resources for Feminist Research* 33, no. 1 (2008): 45–61.

Whitzman, Carol. *Suburb, Slum, Urban Village: Transformations in Toronto's Parkdale Neighbourhood, 1875–2002.* Vancouver, BC: UBC Press, 2009.

Wise, Sarah. *The Blackest Streets: The Life and Death of a Victorian Slum.* London, UK: Bodley Head, 2008.

Wolfe, Patrick. "Settler Colonialism and the Elimination of the Native." *Journal of Genocide Research* 8, no. 4 (2006): 387–409.

Concluding Thoughts

ANDREA DALEY, LUCY COSTA, AND PETER BERESFORD

We wanted to bring this collection of writings together for a number of reasons. These include the increasing discussion, and often insubstantial or sensational accounts of "the mentally ill" in relation to criminalization, police interventions (gone wrong), and institutional trauma, as well as political and structural conditions that contribute to mental health vulnerabilities. These range from deportations of refugees, the impacts of colonization on Indigenous communities, and chronic illness and early death by poverty as a result of neo-liberal economic policy. We sought contributions that would serve critically to question the relationship between power and the nuanced means by which violence is manifest in the lives of mental health service users/survivors through dominant biomedical discourses and diagnoses, institutional practices and policies related to "treatments" and "interventions"; governmental legislations and laws, legal processes, research practices, and public policies; and the changing nature of community, among other means. In doing so, we conceived the relationship between power and violence as underpinned by a neo-liberal rationality that individualizes and pathologizes pain and suffering and emphasizes individual responsibility to the peril of recognizing the role of social structural inequalities in producing and perpetuating mental and emotional distress, and the need for collectivized political responses.

To this end, we hope that this book offers a helpful contribution that challenges the narrow positioning of mental health service users/survivors as merely more likely to enact violence or, alternatively, be victims of violence than are other people. Rather, the contributions outline significant theoretical frameworks and pedagogical tools, drawing on feminist, queer, critical race, disability, postcolonial, political economy, and intersectional frameworks to illuminate a range of interpersonal, structural, and symbolic violence in the lives of mental health service users/survivors. The chapters forming this collection of writings coalesce to illustrate how madness and gender, race, culture, sexuality, class, disability, and refugee and immigration status, among other subject positions, intersect at points of oppression and social exclusion. We also hope that the book contributes to what might now be a broad and growing sense internationally of the need for change away from the neo-liberal ideology that has so far dominated twenty-first century politics and policy. In the United Kingdom, one tragic scandal came to symbolize and make highly visible this need for change and challenge. This was the terrible fire at Grenfell Tower, a high-rise council housing block, largely for low-income people, which caught fire in June 2017, resulting in at least seventy-two deaths. The burned out tower stood as a blackened landmark of this tragedy for months, visible to many thousands daily passing by, by train, by car, on foot, even in the air coming in to Heathrow Airport. It became a byword for exploding all the excuses, rationales, and dishonesties of neo-liberalism and political austerity policy: that there is no public money, that what money there is has to be taken from those with the least, and that the future has to be cuts and regressive redistribution, making for more poverty and inequality.

When we set out to produce this book, although we had hopes, visions, and goals, we had no idea where contributors would take us. Of course, we had some initial ideas for issues we felt needed to be addressed and people who could offer insights into them from different perspectives. But putting this book together was also a mystery tour for us. We didn't know what priorities contributors would identify, where they would take us, the thrust of their arguments, or what unexpected or important issues might emerge. Notwithstanding the critical richness of this collection of writings, we understand it as both an incomplete and a perilous project. Our intent was not to achieve "completeness" but rather to offer various points of entry into ongoing exchanges of experiences, knowledge, opinions, and ideas about violence in the lives of mental health service users/survivors across societies, communities, institutions, and academic settings. We imagine the contributions as holding the potential to be critical meeting places, of sorts, where ideas can be further expanded upon to broaden and complicate conceptualizations of the relationship between madness, violence, and power. Importantly, however, we have been cautious, as urged by the anonymous author of chapter 1, that the inclusion of some issues may risk exacerbating dangerous associations between madness while the exclusion of other issues may risk exacerbating violence in the lives of Mad people by not talking about them. Here, we note that there is potential risk associated with both representation and lack of representation. At the same time we feel that we were vindicated in our belief that violence is a pivotal issue in relation to mental health service users/survivors, although still in many ways a taboo one. In these contradictory days, when there is an ostensibly benign policy enthusiasm for challenging stigma and for encouraging service users to talk about their lives, experience, and recovery, violence remains a subject few dare speak about. Association with a diagnostic category linked with violence puts people into a different camp and resurrects all the folk fears of *insanity*, irrationality, and threat.

We are also pleased that many of the contributions to the book are based on lived experience and experiential knowledge and that many people who identify as mental health service users/survivors contributed. At a time when traditional biomedical perspectives continue to dominate prevailing discourses about mental health policy and practice, this offers yet further confirmation that there is no longer any excuse for ignoring or marginalizing such perspectives. Our view was that the way forward was engaging with the ideas and knowledge of the key actors in the issue: service users and indeed providers. We didn't want just to offer another set of our own personal prescriptions.

We appreciate that a number of contributors wrote from their perspectives of lived experiences of violence in relation to institutions and, in doing so, may have contended with imaginable and real concerns about their vulnerability to further pathologization, regulation, and surveillance. We note that all contributors who offer first-hand accounts of madness, violence, and power in Part I, *Dispatches on Violence*, are women. Our efforts to include the first-hand accounts of men and people with experiences of marginalized identities (i.e., people of colour, LGBTQ2S+) were met with only limited success. This raised questions for us about representation in first-hand accounts of madness and violence and the gendered, racialized, and sexualized nature of risk associated with identifying oneself with madness and violence. However, we do believe our desire to foreground such diversity has realized some helpful effects. It certainly adds weight to the view that violence affects different groups differently and is particularly oppressive to those already facing oppression and discrimination.

Further considerations of the critical issue of madness, violence, and power needed to extend and sustain this discussion include police violence against mental health service users/survivors; the criminalization of "mental illness" and incarceration; discriminatory housing and employment practices and policies implicitly and explicitly acting upon mental health service users/survivors; and lack of political will to address seriously inadequate social assistance rates. It is our hope that the book serves to spur ongoing interrogation of these issues by academic and non-academic community members, activists, and allies within the consumer/survivor, ex-patient, and mad movements thinking, researching, writing, and taking action about new considerations of power, violence, systems, and institutions in relation to mental health service users/survivors.

We also created this book to facilitate the advancement, solidification and mobilization of knowledge required to make real the terms for self-determination and social justice, restorative justice and reconciliation for those people impacted by the violence of systems and institutions. In other words, our hope is that the book serves to answer, at least in part, the question of what now? or, alternatively, serves as a call to action. Our contributors' analyses raise a number of questions that suggest the need for action towards the goal of systems and institutional change. For example:

- How and where are de-medicalized accounts of madness and mental distress prioritized in order to more authentically take account of the range of experiences and concerns of mental health service users/survivors?
- How can the process of seeking support for mental and emotional distress be made less distressing, or violent, and gain a more holistic and just response?
- How do community, mental health workers, researchers, and scholarship activists work in solidarity to resist the medicalization of poverty, racism, sexism, and homelessness, among other structural inequalities? That is, to problematize the *mental health crisis* in different ways that lead to different solutions to madness?
- Similarly, how do these groups work in solidarity to re-imagine practices of inclusion and participation that do not enact state violence through research processes?

Finally, we perhaps need to update the book's context. Since we first got together at the end of 2013 with the idea for this book, a major shift to right-wing populist politics has occurred internationally, most conspicuously with the UK Brexit decision to leave the European Union and the election of the neo-con Donald Trump. Underpinning both of these seems to be a strong sense of exclusion and disaffiliation. Brexit and Trump have both found support from marginalized people who feel disempowered and marginalized – the very conditions that such politics seem to create and perpetuate. Meanwhile those who have rejected and opposed such politics also feel disempowered and marginalized by the divisive and conflictful forces that they seem both to trade on and exacerbate. Meanwhile, as the threats of inequality, poverty, conflict, climate change, and forced population movement seem daily to increase, we may wonder what their implications are for all our physical and mental well-being and the issues which are the direct focus of this book. Put simply, things are likely to have been made worse rather than better since we started on our task, and therefore the need for such exploration and discussion is likely to be even greater.

However, over this same period, while we have seen the continuing dominance of biomedically based psychiatric system, something else more positive has also been stirring. This is the emergence of Mad Studies. The year we linked up on this project, 2013, was the same year that *Mad Matters*, the first major publication bringing together discussion on Mad Studies was published. This was a self-consciously Canadian study. Five years later, there has been a massive increase in action and discussion taking place under this heading. There have been many events, conferences, books, and articles on the subject. Perhaps even more important, Mad Studies has emerged as an international movement. From the start we saw this book as having a role within the Mad Studies project, even if it was not boundaried by it. Now Mad Studies is itself having to grapple with the complexities of issues raised by the association of madness and violence. We hope that this book can be helpful in taking forward that discussion. But in turn we believe that the challenge to the increasing informal alliance between biomedical psychiatry and neo-liberalism has the real potential to be strengthened through the development of Mad Studies action and critiques. We hope it will also be a powerful vehicle for taking forward the issues and ideas that found expression within these pages.

Glossary

adiaphoria: insensitivity and even nonresponse to pain stimuli as a result of previous exposure. Also used to describe a society's loss of sensitivity to perceive and react to early signs of dysfunction.

Assertive Community Treatment (ACT): a widely implemented evidence-based mental health intervention that targets individuals living in the community who are said to be struggling with severe mental illness. ACT teams employ an interdisciplinary staffing model that includes psychiatrists, social workers, physicians, and nurses. Although engagement in treatment offered by ACT teams is said to be voluntary, their interventions often use coercive methods, and practices of health care surveillance are built into the model.

best practice: a depoliticizing discourse often associated with neo-liberal rationalities. Best practices are referenced and enacted in diverse arenas, including academic research communities, the banking and finance sector, non-profit management, and government health care organizations. Discourses of best practices depoliticize through supposedly neutral and consensus-establishing practices – such as auditing and outcome measuring – that enact particular kinds of political relations. Best practices are generally only recognized as such if they are created and reflect research carried out by experts. They thus place other people and ways of knowing in subordinate positions.

bill of client rights: a statement developed by an organization outlining the rights of the clients it serves. Typically developed as a collaboration between those who use services and whose who provide them, they remind all of the fundamental rights clients have.

coercion: persuading someone to do something by using force. In this context a range of coercive practices are in use within psychiatric services, including physical restraint, seclusion, etc.

colonialism: refers to the specific form of colonization that occurred through the expansion of Europe over the last 400 years. Colonization refers to a historically established and enduring process whereby colonies were built in one territory by people from another territory and the dominating territory changed the social structure, government, and economics of the colonized territory. This colonization usually occurred to increase profits or economic gains through exploitation, to expand power through land appropriation or to expand religious domains. Colonization depended upon the subjugation of Indigenous people, slaves, or indentured labourers, as violence was integral to colonialism. This occurred through physical violences, colonial classification, the erasure of histories and languages, and the inferiorizing of practices, knowledges and beliefs.[1]

compulsion: in this context, using the law to bring someone into hospital against their will.

community treatment order (CTO): a legal instrument that enables forced treatment in community settings and provides for compelled hospital admission if community treatment is resisted.

democracy: there are different forms of democracy, which are more or less participatory. In mental health settings this often refers to efforts to equalize power relations and open opportunities to exert autonomy and voice within decision-making processes. Arguably, deliberative forms are better suited to progressive change in services.

depot medication: medication given by injection that is then slowly released into the body over a number of weeks.

direct violence: violence against an identifiable individual or group enacted by an identifiable individual or group. This type of violence is often intertwined with structural violence. (Also see **violence** and **structural violence**)

electroconvulsive therapy (ECT): a type of therapy in which electric currents are passed through the brain. This can cause brief seizures and changes in brain chemistry; also known as shock therapy.

emotional hijack: a term used here to identify a situation in which a perceived threat triggers a strong reflex physiological response that includes a sudden rise in heartrate and levels of certain chemicals in the blood. Thinking processes are typically overwhelmed and the individual in hijack is unable to consider the situation from a more rational perspective. It is hardwired into our nervous system and difficult to avoid, but it can be managed to some degree when a person is very aware of it and how to control it.

employment relations: the social relations and dynamics between workers and employers, often but not exclusively the province of trade unions.

epistemic violence: the discrediting of the world view and experiences of certain groups through particular knowledge claims and practices. In mental health policy and practice this is often achieved through biomedical frameworks and neo-liberal rationalities that impose particular understandings of the causes of and solutions to mental distress. Epistemic violence delegitimizes and erases Mad people's understandings of their own experience.

epistemology: a philosophy or theory of knowledge, its nature and how we come to understand or acquire it.

essentialize: to generalize characteristics, traits or perceptions of individuals within an identifiable group or community to all members of that group or community.

eugenics: a term coined by a cousin of Charles Darwin, Francis Galton, in 1883. Galton defined eugenics as "the study of the agencies under social control that may improve or impair the racial qualities of future generations."[2] Eugenicists argue that "the sterilization and institutionalization of the mentally disabled as well as laws restricting immigration and marriage would improve public health."[3]

feminist political economy: a theoretical approach to social analysis that examines the interrelated, and deeply gendered, processes of production for surplus, subsistence, and social reproduction. Distinct from *political economy* in that social reproduction is considered a part of the capitalist relations of production. Feminist political economists examine how the processes of production structure how and where we work, eat, play, learn, care, reproduce, parent, consume, and interpret the world.[4]

hegemony: a ruling order. According to Antonio Gramsci, the political, social, cultural and/or economic dominances of one power over others usually achieved and sustained through consent; i.e., the ruling power often achieves some sort of agreement from many of those who are subjugated. This differs from cultural imperialism where this imposition is without consent.[5]

heteronormativity: the cultural bias in favour of opposite-sex relationships of a sexual nature, and against same-sex relationships of a sexual nature. Because the former are viewed as normal and the latter are not, lesbian and gay relationships are subject to a heteronormative bias.[6]

imperialism: refers to the formation of empire. Edward Said describes imperialism as "the practice, theory, and the attitudes of a dominating metropolitan center ruling a distant territory."[7] It differs from colonialism in that imperialism does not require actual settlements in the subjugated or dominated territory.

intra-muscular (IM) medication: an injection of medication directly into a large muscle. Includes depot medication but can also be medication (usually sedatives) administered via injection without consent.

just culture: an approach to improving services by reviewing errors that focuses on systems and management of practice rather than on the outcomes and individuals who might have made mistakes in judgment or process. The idea is to focus on where the system failed to support the individual in making the right choice or a better judgment. The notion of just culture also suggests openness, transparency and a non-judgmental ethos. Individuals are accountable for their own choices but not for the system that might restrict their ability to make other choices.

law reform: activities that hold as their primary objective changing laws and/or the impact of current laws. Examples of law reform activities may include government submissions, community meetings, workshops, or public legal education. Activities that fall within the scope are often distinguished from direct legal services and litigation due to the emphasis on addressing systemic rather than individual legal issues.

legal consciousness: the background assumptions about legality that structure and inform everyday thoughts, actions, and practices expressing the attitude of people towards law, legality, and justice and their concept of what is lawful and unlawful. It is how the law sustains its power despite dissonance between the law on the books and the law in action.

legitimacy: the right and authority to assume a powerful position; usually this assumes a settled consensus yet is always open to question and resistance.

lived experience: a concept that developed out of feminist thought to describe the first-hand accounts and impressions of living as a member of a minority or oppressed group. Feminist theory has emphasized the legitimacy of this concept as a means of providing vulnerable communities the opportunity to be heard.

managers' hearing: a form of formal appeal against detention, made to hospital managers, allowed under the prevailing English mental health legislation.

moral distancing: the process of creating detachment between individuals and/or groups it is characterized by inattentiveness, unreceptiveness, and unresponsiveness to the immoral treatment endured by others. It affects one's awareness, judgment, intent, and behaviour towards others.

moral repair: coined by Margaret Urban Walker, the term refers to the process of attempting to restore (or create for the first time) trusting human relations between parties where behaviour has been marked by moral wrongs – from oppressive actions to physical or emotional harm and even torture. Urban Walker describes a number of conditions that must be met before moral repair can begin to take hold.

mortification of self: the process by which an individual's original identity is lost or attacked through being subjected to the restrictions of an institution.

neo-liberalism, rationalities of, practices of: a rationality and set of practices that entails a particular way of conceptualizing the political, the economic, and the social and the relationships among them. In relation to mental health services and policies, neo-liberal rationalities and practices often privilege economic efficiencies and discourses of risk and responsibilization at the expense of social justice commitments.

OBS: short for observations; various degrees of intrusive watching of patients by mental health staff, ostensibly to ensure safety.

physical restraint: physically holding someone to prevent movement; mental health staff are trained in specific methods for physical restraint, similar to those used by police and prison officers.

problematization: a term that reflects an understanding of problems as *constituted* rather than as *given*. It refers both to the practices through which a set of circumstances come to be constituted as a problem and to what emerges from those practices. Circumstances can be problematized in a variety of ways and different problematizations will have different effects on groups of people and populations. Problematizations can invite violence when they constitute certain populations, such as psychiatrized people, as dangerous to the public and thus requiring coercive / or potentially harmful interventions.

psy-complex: a mechanism that helps to construct new subjectivities and identities through the regulation of the psychological self.

psy-discourses: heterogeneous knowledges or ways of knowing developed from the psychological sciences including psychology, psychiatry, and behavioural sciences.

psychiatric intensive care unit (PICU): a secure environment aiming to provide a short-term alternative to standard acute inpatient environments; violence and aggression can form a rationale for PICU use.

psychiatrization: a set of practices that explain and respond to certain thoughts and behaviours in psychiatric terms, often in ways that ignore the complexity and context of the social world. Within the logic of psychiatrization, biomedical knowledge is held as truth and reaffirms itself as what should constitute practices and policy responses to mental distress.

psychiatrized person: an individual who has lived experience as a mental health services user; person with psychiatric disabilities or psychosocial disabilities; psychiatric survivor/consumer, and neurodivergent. The term acknowledges the system's active role in labelling an incarcerated person as "mentally ill."

recalcitrance: a disposition or acts of resistance in the context of psychiatric or other oppressions. Within psychiatric services, recalcitrance can be both a pejorative, applied by staff to challenging patients, or a nobler ideal, framing dissent and reaction to coercive practices – often in the face of few alternatives.

recovery: a process of change through which people improve their mental health, striving to reach their full potential. It is conceptualized in different ways, including as a personal journey; as a social process that includes access to jobs, income, education, housing, and safety; and as critique of professional discourses of good mental health.

sanism: generally, the "systematic subjugation of people who have received 'mental health' diagnoses or treatment".[8]

slow justice: justice that emerges from practices and understandings that challenge dominant representations of problems and the assumptions that they reflect. In relation to mental health policy and services, slow justice develops when actors challenge and offer equitable alternatives to biomedical, police, and neo-liberal problematizations and practices.

slow violence: a theoretical concept used by Rob Nixon to call attention to practices of violence that are incremental and reproduced through a broad time frame but are rarely recognized *as violence.* Slow violence produces human or ecological suffering that is obscured, rationalized, denied, or ignored. The histories of psychiatrization, of colonization, and of government policies that sustain inequalities and poor health for marginalized populations can all be viewed as slow violence. Slow violence is often not visible or obvious.

social reproduction: the necessary daily and intergenerational paid and unpaid work of fulfilling bodily, emotional, and social needs that is disproportionately performed by women. Social reproduction contributes directly to the creation of value through the acts of purchasing resources to maintain daily life, the reproduction of workers, and the care of and social provisioning for those people who are not participating in wage labour and by reproducing dominant social norms. Social reproduction is not limited to the domestic realm but is completed in the home, at school, in community spaces and at the level of the government etc.[9]

spaces of power: Janet Newman's term for temporally situated spaces within which multiple political projects come into contact to produce contradictions, tensions, and reconfigurations of power relations over time. Analysis of such spaces can trace how certain forms of violence have been troubled by locally situated actors and suggest possibilities for political action.

structural violence: violence that results from social arrangements that cannot be easily associated or attributed to a specific individual or social practice and that results in individuals and groups experiencing harm, disadvantage, or injury. This type of violence is often subtle and intertwines with direct violence. (Also see **violence** and **direct violence**)

subjective violence: the most visible forms of violence, including physical, verbal violence, and organized violence perpetrated by individuals, states, and groups.[10]

symbolic violence: a form of objective violence according to Žižek. Symbolic violence is embodied in language and its forms. It "is not only at work in the obvious – and extensively studied – cases of incitement and of the relations of social domination reproduced in our habitual speech forms: there is a more fundamental form of violence still that pertains to language as such, to its imposition of a certain universe of meaning. i.e. sanism."[11]

systemic violence: a form of objective violence according to Žižek: "the often catastrophic consequences of the smooth functioning of our political and economic systems."[12] Systemic violence is "violence inherent in a system: not only direct physical violence, but also the more subtle forms of coercion that sustain relations of domination and exploitation, including the threat of violence";[13] that is, capitalism produces war through expansion requirements and requires unemployment, depends on exploitation, etc.

section: a term that has entered popular jargon to refer to the use of the Mental Health Act – for instance, a person is on a section or has been sectioned when subject to particular provisions of the Act.

secure unit: a secure (low, medium, or high) environment providing assessment and treatment for individuals experiencing severe and enduring mental health conditions who may pose a risk to others.

trauma-informed approaches: methods that acknowledge the prevalence of trauma in particular communities and emphasize the importance of the accurate identification of trauma and related symptoms when training all staff. The goal of these approaches is to prevent re-traumatization being imposed on vulnerable communities by institutions and service providers.

trauma-informed care: "an organizational structure and treatment framework that involves understanding, recognizing, and responding to the effects of all types of trauma. Trauma-informed care also emphasizes physical, psychological and emotional safety for both consumers and providers, and helps survivors rebuild a sense of control and empowerment."[14]

treatment failure: a treatment is unsuccessful in providing the client/ patient with the desired outcome. The parameters for what constitutes a treatment failure are typically situation specific and can be defined in many ways. In the context of restraint and seclusion, the treatment plan ought to include measures to maximize the factors that can prevent the perceived need for restraint or seclusion. Where this plan is inadequate, there is a treatment failure – often resulting in the use of restraint or seclusion.

violence: defined by the World Health Organization as "the intentional use of physical force or power, threatened or actual, against oneself, another person, or against a group or community, which either results in or has a high likelihood of resulting in injury, death, psychological harm, maldevelopment, or deprivation."[15]

violence of neglect: the intentional lack of action or support to prevent an individual or a group from experiencing injury, death, psychological harm, maldevelopment, or deprivation.

whiteness: a defining racial category, "naturalized as an always already-given category against which other races could be distinguished and so not needing to be constituted in a specific way as a separate race grouping."[16] Histories, philosophies, modes of productions, social relations and social orders, religions, languages, and methods of taxonomy associated with whiteness are also positioned as superior and defining of whiteness; i.e., Greek and roman antiquity related philosophical idea, the industrial revolution, the rise of capitalism, English, Christianity, democracy, liberalism, empiricism, etc., are all associated with whiteness and therefore supremacy.

NOTES

1 Césaire and Pinkham, *Discourse on Colonialism*; Fanon, *The Wretched*; Gandhi, *Postcolonial Theory*; Joseph, "Ancestries of Racial"; Loomba, *Colonialism/Postcolonialism*; Said, *Orientalism*; Young, "Colonialism."
2 Dowbiggin, *Keeping America Sane*, 17.
3 Ibid., vi.

4 Vosko, "The Pasts."
5 Ives, *Language and Hegemony.*
6 Head, "What Does Heteronormativity Mean?"
7 See Said, *Culture and Imperialism*; Ashcroft, Griffiths, and Tiffin, *Post-Colonial Studies* (specifically Said, page 8 cited in Ashcroft, Griffiths, and Tiffin).
8 Poole et al., "Sanism, 'Mental Health,'" 20.
9 Cameron, "Social Reproduction."
10 Žižek, *Violence.*
11 Ibid., 2.
12 Ibid., 2.
13 Ibid., 9.
14 Trauma Informed Care Project.
15 Violence Prevention Alliance and World Health Organization, "Definition and Typology of Violence."
16 See Ashcroft, Griffiths, and Tiffin, *Post-Colonial Studies*, 272.

BIBLIOGRAPHY

Ashcroft, Bill, Gareth Griffiths, and Helen Tiffin. *Post-Colonial Studies: The Key Concepts.* Abingdon, UK: Routledge, 2013.

Cameron, B. "Social Reproduction and Canadian Federalism." In *Social Reproduction: Feminist Political Economy Challenges Neo-Liberalism*, edited by K. Bezanson and M. Luxton, 45–74. Montreal, QC: McGill-Queen's University Press, 2006. http://www.jstor.org/stable/j.ctt80rzb.7.

Césaire, Aimé, and Joan Pinkham. *Discourse on Colonialism.* Marlborough, UK: Adam Matthew Digital, 2007.

Dowbiggin, Ian Robert. *Keeping America Sane: Psychiatry and Eugenics in the United States and Canada, 1880–1940.* Ithaca, NY: Cornell University Press, 1997.

Fanon, Franz. *The Wretched of the Earth.* New York: Grove Press, 1965.

Gandhi, Leela. *Postcolonial Theory: A Critical Introduction.* New York: Columbia University Press, 1998.

Head, Tom. "What Does Heteronormativity Mean?" ThoughtCo. 2014. https://www.thoughtco.com/what-is-heteronormativity-721266.

Ives, Peter. *Language and Hegemony in Gramsci.* Halifax, NS: Fernwood Publishing, 2004.

Joseph, Ameil J. "Ancestries of Racial and Eugenic Systems of Violence in the Mental Health Sector." In *Proceedings of the Third International Conference on Violence in the Health Sector, Vancouver, BC*, edited by I. Needham, K. McKenna, M. Kingma, and N. Oud, 234–8. Amsterdam: Kavanah, 2012. http://www.oudconsultancy.nl/Resources/Proceedings_3rd_Workplace_ Violence_2012.pdf

Loomba, Ania. *Colonialism/Postcolonialism*. London, UK: Routledge, 1998.

Poole, Jennifer M., Tania Jivraj, Araxi Arslanian, Kristen Bellows, Sheila Chiasson, Husnia Hakimy, Jessica Pasini, and Jenna Reid. "Sanism, 'Mental Health,' and Social Work/Education: A Review and Call to Action." *Intersectionalities* 1 (2012): 20

Said, Edward W. *Culture and Imperialism*. London, UK: Chatto & Windus, 1993.

Said, Edward W. *Orientalism*. New York: Pantheon Books, 1978.

Trauma Informed Care Project. http://www.traumainformedcareproject .org/.

Violence Prevention Alliance and World Health Organization. "Definition and Typology of Violence." 2018. http://www.who.int/violenceprevention/ approach/definition/en/.

Vosko, L. F. "The Pasts (and Futures) of Feminist Political Economy in Canada: Reviving the Debate." *Studies in Political Economy: A Socialist Review* 68, no. 1 (2002): 55–83.

Young, Robert. "Colonialism and the Politics of Postcolonial Critique." In *Postcolonialism: An Historical Introduction*. Oxford, UK: Blackwell Publishing, 2001.

Žižek, Slavoy. *Violence: Six Sideways Reflections*. New York: Picador, 2008.

Contributors

Artwork Contributors

Ruth Beresford is the creator of the image used at the beginning of Part I of this volume.

Jaene F. Castrillon is a multi-disciplinary artist who explores her relationship to the world through various spiritual teachings and the wisdom of the land. As a mixed race (Indigenous Colombian/Hong Kong Chinese) queer woman of color living with disabilities, her work combines art and activism with spirituality to open a dialogue on ideas of wellness and illness. Jaene believes in sharing the brilliance and heartbreak of living a life less ordinary. Her photograph *Still Life*, which appears on the cover of the book, was taken during 2015–16 while she was media artist in residence at Workman Arts. Of the photograph, she says: "I was ruminating on the idea of institutional violence and its long-term impact on my identity. Using a historical loan from CAMH and my own psychiatric and police records, I attempt to untangle the effects of institutionalization on my psyche through *Still Life*."

Jennifer Crosby is a multifaceted artist based in Toronto, Ontario. Her creative nature has been well established over the past decade. As a self-taught visual artist, she began using canvas as a form of therapy and continues to do so to this day. Art was a very silent and private form of expression for her for many years. She became more noticed throughout Toronto after founding the Crowsnest, a company that dealt with artist representation and relations for musicians and visuals. For more info: www.crosbygallery.ca.

Rachel Rowan Olive lives and draws in London, United Kingdom, where she also writes and studies linguistics. She is a mental health service user/survivor and uses her artwork to campaign for change in how madness and distress are perceived and treated. She has created several zines on this including *A Is for Awkward* and *Goldilocks and the Three Therapists*. Rachel also exhibits regularly with Studio Upstairs, a therapeutic artists' community. You can find more of her work online as @rrowanolive on Twitter and Instagram.

Chapter Contributors

Will Aindow is a former mental health patient who enjoys watching *Columbo* repeats. He is currently outside the system working on his memoirs.

Liat Ben-Moshe is an assistant professor of disability studies at the University of Toledo. She is the co-editor (with Allison Carey and Chris Chapman) of *Disability Incarcerated: Imprisonment and Disability in the United States and Canada* (Palgrave McMillan, 2014) and *Building Pedagogical Curb Cuts: Incorporating Disability in the University Classroom and Curriculum* (Syracuse University Press, 2005); as well as special issues of *Disability Studies Quarterly* on disability in Israel/Palestine (Summer 2007), *Disability Studies Pedagogy* (2015), and *Women, Gender and Families of Colour* on race, gender, and disability (2014). She has written on such topics as prisons and asylums; the politics of abolition; disability, anti-capitalism, and anarchism; inclusive pedagogy; academic repression; and representations of disability. Dr Ben-Moshe is currently finishing a book examining the connections between prison abolition and deinstitutionalization in the United States

Peter Beresford, OBE, is a professor of citizen participation at the University of Essex and emeritus professor of social policy at Brunel University London. He is a long-term user of mental health services and lived for eight years on welfare benefits. Peter is also co-chair of Shaping Our Lives, the UK user-controlled organization and network concerned with the strategic development of user involvement and improving the quality of life of disabled people and service users. He has an extensive background of involvement in issues of participation as writer, researcher, activist, and teacher. He has published widely and writes regularly for the *Guardian* newspaper. His most recent book is *Social Policy First Hand: An International Introduction to Participatory Social Welfare* (Policy Press, 2018),

Mary Birdsell is the executive director of Justice for Children and Youth. With Karen Spector and Tess Sheldon, Mary was co-counsel to the Empowerment Council at the Inquest into the Death of Ashley Smith. Mary has been a child and youth rights lawyer for 20 years and has pursued those rights across a range of legal subjects at every level of court, including the Supreme Court of Canada. She helped to found Street Youth Legal Services, is currently the Chair of the Ontario Bar Association Child and Youth law section, and has recently co-authored a book on the representation of young people in the criminal justice system.

Lucy Costa is the deputy executive director of the Empowerment Council, an independent service user rights-based organization in Toronto, Canada. She works as a community activist and advocate promoting the rights of mental health service users/survivors, as well as encouraging critical analysis about service user inclusion in the mental health sector. She has developed education curriculum for many stakeholders, including psychiatry residents at the University of Toronto. She has written a number of articles and blogs and is co-editor to a special edition of the *Journal of Ethics and Mental Health*. Lucy is Azorean-Portuguese and speaks both English and Portuguese. Her work stems from and is informed heavily by personal experiences growing up in a working-class immigrant family.

Andrea Daley is an associate professor at the School of Social Work, Renison University College (affiliated with the University of Waterloo) in Canada. She has published on social justice issues, including those impacting sexual and gender minority communities with a particular focus on access to equitable and good quality health care; lesbian/queer women's experiences of psychiatric services; and gender, sexuality, race, and class and the interpretative nature of psychiatric chart documentation as it relates to psychiatric narratives of distress. She practices critical research methods to engage politics of knowledge building with communities towards the goal of social transformation. Andrea's work as a community mental health worker has been particularly influential in shaping her commitment to addressing the issues of madness, violence, and power.

Fiona Jones has significant experience of compulsory and coercive mental health services. For six years she has been employed in a research role working alongside colleagues at the University of Central Lancashire in the United Kingdom.

Ameil J. Joseph is an assistant professor in the School of Social Work at McMaster University. He draws on perspectives of critical forensic mental health, Mad Studies, postcolonial theory, critical race theory, and critical disability studies to analyse the historical production of ideas about difference, normalcy, sexuality, eugenics, race, ability, and mental "illness" as they cohere, diverge, interdepend and perform within policy, law, and practice. One of the broad areas he has focused on is the confluence of colonial racialized violence within criminal justice, mental health, and immigration systems. Ameil is also the author of *Deportation and the Confluence of Violence within Forensic Mental Health and Immigration Systems* (Palgrave Macmillan), a historiographical postcolonial analysis of the practice of deportation in Canada for those identified as "undesirable."

Jennifer M. Kilty is associate professor in the Department of Criminology, University of Ottawa. Her research has examined self-injurious behaviour in carceral settings; criminalized women's experiences of psychiatrization; and the criminalization of HIV/AIDS nondisclosure. In addition to numerous refereed journal articles and book chapters, she has edited two books, *Within the Confines: Women and the Law in Canada* (Women's Press) and *Demarginalizing Voices: Commitment, Emotion, and Action in Qualitative Research* (UBC Press). She recently authored *The Enigma of a Violent Woman: A Critical Examination of the Case of Karla Homolka* (Routledge). Dr Kilty was the 2016–2017 Fulbright Visiting Scholar at Kennesaw State University, Georgia, where she examined the effects of criminalizing HIV nondisclosure on the front-line practices of AIDS service organizations.

Azeezah Kanji is a legal academic and writer based in Toronto. She received her Juris Doctor from University of Toronto's Faculty of Law and her LLM specializing in Islamic law from the School of Oriental and African Studies, University of London. Azeezah is director of programming at Noor Cultural Centre, a Muslim religious, educational, and cultural institution in Toronto. She is also a regular opinion writer for the *Toronto Star*, focusing on issues related to racism, law, national security, and social justice.

Tobin LeBlanc Haley is a critical political economist and feminist, and a white, normatively able-bodied, Mad-identified ciswoman. She is currently the Ethel Louise Armstrong postdoctoral fellow in the School of Disability Studies at Ryerson University, where she is conducting research on psychiatric deinstitutionalization in New Brunswick, Canada, and processes of transinstitutionalization impacting Deaf/Mad/Disability communities. She also teaches in the disability studies program at King's University College. Tobin is interested in all things related to disability and social reproduction. She is committed to the project of generating greater conversation between the fields of Disability and Mad Studies and critical political economy.

Janet Lee-Evoy lives in Toronto, Ontario, and is completing her medical training in psychiatry at the University of Toronto. She is interested in the intersections between trauma, culture, and mental and emotional wellness. She writes comics as a medium to explore and reflect.

Sandra Lehalle is an assistant professor in the Department of Criminology in the University of Ottawa where she has taught since 2007. Holder of a European doctorate in law and of a Canadian PhD in criminology, her research interests lie in the policies and practices of detention by the state, including the ill-treatment and torture of prisoners. Through her research, Sandra Lehalle unveils the complex relations between state authority and society by focusing on the role played by politics and the law (at the national and international level) in the legitimizing process of state power and of its privileged repressive device: the prison

Ben Losman holds a masters in social justice education from the Ontario Institute for Studies in Education at University of Toronto. Ben's research and pedagogical interests include anti-oppressive education, community development, and anti-colonial solidarity activism.

Sarah Markham was educated at the University of Cambridge and has a PhD in mathematics. Currently she is a visiting researcher in the Department of Biostatistics at the Institute of Psychiatry, Psychology and Neuroscience, King's College London. She is pursuing a (second) PhD in the Department of Computer Science and IT, Birkbeck College London and developing knowledge representation for intelligent support in military settings. Her research is sponsored by Defence Science and Technology Laboratory (Ministry of Defence).

Mick McKeown is a professor of democratic mental health, School of Nursing, University of Central Lancashire, and a trade union activist with Unison, playing a role in union strategizing on nursing. He has taken a lead in arguing the case for union organizing to extend to alliance formation with service users/survivors.

Brigit McWade is a sociologist from Lancaster, United Kingdom. Her work to date has explored recovery in mental health policy and practice, mental health stigma in the context of neo-liberal capitalism and austerity measures, and the politics of representation of madness and distress in popular culture and academic discourse. In addition, she has contributed to the organization of several Mad Studies and survivor research events in the United Kingdom.

Marina Morrow is a professor and the chair of the School of Health Policy and Management at York University. In her work, Marina is interested in better understanding the social, political, and institutional processes through which health and mental health policies and practices are developed and how social and health inequities are sustained or attenuated for different populations. Marina's research interests have several focuses: critical health policy and the utilization of intersectional theory and approaches in mental health, the impact of neo-liberal reforms on health and social policy, and the role of citizen engagement and social justice in mental health. Marina's research has been published in a wide range of academic journals, including *Studies for Social Justice, Journal of Critical Social Policy*, and the *Canadian Journal for Community Mental Health*. She is lead editor (with Lorraine Halinka Malcoe) of *Critical Inquiries for Social Justice in Mental Health* (forthcoming from U of T Press).

Meghann O'Leary is currently a PhD candidate in disability studies at the University of Illinois in Chicago. She holds a masters degree in special education from the University of New Mexico and a bachelor degree from Vassar College in English literature. Her research interests include the intersections of Mad Studies and disability studies, as well as the intersectional lens on the study of life writings by women diagnosed with psychiatric disabilities. Her current work involves placing life writings by women with psychiatric disabilities in a historical, cultural, and political context to frame the relationship between disability, madness, and gender.

Nicole Penak is a member of the Eagle Clan, and a Maliseet and Mi'kmaq First Nations Woman with mixed Acadian and Ukrainian heritage. Her family is from the territory stretching through what is now known as the Gaspé Region in Quebec and New Brunswick. Born and raised in the Greater Toronto Area, Nicole lives and works in the vibrant Indigenous community of Toronto. Her traditional name, Kiishickokwe, relates to her healing work with the community. A registered social worker and social work educator, Nicole has worked in the areas of mental health, community development, adoptions, and criminal justice. Nicole works as a counsellor providing therapeutic services to Indigenous community members at Anishnawbe Health Toronto. She is also working to complete her PhD at the Ontario Institute for Studies in Education with a focus on Indigenous approaches to social work and social work research.

Merrick Pilling holds a PhD in gender studies and is currently a project coordinator on a study that is analysing psychiatric inpatient chart documentation to examine cultural narratives on gender using an intersectional lens. A second project includes collaborative work as a member of a research team that is using mixed methods to explore the community participation experiences of lesbian, gay, bisexual, queer, and trans people with a diagnosis of schizophrenia or bipolar disorder.

Priya Raju was born on the territory now known as Canada, in the city of Ottawa. Her family is from a rural Telugu-speaking region near the southeastern coast of India, where they have lived for at least the last six generations. She is a psychiatrist who works with marginalized populations across downtown Toronto, including immigrants and refugees, Indigenous people, and other groups often affected by colonialism and capitalism/poverty. She also consults to communities in northern Ontario and Nunavut. At Anishnawbe Health Toronto, she joins counsellor, healer, and primary practice colleagues to work with urban Indigenous families. She is on faculty in the Department of Psychiatry, Faculty of Medicine, University of Toronto.

Kevin Reel studied occupational therapy a long time ago in Toronto and remains a registered occupational therapist. He then worked, lived, and studied in the United Kingdom for 16 years where he got his MSc in medical ethics from Imperial College, London. He returned to the University of Toronto in 2008 to do a Fellowship in clinical and organizational ethics at the Joint Centre for Bioethics. He is currently the ethicist at the Toronto Central Community Care Access Centre, having performed the same role at the Centre for Addiction and Mental Health, Southlake Regional Health Centre, and Mackenzie Health. Kevin is an assistant professor in the Department of Occupational Science and Occupational Therapy, an associate professor in the Dalla Lana School of Public Health, a faculty member with the Global Institute for Psychosocial, Palliative and End-of-Life Care, and a member of the Joint Centre for Bioethics at the University of Toronto. He has co-authored numerous resources on medical assistance in dying for the Joint Centre for Bioethics, as well as a chapter on the topic in the book *Ethics in Mental Health – Substance Use*. He co-authored another chapter in the same book on medical cannabis. Kevin also has a keen interest in enabling sexuality and sexual expression and is a member of the Sexual Health and Disability Alliance International (SHADA International). In his spare time, he likes to play with power tools and kitchen appliances, usually to separate ends.

Jen Rinaldi is an assistant professor in the legal studies program at University of Ontario Institute of Technology. Her current work engages with narrative and arts-based methodologies to deconstruct eating disorder recovery and to reimagine recovery in relation to queer community. Rinaldi also works in collaboration with Recounting Huronia, and has coordinated presentations and interviews across Canada on behalf of the Huronia Survivors Speakers Bureau.

Kate Rossiter is an associate professor at Wilfrid Laurier University where she teaches in the community and public health, and social justice and community engagement programs. She received her PhD from the Dalla Lana School of Public Health at the University of Toronto in 2009 and her MA in performance studies from New York University in 2002. Dr Rossiter's work is highly interdisciplinary and lies at the intersection of bioethics, critical social science, arts-based research practice, and disability studies.

Amy Scholes has experience conducting research within adult inpatient mental health services, and is currently an assistant psychologist within a child and adolescent mental health service. Amy is particularly interested in psychosocial approaches to mental health and distress.

C. Tess Sheldon is an assistant professor at the Faculty of Law at the University of Windsor. With Karen Spector and Mary Birdsell, Tess was co-counsel to the Empowerment Council at the inquest death of Ashley Smith. She recently completed her doctorate at the University of Toronto, exploring the legal issues raised by covert medication administration practices in psychiatric settings.

Karen R. Spector is a staff lawyer at ARCH Disability Law Centre. While working at Justice for Children and Youth, Karen, along with Tess Sheldon and Mary Birdsell, was co-counsel to the Empowerment Council at the inquest into the death of Ashley Smith. Karen has also represented interveners on constitutional and human rights cases before all levels of court, including the Ontario Court of Appeal and the Supreme Court of Canada.

Katherine Teghtsoonian has taught in several interdisciplinary programs at the University of Victoria (Canada) and is professor in its Faculty of Human and Social Development. Her interests in feminist and post-structural approaches to public policy and policy analysis have informed her teaching, her research, and her involvement in equity struggles – particularly in relation to gender and disability – in university settings. Her recent scholarship has involved a critical analysis of initiatives that problematize "depression" within workplaces and as a public health issue. Like her earlier work on women's policy agencies and gender mainstreaming initiatives within the governments of British Columbia (Canada) and Aotearoa/New Zealand, this research is centrally concerned with an analysis of neo-liberal policies, governing practices, and their effects. She has published her work in disciplinary and interdisciplinary journals, including *Critical Policy Studies*, the *International Political Science Review*, *Signs: A Journal of Women in Culture and Society*, and *Social Science and Medicine*.

Christopher Van Veen is a municipal urban health planner and doctoral candidate in the Faculty of Health Sciences at Simon Fraser University. Much of his career has been spent working in a variety of community-based mental health, addictions, and non-profit housing programs in Vancouver's Downtown Eastside. Drawing on practice experience, Chris is interested in uncovering the taken-for-granted assumptions and political rationalities at work in contemporary mental health and addictions policy and practice. His doctoral research uses discourse analysis to examine the emergence of Assertive Community Treatment (ACT) teams and their role in the governance of the severely mentally ill and hard to house in Vancouver.

Jijian Voronka received her PhD from the Department of Social Justice Education at the University of Toronto. Informed by Mad Studies and drawing on principles of survivor research, her current work uses critical theory to query the possibilities, conditions, and limits of service user involvement in mental health and homeless research and service systems. Her forthcoming book *Peer Work: The Value of Mad Labour* (University of Toronto Press) explores the terms of engagement that govern participatory practices. She is an assistant professor at the School of Social Work, University of Windsor, where she teaches for their Disability Studies program.

Carlyn Zwarenstein is a Toronto writer and the author of *Opium Eater: The New Confessions*, a *Globe & Mail* best book of 2016, and a text on university literature and addiction studies courses. Since 2001 she has freelanced for numerous publications, often covering issues of medicine, social justice, and mental states.

Index

models, 108; homophobic and transphobic violence, 60–1, 97, 101, 105–6; individualization, 103, 107; It Gets Better campaign, 128–9, 133n30; Mad Studies, 108; national mental health strategy, 60–1, 104–8; organizations, 105–6; pride discourses, 129; queer, 104; recovery, 60–1, 107–8; rights-based movement, 107; same-sex marriage, 98; stigma and discrimination, 104–5; systemic violence, 60–1; trans people, 103–5. See also *Changing Directions, Changing Lives* (mental health strategy)

Li, Vince, 6

Liegghio, Maria, 64, 70, 205

lived experience: about, 15, 352; epistemic violence, 205; as expertise, 166, 197–200, 205–10; feminist legal scholarship, 209, 215n79; marginalization of, 71–2; personal accounts, 352; and psychiatric assessments, 140–1; as slow justice, 73–5; Vancouver's DTES task force, 71–4

Lukes, Steven, 11

MacMurchy, Helen, 170, 176, 177

Mad in America blog, 158

Mad Matters (Lefrançois, Menzies, and Reaume, eds.), 50, 344n17, 354

madness and Mad people: about, 3–5, 9–10; and class, 128; historical background, 6, 121, 126; key questions, 353; LGBTQ2S people, 108, 352; peer support, 29, 52, 55n6, 73–4; and power, 10–12; terminology, 9–10, 191, 344n17;

and violence, 12–13, 350–4. *See also* mental distress; mental illness; power; terminology; violence

Madness Network News, 158

Mad Studies: about, 9, 354; community voices, 8; as interdisciplinary, 9, 108; as international, 354; *Mad Matters,* 50, 344n17, 354; medical education, 51; psy-knowledges as stigmatizing, 157–9; terminology, 344n17

Malacrida, Claudia, 226, 228

marginalized people: coercion of inpatients, 267; gentrification, 330–2, 338–40; as "hard bodies," 90; populist politics, 354; rights-based analysis of research, 88–90; slow death, 60, 82–5, 90–2; slow violence, 296–7; subconscious assumptions about, 299–300; Toronto's history, 335–40. *See also* ethics and morality; human rights; race and racism; slow justice; slow violence; social justice

Maté, Gabor, 55n5

May, Rufus, 272

Mazer, Katie, 340–1

McLaren, Angus, 170, 176

McLellan, Anne, 240

McWilliams, Wilson Carey, 271–2

media: about, 62, 150–9; alternative representations, 158–9; and Ashley Smith, 216n92, 216n94, 320–1, 325n52; conflation of violence and mental illness, 153–4; diversity of madness and distress, 152; focus on individual violence, 152; guidelines for, 151; gun control and "mental Illness," 31; law and order, 156–7; media effects model, 151–3,

eugenics, 170; inquests into deaths of psychiatrized persons, 204–5; law on the books vs. in action, 203, 213n43; Mental Health Act, 171, 197, 200, 203, 212n21; segregation, 321–2. *See also* gentrification, Toronto (Queen Street); Huronia Regional Centre (HRC); Smith, Ashley; Toronto

Ontario Disability Support Program (ODSP), 136–49

organized violence, 172–3, 179. *See also* violence, types of

Othering process: colonialism, 335–6; epistemic violence, 315–16, 322; vs. kindness and empathy to, 47–8, 50–1; Other as category, xii; power differentials, xii; respectability vs. degeneracy, 333, 335–8, 342–3; stereotypes, 30, 31, 105, 246, 267, 299; tribal instincts, xii; welfare system, 61–2. *See also* dehumanization; ethics and morality

patients: analogy with neonatal intensive care patients, 48–9; kindness and empathy, 47–54, 55nn5–6; research on experiences, 50; self-empowerment in forensic settings (UK), 39–46; terminology, 10. *See also* madness and Mad people; mental distress; mental health systems; mental illness; psychiatric system and psychiatrists

Patton, Cindy, 87–9

peer support, 29, 52, 55n6, 73–4

personal accounts, 352

personal responsibility. *See* individualization; responsibilization

Philo, Greg, 150–5, 157, 159

physical restraints. *See* coercion; restraints, chemical and physical

physical violence, 172–3, 179. *See also* coercion; subjective violence; violence, types of

PICU (psychiatric intensive care unit), 264–5. *See also* psychiatric system and psychiatrists

Pinel, Philippe, 121, 126, 249

police interactions: ACT orders, 68, 69–70; killings of Mad people, 47, 205, 214n59, 334; power relations, 11

political economy, feminist. *See* feminist political economy

politics: ATRS radicalization scale, 245–6. *See also* terrorism

Pollack, Shoshana, 201, 209, 210, 216n88

poverty: incarceration, 126; Indigenous vs. mainstream, 145–6; and Mad identity, 128; Othering process, xii; personal accounts, 116–18, 126, 131–2; as slow violence, 64

power: about, 3–5, 10–12; biomedical model, 106, 107; biopolitics, 82–5, 123–4; CTO cycles of power, 51; hard vs soft, 310, 323n5; legitimacy of, 268, 270–1; media reproduction of structures, 156–7; psychiatric system, 120–2, 131, 141, 269, 271–2, 280; psychopolitical framing, 271; and psy-discourse, 155; regimes, 16; terminology, 10–12; and violence, 12–13; violence where power in jeopardy, 276–7. *See also* madness and Mad people; neoliberalism; terminology; violence